Engaging Parents in Adolescent Therapy

Engaging Parents in Adolescent Therapy

Beyond the Waiting Room

Amie C. Myrick

ROWMAN & LITTLEFIELD
Lanham • Boulder • New York • London

Published by Rowman & Littlefield
A wholly owned subsidiary of The Rowman & Littlefield Publishing Group, Inc.
4501 Forbes Boulevard, Suite 200, Lanham, Maryland 20706
www.rowman.com

Unit A, Whitacre Mews, 26-34 Stannary Street, London SE11 4AB

British Library Cataloguing in Publication Information Available

Library of Congress Cataloging-in-Publication Data

Names: Myrick, Amie C., author.
Title: Engaging parents in adolescent therapy: beyond the waiting room / Amie C. Myrick.
Description: Lanham: Rowman & Littlefield, [2017] | Includes bibliographical references and index.
Identifiers: LCCN 2016057698 (print) | LCCN 2017000116 (ebook) | ISBN 9781442250000 (cloth : alk. paper) | ISBN 9781442272545 (pbk. : alk. paper) | ISBN 9781442250017 (electronic)
Subjects: LCSH: Adolescent psychotherapy—Parent participation. | Mental health consultation. | Adolescent analysis.
Classification: LCC RJ505.P38 M97 2017 (print) | LCC RJ505.P38 (ebook) | DDC 616.89/140835—dc23
LC record available at https://lccn.loc.gov/2016057698

™ The paper used in this publication meets the minimum requirements of American National Standard for Information Sciences—Permanence of Paper for Printed Library Materials, ANSI/NISO Z39.48-1992.

Printed in the United States of America

To my mom and dad: More than ever before, I realize that parenting is not nearly as easy as you have always made it look. I carry your unconditional love and support with me in everything I do. Love you … you know how much.

Contents

Acknowledgments

Taking a year to write a book while working full-time and staying engaged with those around you is no small feat. I could not have done it without the following people—THANK YOU!

- My supportive family and closest friends, who watched and listened to me tirelessly talk and research for these chapters. I know there were points when you wanted me to stop talking, but you never told me to, and for that, I will be forever grateful. I love you all.
- My beautiful little boy, who makes me strive to be a better parent every single day. So many of favorite memories begin with you, and I will feel forever blessed that I get to be your mommy, no matter how imperfectly I do the job.
- My mentors and "work friends," who showed me what being a counselor is all about, every day. Bethany and Victor, I can never repay you for holding my hand every step of the way as I entered the world of academic writing and professional counseling. I am so inspired by you both, every day. Eric, thank you for being my "writing partner-in-crime." We've been through the ups and downs of writing together, and, somehow, we have managed to keep cranking out the goods!
- My editor, Kristina, who never complained when I sent her a seventy-five-page document at midnight. Thank you for reading and rereading, and then rereading again, each and every page of this book. It is better because of you, so I will allow you to plan that Mexican feast to celebrate its publication.
- My assistants, Lauren and Gabrielle, who never backed down from an index challenge! Every time I search the pages in the back of this book to easily find a topic, I will think of you.

- My local Panera staff, who never kicked me out of my booth, even when I had been there for six hours and was on my fourth cup of coffee. Thank you for vacuuming around me.
- Last, but in no way least, my clients and their parents over the years. To say that this book would not have been possible without you is an understatement. Thank you for allowing me to enter your worlds during some of your most difficult days and, parents, for trusting me with your children and teens. I will never forget a single one of you.

Introduction

The idea to write this book first occurred to me after a mother left my office, frustrated and discouraged. Despite nearly a year of weekly individual therapy, her daughter, Maggie, was continuing to struggle with anxiety, depression, and self-injury. She told me that she was paying me to "fix" Maggie and that clearly I was failing. Although most therapists can think of a client (or two, or three) who, in retrospect, they wish they had treated using a different approach, Maggie was not one of those cases for me. I felt confident in our treatment approach, my alliance with Maggie, and Maggie's motivation for therapy. I also felt quite confident that Maggie's mother's approach to therapy, which included unreasonably high expectations of both her daughter and me, minimal follow through with recommendations, and complete disengagement from therapy sessions, was affecting Maggie and her continued symptoms.

At the time, I looked for articles, books, and webinars to help me work with parents of adolescent clients, and I was disappointed when I found nothing to meet my needs. It was then that I decided that one day I would write a book to help clinicians navigate the murky waters of parental involvement in adolescent therapy. A few years, and many, *many* adolescent clients later, I finally felt ready to take the leap and submit the proposal to a publisher. One of my proudest career moments so far was the day that Rowman & Littlefield graciously accepted my book proposal. Another is knowing that I can share this book with you now.

The topics I discuss throughout the book are not separate entities, and they each interact in fascinating and challenging ways. Nevertheless, I organized them into nine chapters. In the first two chapters, I discuss what brings parents to a child therapist's office and, once there, how you work to understand the parent–teen relationship while developing alliances with both parents and teens. In the next two chapters, I dissect complicated issues such as confidentiality and digital media, two areas that can be particularly difficult when you are seeing teen clients. In chapters 5 and 6, I tackle "tough" teen problems and parental issues that interfere with treatment progress. Chapter 7 addresses nonoffending parents of traumatized adolescents, a population that requires more patience, empathy, and self-care than any other with whom I work. I finish the book with two chapters about limits; specifically, when it is time to refer parents and their teens for family therapy and how to say good-bye when treatment is complete. Interwoven throughout the book are frank discussions about countertransference, ethical obligations, and mandated reporting, along with ways to manage these issues with parents.

I am a research nerd at heart; I love to read about new studies that confirm or differ from clinical experiences. Over twelve years of working on research studies has greatly shaped the way I do therapy; I often share the things I read and learn with my clients and their parents. I have written this book much in the same style—every topic has been thoroughly researched and heavily cited so that you can feel up to date on the research about the topics that I discuss in this book without having to spend hours in an online library database.[1] My hope is that whether you love or merely tolerate research, you will be able to use this book and the mixture of case examples,[2] research, and clinical approaches I've provided to inform your own work with adolescents. If you do not currently work with teens and their parents, I hope this book motivates you to try out this exciting population (and does not scare you off!).

NOTES

1. Unfortunately, there are aspects of these issues that I could not get into in as much detail as I might have liked (e.g., cultural differences) or even at all (e.g., eating disorders). I would certainly encourage you to delve further into the literature to learn more.

2. All identifying information has been removed and details of treatment have been disguised to protect parents and teens' confidentiality.

Chapter One

"Meeting the Parents" and the Decision to Seek Help

"Hi, I'm looking for treatment for my teenage daughter. She is having some trouble, and I'm wondering if you are taking new clients." I listen to a voicemail that begins with this statement at least once a week, and sometimes more often. If you are well known among referral sources as someone who accepts adolescent clients, you probably receive similar phone calls. When I first began building my practice, I thought of this phone call simply as the first step in treatment. As I gained more experience working with these families, however, I came to value this phone call, not only as the beginning of a treatment episode for the teen, but often as the end product of a longer journey for the parent.

For some parents, the process is a relatively straightforward, linear progression that begins with the recognition of a problem and ends with a scheduled intake. Other parents seek treatment following the emergence of multiple comorbid symptoms or because they have been required to do so by another provider or agency. Regardless of the precipitants, however, a parent's decision to pursue treatment for his/her teen can be a difficult one, wrought with emotional and pragmatic barriers. More than once, I have heard parents tell me that they feel guilt for not being able to help their children or for failing to notice that there were issues at all.[1] When parents call me to initiate treatment for their teens, I keep in mind that they have likely been working through a process involving some combination of gaining awareness, observation, Internet research, and/or consultation with other professionals. After coming to the conclusion that their teen needs counseling, parents are charged with the frustrating task of finding a competent therapist. From there, they must schedule an appointment within the limited confines of the provider's hours, communicate with insurance companies, and rearrange schedules to actually get themselves and their teen to the intake appointment. All of this occurs while balancing other family responsibilities (including other children), attending work, and supporting the teen for whom they are seeking treatment. By the time an adolescent officially begins counseling, the parents may already feel exhausted and as though they have barely survived the process. But, of course, the fun is only just beginning.

ADOLESCENT MENTAL HEALTH ISSUES WARRANTING TREATMENT

Despite the arduous process involved, parents across the country seek treatment for their teens every day. Studies have approximated that as many as one quarter of adolescents receive specialty mental treatment (Costello, He, Sampson, Kessler, & Merikangas, 2014). Why? In short, about one in five adolescents meet the criteria for a psychological disorder that causes severe distress and/or impairment (Merikangas et al., 2010), and as any counselor who works with adolescents can attest, these mental health symptoms can drastically influence mood, behavior, and choices.

Mood Disorders

Teens report a great need for treatment that addresses symptoms of depression and other mood disorders (Wu et al., 1999). Statistics agree: one study estimated that over one year, one in a hundred youth received outpatient treatment for depression (Olfson, Gameroff, Marcus, & Waslick, 2003), and even more (14.3 percent) experience symptoms of major depressive disorder (MDD), dysthymia, and bipolar disorder (BD; Merikangas et al., 2010), according to the National Comorbidity Survey Replication—Adolescent Supplement (NCS-A) study.[2] According to this study, mood symptoms tend to onset around age thirteen and increase steadily as adolescence progresses into young adulthood. Mood disorders are more prevalent among adolescents who are older, female, and Hispanic; symptoms frequently co-occur with those of anxiety disorders, behavioral disorders, substance use, and eating disorders (Merikangas et al., 2010; Olfson et al., 2003). Identifying and treating these symptoms early is important, as teens with mood disorders are at increased risk for suicide and substance abuse, and relapse of MDD in young adulthood is common (Lewinsohn, Pohde, Klein, & Seeley, 1999).

Anxiety Disorders

Research has demonstrated that anxiety disorders are the most common ones among adolescents (Kessler et al., 2012), with nearly one in three teens

(31.9 percent) meeting the diagnostic criteria (Merikangas et al., 2010). Anxiety is probably the most frequent presenting symptom that I hear from parents and their teens. Symptoms often follow a persistent course that begins at a young age; the NCS-A study found that half of the teens experienced onset of symptoms at age six, and prevalence remained relatively consistent when assessed at one-month, one-year, and lifetime intervals (Kessler et al., 2012; Merikangas et al., 2010). All of the subtypes, which include agoraphobia, generalized anxiety disorder, social phobia, specific phobia, panic disorder, post-traumatic stress disorder (PTSD), and separation anxiety, tend to be more frequent in females, older adolescents, and non-Hispanic ethnic minorities (Merikangas et al., 2010). Although comorbidity with other categories of disorders is reported by some teens, the NCS-A study reported that anxiety disorders were the most frequent disorders to occur alone, without the presence of mood or behavioral disorders (Merikangas et al., 2010).

Behavioral and Substance Use Disorders

Attention deficit hyperactivity disorder (ADHD), conduct disorder (CD), and oppositional defiant disorder (ODD) often first appear in early adolescence (Merikangas et al., 2010), with rates of 8.7, 12.6, and 6.8 percent, respectively. Substance abuse has a later onset than mood, anxiety, or behavioral disorders, increasing rapidly after age fifteen, with rates of 6.4 percent for alcohol abuse/dependence and 8.9 percent for drug abuse/dependence. Males are more likely than females to be diagnosed, and Caucasian adolescents are more likely to struggle with substances than minority peers. You will definitely encounter these issues if you work with teens; high rates of externalizing behaviors are related to greater use of mental health services by youth (Wu et al., 1999). However, teens are less likely than their parents to report them (Younstrom, Loeber, & Stouthamer-Loeber, 2000).

High-Risk and Self-Injurious Behaviors

One of the scariest parts of being an adolescent therapist is the level of high-risk behaviors that some teens exhibit. Nonsuicidal self-injury (NSSI) rates among teens are high, between 12 and 39 percent according to some general population studies (Lloyd-Richardson, Perrine, Dierker, & Kelley, 2007; Zoroglu et al., 2003); NSSI is more common among females. Suicidal behaviors increase in frequency through adolescence before decreasing once teens enter adulthood (Vander Stoep, McCauley, Flynn, & Stone, 2009). Similarly, running away increases in adolescence, peaks at age sixteen, and then decreases significantly (Sunseri, 2003). We will talk a bit more about these difficult topics in chapter 5.

THE PROCESS OF HELP-SEEKING BY PARENTS

The question of which disorders make parents more likely to seek treatment has been a difficult one for researchers to answer. Some studies have suggested that externalized problems—behavioral and substance abuse disorders—are easier to detect and often cause more direct distress for parents and school staff, which in turn increases referrals and help-seeking (Wu et al., 1999; Zwaanswijk, Verhaak, Bensing, van der Ende, & Verhulst, 2003). Parental distress has been linked with the amount of distress they are experiencing in child-rearing, rather than the severity of symptoms themselves. Parents are often unaware of their youth's emotional struggles, and many have a poor working knowledge of warning signs for suicide and other high-risk behaviors (Maine, Shute, & Martin, 2001). This corresponds with my experiences as a therapist; for many parents, it wasn't until their teens explicitly shared information about their anxiety and mood issues or the parents started seeing external signs of distress (e.g., suicidality, self-harm, and academic struggles) that parents entered into the help-seeking process. As a result, many feel tremendous guilt over "not knowing" what was going on with their adolescents.

In addition to the severity of mental health issues, it is important to keep in mind the essential role that barriers and obstacles play in the recognition of symptoms and decision to seek help. In one study, just 16.5 percent of the adolescent sample had used mental health services over the past year, despite all of them demonstrating significant mood, anxiety, and behavioral issues (Zwaanswijk, van der Ende, Verhaak, Bensing, & Verhulst, 2007). Owens and colleagues (2002) have categorized these into three subsets: *perceptual obstacles*, which include failure to detect problems or the severity of the problems; *structural barriers*, which include obstacles such as cost, insurance coverage, time management, and transportation; and *treatment views*, which include negative views about mental health treatment and treatment providers, mistrust of providers or the mental health care system, and concerns about stigma.

The Process

Studies have suggested that parents go through a loosely structured, elaborate process of help-seeking (Chen, Gearing, DeVylder, & Oh, 2016; Logan & King, 2001; Shanley, Reid, & Evans, 2008; Thomson et al., 2014). When changes in behaviors or affect first become apparent, parents may engage in *normalizing*, framing changes as within the range of typical adolescent development or believing that they will be short-lived (Thomson et al., 2014). Once the changes persist, however, parents may experience *ambivalence* and/or *ambiguity*, ranging from denial that there is a problem to the gathering of evidence and increased observation. Parents at this stage may begin consulting websites or books to gain more insight into the potential issue (Thomson et al., 2014). School staff or other third parties may also express concern.

Following these first two stages, parents may reach a decision point where they recognize that their adolescent is struggling in some way, thereby working their way through the perceptual obstacles I mentioned above. Unfortunately, this is often after the behavioral or emotional problem has become serious or presents comorbid with other concerning symptoms (Stouthamer-Loeber, Loeber, van Kammen, & Zhang, 1995; Zwaanswijk et al., 2003).

Barriers to Receiving Treatment

Once the decision to seek treatment is made, parents often begin consulting with others, sometimes for the first time, and often informally with family, friends, or pediatricians during their teen's routine check-ups (Horowitz, 1978; Stouthamer-Loeber et al., 1995). It is important to note that a pediatrician's denial of problematic symptoms can act as a significant barrier to mental health treatment-seeking (Zwaanswijk et al., 2003) and that cultural norms may normalize symptoms (Gerdes, Lawton, Haack, & Schneider, 2014). Furthermore, structural and treatment view barriers greatly influence the help-seeking process at this stage. Pragmatic barriers such as cost, transportation, insurance coverage, and providers accepting new clients may factor into how quickly or easily parents decide to seek treatment (Chen et al., 2016; Raviv, Raviv, Propper, & Fink, 2003; Wisdom, Cavaleri, Gogel, & Nacht, 2011), as can issues such as stigma, beliefs regarding mental health symptoms and treatment, and/or prior negative experiences with the mental health care system. However, fear not! It *is* possible for parents to work through these issues, and some even find that treatment is not so bad. Some studies have found that parents who have used treatment services previously are more likely to pursue services a second time (Carlton & Deane, 2000; Starr, Campbell, & Herrick, 2002), even more so if their previous experience was positive (Deane, Skogstad, & Williams, 1999).

Stigma is a complex, multifaceted issue that involves views of individuals with mental health issues as weak, dangerous, or unpredictable, and someone from whom others would like to keep their distance (Yap, Wright, & Jorm, 2011). Most studies that have examined the role of stigma in parental help-seeking find that the higher the perception of stigma, the lower the likelihood of seeking treatment (Corrigan, 2004; Dempster, Wildman, & Keating, 2013), although some studies have not found a relationship between the two variables.[3] Researchers have discussed *public stigma*, the way people treat others with mental health issues (Corrigan, 2004). Parents may worry that others will judge them as bad parents or treat their teens differently (Dempster et al., 2013).

As opposed to public stigma, others have discussed the idea of *self stigma* (Corrigan, 2004). Nadler and Fisher (1986) propose that for some individuals, seeking help acts as a threat to their self-esteem, and others have spoken about the narcissistic injury that occurs when parents recognize mental health issues in their children (Phares, Ehrbar, & Lum, 1996). Therefore, parents may attempt to defend against these feelings of inadequacy and worthlessness by using mechanisms such as denial, projection of blame onto others, and/or rationalizing reasons why treatment cannot occur. Parents may also worry about exposing their teen's symptoms, family discord, or parenting weaknesses (Raviv et al., 2003). Although parents of teens are less likely to be blamed by others for their teens' behaviors, Hinshaw (2005) reported that those parents who do view themselves as the cause of their teens' problems are less likely to initiate treatment.

Culture plays a role when considering who enters treatment and when. Professionals and researchers have examined the conflict between Western psychotherapy and Asian American values, for example, finding that the more traditional the Chinese values, the higher the feelings of shame and stigma (Lau & Takeuchi, 2001). Similarly, one study of ultra-orthodox Jewish parents concluded that parents seeking treatment may worry about how others view their family (Schnitzer, Loots, Escudero, & Schechter, 2011). Latino parents are less likely than non-Latino parents to seek professional help for their children, particularly when they distrust providers, are not knowledgeable about symptoms or treatment options, and cannot find bilingual services (Gerdes et al., 2014). Social and cultural perceptions of mental health also affect how frequently African American parents recognize symptoms and/or pursue treatment (dosReis, Mychailyszyn, Myers, & Riley, 2007).

Another issue that can affect parents seeking help is their *teens' views* about beginning treatment. Although parents are viewed as the gatekeepers to mental health treatment, many times teens play a larger role than younger children in the decision to pursue treatment (Gaskin, Kouzis, & Richard, 2008). Adolescents tend to prefer informal sources of support, such as family and friends (see Raviv, Sills, Raviv, & Wilansky, 2000, for review), and I know countless teens who fought their parents for months before, finally, unhappily entering treatment. If parents are already ambivalent about starting therapy, their teens' minimization of symptoms and reluctance or outright refusal to attend an intake appointment may be all parents need to drop the subject for a while.

Facilitators for Seeking Help

Although much of the research has focused on barriers to seeking treatment, there are also some great studies that have looked at variables that assist parents in seeking help. I find these particularly helpful to keep in mind. When I hear a parent mention any of the following when discussing their adolescent, I frame this as a positive first step toward developing an alliance and formulating a successful treatment plan.

Chen and colleagues (2016) found that the quality of *communication* between the parent and teen was critical, as difficulties in contact tended to prevent parents from noticing changes and signs of mental illness. *Family history* of mental health issues, including parents' own mental health issues, can assist parents in assessing teens' symptom severity, as well as daily observation of behaviors and vigilance for concerning symptoms, such as self-injury, suicidal ideation, high levels of avoidance, substance use, or severe issues with sleep or food (Chen et al., 2016; Mojtabai & Olfson, 2008; Walker, Moreau, & Weissman, 1990). Related to this, parental detection of high-risk behaviors such as self-harm can increase the likelihood of seeking treatment (Owens, Lambert, Donovan, & Lloyd, 2005). In my experience, it is this latter cluster of "scary symptoms" that prompts parents to seek help and begin considering treatment options.

Finally, after determining that their adolescent has a problem—one that the family cannot manage alone—and deciding (consciously or unconsciously) that the benefits of seeking counseling outweigh the emotional and physical costs (Chen et al., 2016; Raviv, Sharvit, Raviv, & Rosenblat-Stein, 2008), parents reach out for help from the counseling profession. And, after attempting to schedule appointments with several different providers—as many as eleven in one study!—parents are put in contact with you, who schedules them for an intake appointment and ultimately becomes their teen's therapist (Shanley et al., 2008).

FIRST CONTACT WITH PARENTS

Keeping in mind the time-consuming process of treatment-seeking and adolescents' need for treatment, I return phone messages from new, potential parents quickly, usually within twenty-four hours, and only when I know that I have some time to talk. I acknowledge how difficult it can be to find a "good counseling fit" for their family, and I give parents an opportunity to tell me about their teen and how they would like me to help. Then I give them information on my training, typical clients, and treatment approaches; I also answer questions about appointments, billing issues, and experience. If parents are interested in making an appointment, I schedule an intake, where I explain that I will meet with them for half of the session and their teen for the second half. I schedule this as quickly as possible at a time that is convenient for the parent; one study found that the most frequent reason for intake "no-shows" is inconvenience of the time that the intake is scheduled (Kourany, Garber, & Tornusciolo, 1990), and the last thing I want to do is start our counseling relationship with the parent (or teen) feeling flustered, rushed, or resentful. I stress the importance of them feeling comfortable with my treatment approaches and personal style, and I encourage them to think of topics they'd like to discuss during the intake. With this first phone call, usually no longer than thirty minutes, I strive to set two important precedents for treatment. First, I express my expectation for the parent to attend and engage in the intake appointment, and, second, I begin working toward a collaborative relationship built on empathy and understanding.

Finally, I send parents a confirmation e-mail, which includes the date and time of the intake, my contact information, and all of my required forms, including contracts and demographic forms, so that they have time to review them and compile a list of questions or concerns before we meet. I know when I have to schedule my own, personal appointments, I sometimes feel overwhelmed with the amount of information I have received, so the e-mail serves as a summary and a reminder of our appointment and what I need parents to do before the intake. It also gives parents an opportunity to "opt out" if they decide they aren't interested without having to call and risk having me answer. Furthermore, continued contact between the parent and the counselor between the initial phone call and intake appointment decreases "no-shows" and acts as an ongoing confirmation of desire to receive services (Kourany et al., 1990; Wiseman & McBride, 1998).

The Intake

When I walk into my waiting room for that first intake appointment, I tend to greet three types of parents. Of course, every parent and set of parents that I meet is unique, and, as such, each relationship that I form with parents is a little different (more on this in the next chapter). However, most, if not all, fit broadly into the categories of eager, angry, or anxious. The *eager* parents are prepared for their adolescents to start treatment, usually have the forms filled out ahead of time, and present as open to treatment and my treatment approach. Sometimes I don't even need to ask them to give me the timeline I just mentioned, because they have already been thinking about it. These parents are often insightful and give me helpful information about their teens' lives, interpersonal relationships, goals, strengths, and treatment needs. Intakes with eager parents put me in a great position to meet their teens and hopefully forge ahead with treatment.

The second type of parent is *angry*. These parents are usually at their wits' end, frustrated by their adolescents' behaviors, previous treatment attempts, perceived failure by the school to help, medication challenges, the toll the mental health issues have taken on the rest of the family, or some combination of all of these. As we have spent much of this chapter discussing, I can empathize with these parents. The treatment-seeking process is difficult, seeing their children suffer is painful, and admitting that they need help can bring up a lot of unresolved personal issues. Many times these parents are struggling with teens whose symptoms are making them terribly unlikeable. I once had a mother lower her eyes and, with a shaky voice, tell me that she didn't like her son very much anymore. The tears in her eyes and the relief on her face when I told her that we were going to work on separating the son she loved from the symptoms she hated made me realize just how long she had been hiding that shameful thought. After that, I began initiating that conversation with parents, in effect giving them permission to share how unlikeable their symptomatic children could be at times.

The third type of parent is *anxious*. These parents, like eager parents, may come in prepared for the intake, poised with forms, questions, and history. These parents may also come in feeling totally overwhelmed by their teens' behaviors, like angry parents. What sets anxious parents apart is that their preparedness and/or feelings over being overwhelmed are due to their own personal feelings of anxiety. Anxiety and depression run in families, so sometimes the anxiety is an undiagnosed (or diagnosed) anxiety disorder, whereas other times the anxiety stems from bringing their children in to "see someone." As we've discussed, there is a lot of stigma still attached to child psychotherapy, particularly if the parents think that they are being judged for needing to seek a formal source of help.

Let Them Tell Their Stories

During the parents' half of that first intake appointment, I have two goals. First, I aim to continue the process of rapport building, and second, I aim to understand the parent's conceptualization of their teens' mental health and behavioral needs. Although every therapist has a way that they prefer to do intakes (or a way that their agency prefers they do intakes), I cannot stress enough the importance of allowing parents to *tell their stories*. Parents' feelings of being respected and treated kindly go a long way at this stage of treatment and can actually assist parents in overcoming barriers to treatment (Kerkorian, McKay, & Bannon, 2006). Never was this clearer to me than when I became a parent and began navigating the health system as my son's advocate.

One morning, when my son woke up sick and feverish, we spent close to an hour waiting for a doctor to come in and examine him. Unfortunately, because it was a weekend, we could not see his regular pediatrician. When the doctor finally came in, he made no mention of the wait, barely said hello to me or introduced himself, and began his examination. Throughout the brief time he was in the room, he asked me minimal questions and cut me off before I could answer any of them. He rattled off some instructions, made eye contact with me for the first time, and, preparing to leave the room, mumbled, "Okay?" Angry and feeling completely disrespected, I said, "No, not okay. I have some questions, and I need you to repeat those instructions so that I am sure that I have it right." Needless to say, we did not return to that doctor. This experience comes to mind whenever new parents come to my office. Even when parents are giving me information that I do not necessarily need, I listen to their story anyway. This is *their* session, possibly one they worked for months to get, and these minor details are part of their story. Listening, instead of cutting them off and pretending I know their teens better than they do, helps me demonstrate my genuine caring for them and their teens. It also establishes parents' position as the "expert" on their teens, a first step in (hopefully) decreasing power struggles between you and them down the line. Humility is key.

Some other reasons why parents' stories are critical clinical information include the following:

1. Understanding the history of your clients' symptoms is useful for treatment planning. At some point, you will need to piece together the course of symptoms, which teens may or may not be able to verbalize and parents may forget over time. During the intake, at the peak of the treatment-seeking process, is when I find parents to be most prepared to offer their observations and timelines of events.
2. Understanding the process by which parents first noticed symptoms will give you information about the parent–teen relationship and levels of attunement. As mentioned previously—and as we will discuss in chapter 2—the parent–teen relationship is paramount in your work with parents.
3. Hearing about parents' path to finding you, including what the "final straw" was before deciding to seek professional help, why they chose you over other therapists, and previous attempts to seek treatment, gives you clinical information about the family's decision-making, follow through with recommendations, and motivation for treatment. For example, if a parent tells you that the only reason she is in your office is because Susan's school counselor insisted on it and no one in the family understands why, you will likely tackle therapy a little differently than if a parent tells you he became concerned when Joe's grades started dropping and he began spending all of his free time sleeping. Similarly, I always want to know ahead of time if parents chose me because I was referred to them, if they

just liked my profile online, or if I was the only therapist to return their phone call.

4. Many parents who have struggled to get this far in the treatment-seeking process want to tell their story. They have experienced a range of emotions, from sadness and grief to anger and embarrassment to hopelessness and frustration. It is possible that their friends and family are supportive; it is possible they are not. It is possible that the school knows what is going on; it is possible the family wants to maintain as much privacy as possible. You may, quite literally, be the very first person they can truly talk to about their family's difficulties. For me, there is no better way to show them that I genuinely care about helping their family then to bear witness to their experiences.

A Word about Blame

Before I realized how much I loved working with teens and their families, I was trained to work with young children using play therapy. I also enjoy that work very much, but the entire process, from the recognition of symptoms to the intake itself, looks very different. In those intakes, I tend to meet parents who view their children's symptoms as a product of their environment, genetics, or both. Blaming of the child is often minimal. In comparison, I notice that preteens and then teens are increasingly expected to be more effective at managing their symptoms, no matter what the cause or level of impairment. I hear a lot more about adolescent clients being "lazy," "unmotivated," and "manipulative."

This experience was validated when I was working on an article about trauma treatment with nonoffending parents (Myrick & Green, 2013). Multiple articles I read spoke about the higher level of blame that parents placed on their traumatized teens, often because the abuse situation occurred due to choices that the teen made, such as lying about going to a party where she knew there would be drinking and sexual activity (Davies, 1995; Regehr, 1990; Turner et al., 2012). In contrast to parents of younger children, who rarely suggest that their child should have "fought back," I do hear this from parents of teens sometimes. One mother, whose daughter was sexually assaulted by a longtime male friend after school, told me that she was surprised her daughter "hadn't yelled or hit him or *something*."[4]

We will talk more about how to handle the issue of blame, but I mention it here because if the parent truly believes that the teen could stop the behavior "if he really wanted to," you are going to hear about it during the intake. You probably have your own way of deflecting unhelpful statements in therapy already, but I tend to ignore the blaming part of the statement and empathize with the feeling instead. After all, this is part of their story, and if you were trained in psychodynamic theory like I was, one of those pieces of information that you will tuck away and understand more clearly as you get to know the parents and their teens better over the course of treatment.

The Wish List

I end parents' half of the intake appointment by completing their wish lists. I actually got the idea for this activity from a colleague who does amazing work with couples. The concept comes from the *prepare-enrich* couples therapy model and involves each partner making a list of things he/she would like more or less of from the other. Although I sometimes use the wish list later in therapy, and both the parent and the teen completes his/her own list, I often have parents complete an initial one during the intake. It's similar to the "miracle question" utilized in solution-focused brief therapies. With the miracle question, the therapist asks the client, "Suppose tonight a miracle occurred. When you wake up tomorrow, what will have suddenly gotten better?" As the client talks, the therapist gains more information: what would be different if this issue improved and what are some ways to work toward those gains. I love doing the wish list (or miracle question) exercise with parents because it helps me understand the focus of their concerns, their hopes (implicit or explicit) for treatment, and how realistic their goals are. Once I know what parents' therapy wish list is, I can devise a treatment plan that incorporates their concerns. Most often, I engage in similar interventions with each teen at the start of therapy, but the wish list allows me to customize these interventions to fit the concerns parents have expressed. This process also allows parents to feel like they are leaving the intake with something. I have had parents express their disappointment that therapy wasn't beginning on the day of the intake, which makes sense when the help-seeking process has been long and parents see their teens suffering. The wish list allows me to give parents a "game plan" to hold on to while treatment is initiated, and it acts as one final "brick" in the foundation of a working relationship between them and me—their teen's new therapist.

Is This Really Possible in Fifty Minutes?

Obviously everything I just outlined is *a lot* to cover in one intake appointment, so plan carefully to allow for this process to unfold. Because of the way I structure my intake process, with parents reviewing consent forms and completing basic demographic and development forms before the actual intake appointment, the consent form and policies review process is relatively smooth. Then I am able to devote most of the time I spend with parents to simply hearing their story. A great mentor, who taught me so much about the therapeutic alliance and process, once told me that I needed to take the pressure off of myself to get every piece of relevant data in that first intake appointment. He told me that the intake is about giving new potential clients a chance to experience what working with you would be like. That advice has largely driven the way in which I work with parents during that first intake appointment, and I wholeheartedly encourage you to do the same, no matter what type of parent sits down on your couch.

CONCLUSION

Help-seeking is stressful and challenging for parents and often follows the difficult realization that their teen is in trouble and in need of counseling. Understanding and empathizing with the multifaceted process of help-seeking, which includes overcoming pragmatic and emotional obstacles, enduring wait lists and unreturned phone calls, and managing insurance and scheduling requirements, is paramount when you are contacted by potential clients' parents. Starting with the first phone call, your way of handling parents' concerns, frustrations, and personality styles sets the stage for a successful intake appointment and treatment process. Allowing parents to tell their stories, to identify their hopes and goals for treatment, and to feel valued and understood will increase the likelihood that your intake and initial treatment process will begin smoothly. The success of the intake appointment is important, because the next time you see these moms and dads, you will be their son or daughter's counselor. Your job will involve simultaneous rapport building with both parents and teens, two groups who are often on opposite sides.

NOTES

1. Research has demonstrated that parents are not always aware of their children's high-risk behaviors (see Mojtabai & Olfson, 2008).
2. This study collected data from over ten thousand adolescents aged thirteen to eighteen and was the first to provide lifetime prevalence rates for mental health disorders experienced by teens.
3. Dempster, Wildman, and Keating (2013) suggest that these discrepant findings are likely due to the many ways that stigma is defined and measured in studies.
4. Nonoffending parents' experiences after their children are traumatized are like nothing else you will encounter, so I've devoted chapter 7 entirely to this topic.

Chapter Two

Achieving the Relationship "Trifecta"

"No matter what I do, I am the worst mother in the whole world." Ah, the parent–adolescent relationship. Popular media likes to portray this time in parents' and teens' lives as conflicted and largely negative, and there is a reason for this. Many parents struggle to maintain a positive relationship with their teen, which is why some seek treatment in the first place. I recall one instance when a father jokingly referred to me as the "teen whisperer" because I was able to help his daughter open up about personal and difficult topics. I am proud of my ability to forge relationships with the adolescents that I treat, but I am even prouder when I can develop those same relationships with their parents.

After the intake appointment, your next order of business is to begin developing a therapeutic relationship. You likely have some methods for building alliances with your adolescent clients, but you may or may not have strategized about how to best build a working relationship with the parents who sit patiently in the waiting room. In adolescent therapy, however, three interactions will weigh heavily on your work: (1) parent–adolescent attachment, (2) therapeutic alliance with the adolescent, and (3) working alliance with the parent(s).[1] If you can understand and utilize each of these multifaceted and complex relationships, you will achieve the relationship "trifecta" of adolescent therapy.

THE PARENT–ADOLESCENT RELATIONSHIP

When you hear the term *attachment*, you may immediately recall a study from one of your many psychology courses. The study included "The

Strange Situation" (Ainsworth & Wittig, 1969) and involved observations of infants and young children's responses when they were (1) with their mothers, (2) with their mothers and a stranger, (3) without the mothers and with the stranger, (4) alone without any adult, and (5) reunited with their mothers. The researchers found that *securely attached* children explored their environments when their mothers were present and were distressed when their mothers left, friendly with the stranger when their mothers were nearby but avoidant of the stranger when alone, and happy when their mothers returned. The mothers were responsive to their children's needs, affectionate, and comfortable giving their children age-appropriate autonomy in the play room.

Children with an *ambivalent attachment* pattern explored the room less with their mothers present, demonstrated intense distress when their mothers left, were avoidant and fearful of the stranger regardless of their mothers' presence, and acted resistant toward their mothers when they returned. These mothers were less responsive to their children's needs and were affectionate but awkward in their interactions with the children. Finally, those children with an *avoidant attachment* pattern explored the room more than ambivalent children but less than secure children, showed no signs of distress when their mothers left, played normally when the stranger was present, were uninterested in their mothers upon their return, and were comforted equally by the mother and stranger. These mothers showed less warmth and affection, were avoidant of their children, and sometimes were even angry or rejecting of their children. A fourth pattern, known as disorganized attachment (Main & Solomon, 1990), was identified later. These children demonstrated a combination of avoidant and ambivalent behaviors, along with confused and anxious affect. Mothers of disorganized children demonstrated a range of troubling behaviors that were perceived as frightening, intrusive, or deferential (i.e., the child was in control).

Along the same lines of Ainsworth and Wittig's (1969) findings, Bowlby (1982) theorized that during early childhood, children develop *secure* or *insecure* attachment relationships with their parents.[2] These relationships encompass proximity seeking, safe haven, and secure base. *Proximity seeking* involves children seeking physical closeness with their attachment figure, while *safe haven* refers to children seeking comfort and support, particularly during times of distress. *Secure base* involves parents providing stability for children to explore and take chances in their environments. Inherent in the concept of attachment is the notion that parents are responsive, appropriate, and able to tolerate distress and other intense emotional experiences their children may experience until their children can do so themselves (Briggs, 2003).

Attachment in Adolescence[3]

Ideally, adolescents develop secure attachments with their parents where they trust that their parents will be readily available, supportive, and responsive to their needs. This is necessary as they embrace their curiosities, develop a positive sense of self-worth, and explore new relationships and experiences in the world around them (Duchesne & Larose, 2007). One study found that teens who reported attachment security were more likely to view the past positively, interpret the present accurately—both cognitively and affectively—and expect positive outcomes in the future (Laghi, D'Alessio, Pallini, & Baiocco, 2009). Securely attached adolescents—having their own needs satisfied and learning prosocial skills from their parents—are responsive to others' feelings and demonstrate empathic understanding of others (Thompson & Gullone, 2008).

Taken together, skills facilitated by a secure attachment relationship protect against anxiety, depression, suicidal ideation, hostility, and high-risk behaviors, so it is not surprising that securely attached teens also report less internalizing (Buist, Dekovic, Meeus, & van Aken, 2004; DiFilippo & Overholser, 2000; Laible, Carlo, & Raffaelli, 2000; Liu, 2007; Vivona, 2000) and externalizing problems (Buist et al., 2004; Howard & Medway, 2004; Laible et al., 2000; Shelton & van den Bree, 2010; van der Vorst, Engels, Meeus, Devokic, & Vermulst, 2006). You will see less of securely attached teens; attachment has been shown to separate youths in treatment and those not receiving treatment (Speltz, DeKlyen, Greenberg, & Dryden, 1995).

You *will*, however, frequently see insecurely attached adolescents. These include ambivalent, avoidant, and disorganized teens. These teens, whose attachment relationship may be characterized by harsh and rejecting parenting styles or parents who are not attuned to their needs, are vulnerable to feelings of worry, hopelessness, and inadequacy (Caffery & Erdman, 2000). They tend to report high levels of internal distress (Berger, Jodi, McElhaney, & Kuperminc, 2005), anxiety about the future, and feelings that they are expendable to their parents (Lyon et al., 2000). Insecurely attached adolescents may put themselves in danger, acting recklessly in an effort to engage parents in caregiving. Theorists suggest that parents who are unresponsive to adolescents' needs, except when the requests are extreme or dangerous, and who then may still respond ineffectively, put their teens in a situation where they must aggressively attempt to force their parents to meet their needs (Caffery & Erdman, 2000; Moretti, Holland, & Peterson, 1994). One of my clients, Gina, repeatedly told her parents that she was worried about her mental health, but no attempts to seek treatment for her were made. It was not until she made a near-lethal suicide attempt that they finally got her into treatment. However, once she was stabilized, they began ignoring her needs again, effectively reinforcing the notion that she would have to make a "grand gesture" to regain their attention.

Utilizing Your Knowledge of Adolescent Attachment

In Gina's case, and so many others, understanding the parent–adolescent attachment will help you conceptualize problems with which your adolescent clients present. Direct observation, as well as conversations with parents and teens about trust, security, and communication in their relationship will give you an impression of the quality of the attachment from both perspectives (Myrick, Green, & Crenshaw, 2013). Let me present another example. Frank was a sixteen-year-old who was struggling academically—with the exception of his creative writing course. His ability to create and write stories was apparent in his work, and he received much praise from his teacher. He struggled to put forth the same effort and focus into his nonwriting courses, however, and it was causing conflict with his parents, who both had successful business careers. They expressed great concern in the intake appointment that he would limit his options in the future if he continued with his present choices. They told me that they were constantly embroiled in power struggles over homework with their son; Frank would tell them that he couldn't focus and didn't care about his future, and they would tell him he was just being lazy. Frank shared similar observations, stating that even when he tried to talk to them about his struggles, his parents tended to be disbelieving and insistent that he complete his work in a timely fashion.

Depending on your theoretical orientation, you might proceed with this case in any number of ways. Some might suggest educational testing; this was conducted and revealed no learning differences or disabilities. Some might suggest Frank is struggling with ADHD; there were some symptoms that suggested the diagnosis, but these symptoms only seemed to affect Frank during noncreative writing assignments and teachers did not see any behaviors indicative of ADHD in the classroom. Taken from an attachment perspective, several issues snap into focus: Frank struggles with (1) completing assignments at home but nowhere else, (2) completing assignments where answers are graded as "right" or "wrong," and (3) considering and planning for his future.

In further discussions with Frank, I learned that he felt immense pressure to get good grades in order to ensure a successful career in adulthood. His parents regarded careers highly, and, according to Frank, above and beyond his happiness in the present. He also felt misunderstood and rejected by his parents when they would call him lazy or when he perceived that they were only focused on the "real" classes, rather than the creative writing courses he identified with and enjoyed. Thus, the failure to complete assignments was due to anxiety and feelings of inadequacy, rather than laziness or a learning issue. Using attachment terms, Frank did not view his parents as a safe haven in which he could manage his anxiety, or a secure base from which he could further develop his interest in creative writing. Treatment approaches such as behavioral charts aimed at increasing his work completion were unlikely to be effective. Furthermore, they were unlikely to help me in forging a therapeutic alliance with Frank, the second and arguably most important relationship in adolescent therapy.

THE THERAPEUTIC ALLIANCE

I could write an entire chapter, or book for that matter, on the subject of therapeutic alliance with adolescents. Since the focus on this book is on parents, I will attempt to keep this section brief.[4]

Importance of the Therapeutic Alliance

Therapeutic alliance has been loosely defined as the collaborative relationship between a therapist and client (Martin, Garske, & Davis, 2000). Hougaard (1994) proposed that a therapeutic alliance incorporates therapist contributions (i.e., empathy, expertise, engagement, and genuineness), client contributions (i.e., motivation, receptiveness of empathy, and working capacity), and therapist–client agreement on therapeutic goals and objectives. Clients may view alliance even more simply than proposed in the literature; one study found that eye contact, encouragement, and remembering/referencing past conversations helped clients feel aligned with their therapist (Bedi, Davis, & Williams, 2005).

The therapeutic alliance is a key component of successful therapy and for adolescents, may well be *the* ingredient that makes therapy work (Shirk, Karver, & Brown, 2011). The concept of alliance building can be tricky with adolescents who rarely refer themselves for treatment. Furthermore, you may face reluctance, failure to recognize a problem, and disparities in parent and teen views of problems (Green, 2006; Horvath & Bedi, 2002). Alliance research in the adolescent literature is limited in comparison to the adult literature, but a few publications have concluded that, as in adult studies (Martin et al., 2000), there is a positive relationship between alliance and treatment outcome (Shirk, Karver, Handelsman, Fields, & Bickman, 2006), where higher perceived alliance is related to greater outcomes. Although teens vary in their alliance-forming trajectories (Hogue, Dauber, Stambaugh, Cecero, & Liddle, 2006), stronger client-perceived therapeutic alliances are related to decreased internalizing problems and increased client-perceived benefits and satisfaction from treatment (Bhola & Kapur, 2013), regardless of the treatment modality used (Martin et al., 2000).

That treatment modality matters far less than the therapeutic relationship is an important point to consider, particularly in today's world of technology and third-party payment. Therapists are feeling mounting pressure to produce fast therapeutic results, and training is becoming increasingly focused on diagnoses and elusive "breakthrough techniques" that promise the quick resolution of complex mental health issues (Crenshaw & Kenney-Noziska, 2014). In my work with traumatized and nontraumatized adolescents, the role that therapeutic alliance has played in our work together is immeasurable, and when I ask them what they like best about therapy—an aspect of "checking it out" discussed more below—I am regularly told that they enjoy having someone who genuinely cares about their well-being, thoughts, and feelings.

What Do Adolescents Want in a Therapist?

Tim, a sixteen-year-old client who began treatment following school suspension for substance use, frequently told me (in more colorful language) that I did not mess around. He knew that I had an expectation that he would come to therapy on time, be honest, and engage in our sessions. This aspect of our relationship held him accountable for his actions, something he later told me was rare in his other relationships. Another client, Elaine, told me that she liked discussing the future in our sessions because I did not regard college as her only option, as guidance counselors at her private school often did. Although she was confident she wanted to go to college, she liked being able to entertain other ideas and could do so freely and without judgment in our sessions. Sarah shared that she thought her best friend was lying to her about dating a boy they both liked. A longtime client who struggled to initiate and maintain friendships, I could tell she was not sure if she could give herself permission to be angry, so I said, "Ugh, that's the worst. I hate when I feel like someone is not being honest with me." She later told me that my identification with her in that moment helped her accept her own feelings.

The importance of the therapeutic alliance is only bolstered by studies that have directly asked adolescents about helpful aspects of treatment. These studies have consistently pointed to qualities such as those mentioned in the examples above: accountability, honesty and directness, listening, openness, offering support (not advice), respect, identification, trust, freedom, and guidance (Church, 1994; Diamond, Liddle, Hogue, & Dakof, 1999; DiGiuseppe, Linscott, & Jilton, 1996; Eyrich-Garg, 2008; Martin, Romas, Medford, Leffert, & Hatcher, 2006; Weiner, 1992). All of these qualities point to genuineness, accessibility, and an active presence on the part of their therapists.

Therapeutic Presence

Developing a therapeutic alliance with adolescents requires a *therapeutic presence* on the part of the therapist. This presence involves being in the moment physically, emotionally, cognitively, and spiritually (Geller & Greenberg, 2002). Working with teens requires far more than simply knowing the literature and understanding development. Therapists need to be attuned with their own selves, keeping countertransference issues in mind and manageable, and they must be open and receptive to what is most relevant for teens in the moment (Geller & Greenberg, 2010; Geller, Greenberg, & Watson, 2010). Research has found that for therapists who can master the art of providing a therapeutic presence, clients report a positive therapeutic relationship and progress in treatment (Geller et al., 2010).

Consider Marcy, thirteen, who comes in for her weekly session. She has a history of self-harm and depression, and she has recently been struggling with bullying at school. Marcy sits down and asks for your opinion about a friend who has been hinting that she might have some mental health issues of her own. Marcy's mother called you earlier this week to let you know that Marcy self-harmed after an argument at home, and a part of you is concerned that Marcy is avoiding the topic by bringing up her friend. Another part of you thinks that Marcy bringing up her friend is a way to talk about a positive relationship she has at school, but you may also be concerned that this friend and Marcy will develop an unhealthy relationship based only on their shared mental health concerns. A fourth part of you may be worrying that if you talk about this too long, you will run out of time to talk about the self-harm, which must be addressed today.

So, where do you begin? This can feel like a pivotal decision, particularly if you do not work with adolescents often. I find this group of clients the most unpredictable when it comes to the topics they bring into therapy, and sometimes it is difficult to decide whether or not to change course. One of my graduate professors once said that no matter where you start in therapy, you will always end up where you need to be with your clients. He encouraged us to "trust the process," a notion in line with therapeutic presence. Therapeutic presence would involve being aware of the many (often loud) thought processes occurring in your mind while being physically, emotionally, and cognitively attuned to Marcy's need to talk about her friend in the moment. Such a decision may delay your ability to talk about self-harm for a bit, but it will make a big difference in terms of therapeutic alliance. This alliance may enable Marcy to feel more comfortable sharing her problems, including self-harm, allowing for countless opportunities to discuss core issues in the future.

Keeping Attachment in Mind

I would strongly urge you to use your knowledge about adolescent attachment to inform your alliance-building with teens. As you engage fully and presently in sessions with your clients, you will become aware of your own reactions to them. An anxious adolescent who struggles or resists any efforts at increasing independence or mastery may trigger feelings of frustration, boredom, or resentment in you. Similarly, you may feel discouraged or inadequate with an adolescent who demonstrates avoidant attachment and fails to develop a traditional therapeutic alliance with you. These countertransference experiences provide you with insights about teens' interaction patterns and can help you to reframe frustrating symptoms as manifestations of insecure attachment rather than resistance or overdependence (Myrick et al., 2013). These reformulations will likely increase your ability to be patient, therapeutically present, and hopeful early in treatment, despite alliance-building obstacles.

Checking It Out with Your Client

Difficulties in the therapeutic relationship can wreak havoc on an adolescent's treatment episode and have been cited as the primary reason for premature termination of therapy (Garcia & Weisz, 2002). Furthermore, your perceptions as the therapist may differ from teens' (Taylor, Adelman, & Kaser-Boyd, 1986), and in general, yours are less predictive of the quality of therapeutic alliance, process, and treatment outcomes than adolescents' experiences (Duncan & Moynihan, 1994). Therefore, I prioritize "checking it out" with my adolescent clients; this includes asking about the therapeutic relationship, goals, and treatment approaches currently being utilized. Safran and Muran (2000) have famously said that a therapeutic relationship is negotiated at the outset of therapy and renegotiated over time. I consider "checking it out" to be a way of facilitating this renegotiation regularly in therapy. Rather than asking adolescents if things are going well—many will just respond "yes"—I ask open-ended questions that require them to really think about their treatment. Some examples might include the following:

- What has been your favorite part about therapy so far?
- What has been your least favorite part?
- Are there any things that you wish we were covering but aren't?
- How are you feeling about your parents' involvement?
- How did you feel after our last session?
- How did you feel as you were coming here today?
- Are you still feeling good about our goal(s) of ____________________?

The last question addresses many adolescents' desire for autonomy and responsibility. These important developmental issues may very well interfere with the therapeutic relationship if adolescents do not feel that they are involved in the setting and execution of therapeutic goals and tasks. If you find yourself viewing initial goals as superficial or trite, remember my professor's suggestion to trust the process, and know that your willingness to collaborate with teens on goal setting is helping to foster the vital therapeutic alliance.

THE WORKING ALLIANCE

Development of the therapeutic alliance on its own is complex, but with adolescents, you do so while also building a relationship with their parents. This final third of the relationship trifecta, called the *working alliance*, is generally discussed less frequently in the literature but is just as crucial to successful adolescent therapy (Taffel, 2005). Naidu and Behari (2010) encourage therapists to make the following assumptions (among others):

- The parent is the catalyst to the success of the child's treatment process, both to initiate and maintain change.
- Therapeutic gains can be "undone" between sessions if the parents are not included in the alliance.
- Most parents are not intentionally "bad" or destructive.

As we will discuss throughout this book, you want and *need* parents on your side in treatment. This does not mean that you always share their perspective. All it means is that you need parents' support of treatment both in and out of sessions. First and foremost, this includes engagement in realistic aspects of treatment, such as transportation and payment. Studies have found that the strength of the parent–therapist alliance is related to attendance and drop out; that is, those who have stronger alliances tend to stay in treatment while lower alliance is related to premature termination (Garcia & Weisz, 2002; Hawley & Weisz, 2005; Kazdin, Holland, & Crowley, 1997). In short, building working alliances with your clients' parents keeps you in business! Having parents on your side in treatment is more likely to translate into parents' willingness to examine and modify the dynamics of their parent–teen relationships, with your guidance and encouragement. Studies have demonstrated relationships between strong parent–therapist alliances and improvement in depressive symptoms, anxiety, and behavioral difficulties (Dowell & Ogles, 2010; Hawley & Garland, 2008; McLeod & Weisz, 2005; Shirk et al., 2011).

The Blame Game

Blame plays an interesting role in adolescent therapy, specifically in your work with parents. As I mentioned in chapter 1, parents often believe that their teens are responsible for their behavior and emotions, contrary to parents of younger children (Morrissey-Kane & Prinz, 1999). I frequently encounter parents who tell me that their teens are "just doing [it] for attention" or "to get their way," and these parents are often struggling with angry, combative interactions with their teens. This makes sense: if my friend cancels dinner plans because she just does not "feel like" going, I am more likely to be angry than if something outside of her control interferes, such as a business meeting that ran over. When parents see their teens as capable of stopping the symptoms whenever they want, of course they are frustrated when their teens do not stop. Furthermore, when parents attribute their teen's struggles to stable qualities, they may be less likely to examine their parenting skills which tend to be more inconsistent and ineffective (Morrissey-Kane & Prinz, 1999). We will discuss blame a bit more in chapter 8.

The other aspect of blame refers to the blame parents place on themselves. Parents who have an external locus of control tend to believe that their teens' behaviors and mental health are outside of parental control. These parents tend to blame chance, other people, teen temperament, and biology. They may come in to your office feeling unsure of their parenting skills, defeated, and ineffective (see Morrissey-Kane & Prinz, 1999, for review). Parents with an internal locus of control, on the other hand, view themselves as at least partially responsible for their teens' behaviors and psychosocial development. These parents often adapt their parenting to meet their teens' needs, but may also blame themselves for causing, contributing to, or exacerbating their teens' problems. This can be true even if parents understand the genetic underpinnings of problems (Moses, 2010). I have had parents express guilt over a strong family history of depression or anxiety or failure to notice symptoms quickly enough. Moses (2010) found that the strongest contributors to parental self-blame included perceived bad parenting, passing on "bad genes," and negative family environment. Society plays a role here too; many parents continue to feel scrutinized and blamed for their children's problems (Williams, 2006). The pressure to be the "perfect parent" has never been more intense.

You will likely see the issue of parental blame manifest itself in a couple of ways. Some parents experience great anger and frustration when interacting with their teens. This feeling alone may cause guilt; many parents are faced with the realization that parenting has not gone the way they had expected (Robinson, 1990). As opposed to parents who aggressively engage with their teens, others withdraw, worried that they will continue to fail as caregivers. One father who worked out of town told me, "At least I know I can't screw up or say the wrong thing if I'm not there." Parents may become passive with minimal expectations for their teens, which in turn perpetuates noncompliance (Morrissey-Kane & Prinz, 1999). These dynamics are important to consider as you get to know parents. Their perspectives on blame will play a role in willingness to engage in treatment, identify goals, work on those goals, and trust in the process.

BUILDING A WORKING ALLIANCE

My method of building a working alliance includes genuineness, collaboration, and transparency. It is loosely based on a three-phase process presented by Bordin (1979): (1) establishing a bond, (2) identifying meaningful treatment goals, and (3) agreeing on how to achieve these goals.

Genuineness

Because many parents are already overwhelmed, angry, or fearful at the prospect of letting a new person into their family's issues, I start out by simply getting to know them. I nurture our new relationship during check-ins before a session, check-outs after sessions, and during between-session contacts (more on these below). Sometimes I schedule parent sessions without the teen present. Depending on the case, these may occur as often as weekly or as infrequently as every few months. I work hard to understand family relationships, parenting styles, and stressors. Sometimes, parents share very personal information during early sessions, such as marital issues or their own mental health issues. I like to point out parents' strengths, too, particularly when it does not seem that the parents themselves are aware of them. I empathize with the difficulties of juggling work and family.

Genuineness, above all else, helps me achieve a comfortable atmosphere in which parents can let me into their world. It involves a careful balance of empathy, self-disclosure, and realism. One of the most therapeutic things I can do is acknowledge just how *hard* it is to be a parent, let alone a parent of a depressed, anxious, or impulsive adolescent. Schimel (1974) muses,

> The therapist generally enjoys his time with his adolescent patient while the parent suffers the tensions, the fears, and uncertainties, and the expense of the situation … I don't know why parents cannot be told that the therapist realizes what an annoyance the kid is and how frustrating it is to live with him. This hardly constitutes a breach of confidentiality since everyone, including the adolescent, knows it. The parents' relief at having the obvious verbalized and validated may be, nevertheless, considerable. (p. 246)

I love this statement because it is so very true. Several difficult clients likely come to mind for you, as they do for me. One of my first clients, Laura, presented herself as spoiled, oppositional, annoying, and awful to her parents. Everyone involved knew it! It helped her parents to know that I saw it too and that similar symptoms were commonly seen among teens struggling with depression and substance use. Laura's mom even managed a small laugh before saying, "So it's not just me?"

I often infuse research to validate what I tell parents; this adds some credence to my statements and often helps parents believe that their problems are not insurmountable or uncommon. Hearing that studies point to child-rearing years as the most challenging in a marriage, for example, somehow strengthens my statement of "It sounds like parenting is really taking a toll on you and your wife right now," possibly by targeting both emotional and intellectual aspects of people's defense mechanisms. It also encourages parents like Laura's to be hopeful and understand that, no, it's not just them.

Inevitably, parents ask me about my own family, and many seem relieved to learn that I, like them, am navigating parenthood. Even though I am not yet (thankfully!) parenting a teenager, some of the challenges of parenting my preschooler are not that different. Recently I read a great article about the similarities between toddlers and teenagers,[5] a fact I gladly shared with several of my clients' parents. In each case, we had a good laugh about their similarities: egocentrism, fierce independence, sensitivity, sense of fairness, intensity, and tendency to be a bit of a know-it-all. In each case, this conversation segued into a discussion about the shared needs at these two developmental stages: reassurance, listening, physical attention, limits, safety, guidance, and freedom. Discussing the challenges of meeting these needs by talking openly and honestly about them can help parents feel less "preached to" and more understood.

The example above is just one of the times that I could not have made progress in building a working alliance without *self-disclosure*. Self-disclosure in the therapy field carries with it a largely negative connotation and is considered the polar opposite of neutrality in therapy. Depending on your theoretical training, you may have even learned that self-disclosure reflects poor boundaries or is an early sign of burnout. However, without it, I do not honestly think I could build the strong working alliances with parents that I often do.

Although self-disclosure varies from case to case, I believe that it is a natural part of therapy. Therapists are people, after all, and as people we are incapable of being blank screens. From this perspective, sharing our thoughts, feelings, or experiences is just another way that we participate in the therapeutic process (Gaines, 2003). If you work with adolescents already, you may find that it is difficult to do so without sharing some information about yourself. I self-disclose with the following in mind: "It is not the content of the disclosure that matters but the willingness to open ourselves up to the child in the same way we are asking him or her to open up to us" (Gaines, 2003, p. 571). The same is true for work with parents. Gaines also goes on to say that all individuals, no matter their age, need help becoming clients; therapist self-disclosure can facilitate the process.

Furthermore, with parents, I find it important to humanize myself. We have already talked about the difficulty some parents have admitting that their teens are in trouble. The self-blame and guilt can act as insurmountable barriers to treatment if not addressed, so I share my own experiences. I tell them about the time that I swore I would not let my son have dessert after he refused to eat dinner, and how hard it was to follow through later. I share with them my wish that someone could create a parenting manual that I could follow dutifully. I grow slightly emotional (every time!) when I tell them about a video of mothers criticizing their own parenting and then their children coming on screen and telling the interviewer about all of the wonderful things their mothers do. All of these things (I hope) let parents know that I am not perfect, I do not expect them to be perfect, and their children do not expect them to be perfect either. At least three times a week I tell a parent, "No one expects you to be a perfect parent. Not me, and, most importantly, not your child. Children just need you to be good enough." This simple statement, which most of my parents hear more than once from me, can be a turning point for them.

Collaboration

Collaboration has been defined as a relationship that successfully assists individuals to accomplish goals that they could not have achieved alone. Understanding, supportiveness in getting services, clear and open communication, and flexibility on the part of the therapist are necessary components of this process (Koren & DeChillo, 1995). Despite the fact that many treatment approaches for adolescents include elements of autonomy, separation, and individuation, collaboration with parents is *always* important and relevant (Gatta et al., 2012). When asked about their relationships with their children's therapists, parents emphasize the importance of acceptance, respect, communication, and the absence of blame. These traits result in feelings of empowerment (Norton, 1998). A collaborative relationship with parents has a positive effect on the outcome of treatment (Gatta et al., 2012), and valuing it directly opposes the notion that you see parents as the cause of their teens' problems. Instead, it promotes a belief that parents can be part of the solution.

The ability to collaborate on goals with parents requires that you are first able to *join* them in their perception of the presenting issues. Joining does not mean that you necessarily agree with parents' perspectives, but it does help you to understand why the problem is so troublesome to them and formulate goals upon which everyone can agree (Minuchin & Fishman, 1981). It allows you to treat the concerns of parents respectfully and, in conjunction with what you are learning in your work with the teens themselves, to achieve the task of fitting therapy to the client, not the other way around (Schimel, 1974).

Delineation of goals encompasses making a "short list" of treatment objectives and determining how progress will be measured. This can be a tricky part of therapy, particularly when there are many areas that need to be addressed or when parents' goals greatly differ from adolescents' goals. After a parent gives me a particularly long list of things to address in therapy, I usually laugh slightly and say, "Oh, is that all?"[6] This often allows parents realize just how much work is ahead. Narrowing the list down is important, however, to give the therapy the best chance at success. I love Ross Greene's (2001) basket method to facilitate the task of prioritization. Here is how I generally explain it:[7]

> We can think of problems in three categories that we'll label A, B, and C. Category A involves behaviors that you will always correct—safety issues mostly. For a little boy, this might be something like running into the street, or touching something hot. Category B behaviors are ones that you will negotiate with your teen to help them build skills, problem solve, or make choices. For that same little boy we just stopped from running into the street, we might choose our battles when it comes to topics such as picky eating or chores. Category C behaviors are ones that you will let go of for the time being. You might let this boy slam the door if he's angry, for example. Perhaps eventually this will be a goal to work on, but for now it will be put aside. The key here is that only you and [partner] can really decide which category each behavior will fit into for your family. Things that I might put into category C might be A or B behaviors for you. So, looking at this list of problem areas, where would each of them go?

Parents and I typically collaborate on three treatment goals to start, one of which is always the development of a therapeutic alliance. I educate parents on the importance of the relationship in therapy, and I tell them how I think the relationship can help us achieve our other goals. Second and third goals are identified from the categories A and B. With the knowledge I have gained so far from the teen and his/her parents, I usually point out two additional goals that are reasonable to target in early therapy. If I have done my job well, parents will be receptive to this and will view these suggestions as genuine, hopeful, and joined with their feelings.

Finally, we must collaborate on our definitions of treatment success. Some parents base progress on objective measures (i.e., improved grades, respecting curfew) while others' measures are more subjective (i.e., better communication, taking more responsibility, maintaining change). I rely on the working alliance platform we have built so far to be honest with them about my expectations of success. You need your and the parents' definitions of success to be synonymous, if not identical. I once had a father who wanted his daughter to complete more of her schoolwork. Additionally, he wanted her to "be happy about it." I gently expressed my concern about the second part of this goal, as I was not sure how reasonable it would be to expect this client (1) to enjoy her schoolwork after a difficult transition to high school and (2) be internally motivated to complete it given her external locus of control. I encouraged her father to focus on objective goals and external motivators and rewards; he refused. Even as she began begrudgingly completing more assignments, he refused to reward her because "she need[ed] to learn that you don't get rewarded just for doing your job." Clearly, his definition of success and my definition were mismatched. Their parent–teen relationship continued to suffer despite her efforts, which frustrated and discouraged her and left her father feeling unsatisfied with treatment.

Transparency

Once you have determined goals and measurable outcomes with parents, your job is to figure out how these goals will be addressed in their teen's therapy. Sometimes, most often when teens come willingly to therapy, goals between parents and teens match up beautifully. Other times, teens do not see problems the same way that parents do or will flat out refuse to work on them. In the latter, intimate relationships come to mind, along with high-risk behaviors and academic achievement. In these cases, your job is a little more difficult. Let's look at two examples of social anxiety.

- Maria asked her mother to find her a therapist to address severe social anxiety and generalized anxiety disorder. Her mother expressed concern over Maria's refusal to attend school or extracurricular activities and difficulty at family functions. Similarly, Maria viewed her social anxiety as the most impairing of her symptoms, so we started working on it immediately and directly. We began identifying anxious thoughts, feelings, and maladaptive ways of coping, a relatively standard cognitive behavioral therapy (CBT) approach.
- Tyler's parents brought him to see me after he was caught drinking at a party. They were concerned about his underage drinking, but he was not. He made it clear to me from the first meeting that he had no motivation to decrease his alcohol use. Instead of talking about his maladaptive coping skills to start, I suggested he tell me about the parties he attended and encouraged him to wonder what about his "typical teen drinking" worried

his parents most. As our therapeutic alliance grew, we started talking more about what would happen if he chose not to drink at the parties he attended. He admitted to me that social situations made him nervous, but his anxiety lessened after having a couple of beers. From there, we were able to start working on adding some other coping skills to help in those situations, without my ever demanding he stop drinking. Gradually, his management of anxiety improved, and we were then able to have a more direct conversation about his drinking behaviors.

Tyler and Maria both struggled with social anxiety; however, their awareness of these issues and willingness to work on them varied greatly. As a clinician, you already know that sometimes the path to problem resolution is linear, while other times the path winds and has many rest stops along the way. Parents are not always aware of the process of therapy, and your approach may be different from that of previous providers. Do not be afraid to be *transparent*. Reveal your processes and treatment conceptualizations to your teens' parents. Prepared parents who understand what you are doing (and why) are more engaged in treatment (Gatta et al., 2012). In my experience, these parents feel comfortable to ask questions or follow up with me when they are clear on the logic behind my treatment of their teen.

I also find that parents are more likely to trust my judgment about when therapy is over, rather than prematurely stopping treatment because the immediate crisis is past. Problem resolution is often a reason that parents terminate treatment; they may fail to see a reason to continue treatment when symptoms subside (Block & Greeno, 2011). Because I have been transparent about my approach from the beginning, the majority of my parents are open to my explanation about underlying issues to symptoms. This explanation generally sounds something like "Mental health treatment is a lot like a bad cut on your arm. It may be minor, requiring only a Band-Aid. Others are deeper. In these cases, it's an antibiotic cream that heals the wound, while the Band-Aid is just there to help the process along. Right now in treatment, we have a 'Band-Aid' on the injury. It will help, but not forever, and not without some antibiotic cream."

Even though most parents understand my perspective, some still struggle to keep therapy from taking a back seat to other priorities once their teen is no longer visibly suffering. This period of treatment tends to be when I encounter the most no-shows and cancellations. Limit-setting as a therapist is important here, and I hold parents accountable when I start noticing the cancellation/no-show pattern. Always striving to be genuine and transparent, I gently tell them that I notice them disengaging and voice my concern over symptoms reemerging if treatment abruptly stops. Despite this conversation, there are certainly times when I "fire" families who consistently no-show or are clearly distancing themselves from treatment. Although those parents have not always been happy with my decision, none of them have ever accused me of being unclear about my treatment approach aimed at treating the issues, not just the symptoms. In that way, transparency plays an important role throughout the entire treatment episode.

Finally, I think it is crucial to solicit and address parents' feedback about each of the steps of this process. I recommend that this be done directly, in a manner similar to the one I outlined above with teens. If possible, I like to include both parents in treatment, and the feedback aspect is no exception. One parent may perceive their alliance differently from the other parent(s) (Ellison et al., 2012), which is particularly important in cases such as noncustodial parents who sometimes bring children to therapy, ongoing financial commitment, and prioritization of treatment over other activities within the family.

Maintenance of Contact

You may be wondering how in the world I have time to build such complex relationships with parents. There are so many working parts; your sessions are primarily with the teens, and there is only so much time outside of sessions to spend on the phone and responding to e-mail. As with the intake process we discussed in chapter 1, you may have a way that you like to engage with parents, and your agency may have requirements as well. I am typically able to create a working alliance using check-ins, check-outs, and between-session contact.[8] Depending on the parents and issues, I may schedule in-person parent sessions, but not often.

During Sessions

I was trained to do check-ins at the beginning of sessions and check-outs at the end, and I truly love engaging with parents in this way. During check-ins, I get to touch base with parents before their teen and I get started. Ninety-nine percent of the time, the check-in occurs with the teen present as well, so I am able to observe their interactions, including tone, nonverbal language, and different perspectives. I hear parents' concerns and their observations. The consistency of the check-ins is also useful. Knowing it will occur each week leads some parent–teen dyads to talk about what they want to bring up on their drive to my office; the check-in encourages them to use therapy as a tool for communication. I also hear about times when one or both parties are using check-ins as a weapon (i.e., "I'm going to tell Amie about this"), and the time set aside for a check-in opens up into a conversation about their conflicts. A check-in can always turn into a parent–child session if needed, but I keep this infrequent; otherwise individual therapy slides into family therapy, which some of my families do eventually need (more on this in chapter 8).

Check-outs occur in the last five to ten minutes of the session. This is an opportunity for me to keep parents involved in the goals of treatment in addition to discussing scheduling and completing payment. Furthermore, I usually gain some trust "points" with my teens during check-outs, as they listen to me give parents updates on treatment without disclosing any of their personal information. Telling a parent that we have been working on "how to manage difficult feelings" encompasses many topics, and by sharing this simple summary of our session, I can collaborate with parents while also maintaining the therapeutic alliance with my teen clients. This is a slippery slope, and we will discuss the challenges of confidentiality in the next chapter.

Between Sessions

I invite parents to call or e-mail me whenever they have any information they want to share with me. Although I have had to set limits with a few families over the years, I find that parents do not usually take me up on this offer very often. Schimel (1974) suggested that the offer might alleviate anxiety or guilt and actually have a paradoxical effect on the number of phone calls therapists receive from parents. When parents do call, I let them know from the start how much time I have to speak with them. This helps them determine whether they continue or schedule a different time, and it usually prevents me from having to interrupt them and/or cut them off mid-thought. Our phone calls rarely exceed thirty minutes, with the exception of crisis calls, which as you know, can take any amount of time.

I aim to check my phone throughout the day for missed calls, voicemails, and the occasional text message or e-mail from parents. A little responsiveness goes a long way. I learned the value of this practice early on when one of my first private practice clients, Laurie, presented with suicidal ideation and was hospitalized. Her mother, June, was one of the anxious parents I described in chapter 1 and one of my more difficult parents in many ways. Early in treatment, June was demanding, wanting to know my statistical success rates and threatening to terminate treatment if sessions with Laurie were not "productive." Some of the issues were cultural; June's family was largely unsupportive of her decision to initiate treatment. Others were personal; she felt as though she had failed Laurie, was worried about her younger son, and was struggling with her own depression following a high-conflict divorce. June had difficulty respecting the limits I set with respect to nonemergency phone calls after hours and frequently missed check-ins and check-outs during sessions. Our working alliance was virtually nonexistent.

So, when Laurie was hospitalized, I was concerned about how her mother would cope. After all, it had only been after I insisted that June take Laurie to the hospital for an evaluation, and she made it clear within a few hours of Laurie's admission that she was unhappy with the staff. June began calling me nightly to complain about the treatment and to demand that I "do something" about it. Meanwhile, I had been very involved with the treatment team, and I respected and agreed with their course of action. Nevertheless, Laurie was not getting better, and no one understood why. I continued returning June's calls and listening to her complaints without seeing an end in sight. I was tired, frustrated, feeling helpless, and beginning to harbor some resentment toward June, who was interrupting my family time on a nightly basis.

I consulted a trusted colleague to get some relief, and he suggested that my own reactions were mirroring June's feelings. She, too, was feeling tired, frustrated, helpless, and resentful, and she was using our phone calls as an outlet. He encouraged me to consider handling her phone calls the way I would with a client, so the next time June called, I suggested we schedule an in-person session to talk. To my surprise, she readily agreed, and when she came in the next day, she tearfully shared how difficult it was to see Laurie in the hospital, how confused she felt that nothing was working in improving her symptoms, and how glad she was that I had suggested the meeting. She felt that the treatment team at the hospital was becoming tired of her and that no one was telling her anything. My suggesting a session had made her feel supported and understood. She told me that she now felt that someone was "on her side."

This moment was a turning point in my working alliance with June. Over the next week, medication issues were worked out, symptoms stabilized, and Laurie prepared for discharge. June no longer called me every night. She seemed to do a complete turnaround, now asking my thoughts on issues and trusting that I was advocating for Laurie with the treatment team. We were able to agree on post-discharge goals, and my sessions with Laurie were no longer categorized as "productive" or "unproductive." My alliance with Laurie grew. The solution to this experience seems so obvious to me now, and it may have been clear to you too. However, I think it is easy to forget that being there to meet some of parents' needs is also part of the job when working with youth. And, many times, work with parents happens outside of the child's sessions.

Keeping Parents' Attachment in Mind

Akin to teens' attachment styles affecting the development of therapeutic alliances, parents' attachment also plays a role in the formation of your working alliances. Caregiving is guided by parents' own attachment experiences, and when parents' emotional needs have never been met, they will carry these needs into their relationships with their children (Frew, 2014). Therefore, when you see attachment-related issues in teens, you will also likely see some similar issues in their parents. Securely attached parents may feel more comfortable engaging in a relationship with you than insecurely attached parents; the latter is more likely to demonstrate avoidance or withdrawal. You may find yourself feeling frustrated with parents who seem preoccupied with their own needs and reject those of their teens; this characteristic may reflect an avoidant attachment pattern (Turney & Tanner, 2001). Avoidant parents are often critical and controlling, and they may be disrespectful of the therapeutic alliance between you and their teens. It may be difficult to collaborate with them on goals aimed at their teen's autonomy or relationships. Overdependence and helplessness, reflecting disorganized attachment patterns, may bring up strong countertransference issues in you. Finally, an inconsistent, insensitive, and permissive parenting style that disrupts efforts in a teen's therapy is similar to behaviors seen in ambivalently attached adults (Neal & Frick-Horbury, 2001). Appreciation of the relationship between attachment and caregiving styles can, and will, help you demystify why parents are parenting and behaving the way they are.

CONCLUSION

Achieving the relationship trifecta takes time, patience, commitment, and the conviction that parents are a central part of adolescent therapy. From the outset of treatment—and concurrently with building the therapeutic alliance and acquiring information about the parent–teen attachment—you construct a working alliance with parents. The three-step process I use and recommend encompasses being genuine and empathic, collaborative and inclusive during goal development, and transparent in your approach; I occasionally use self-disclosure. All of these steps are aimed at a working alliance wherein parents trust me as a person, professional counselor, and most importantly, their teen's therapist. This last point is imperative, especially as you progress in the therapeutic work and issues involving privacy and confidentiality emerge.

NOTES

1. Schimel (1974) suggests using the term "therapeutic alliance" to refer to the therapist–adolescent relationship and "working alliance" for the therapist–parent relationship.
2. Attachment figures are not always parents and can be any caregiving adult.

3. Revised from Myrick, A. C., Green, E. J., & Crenshaw, D. The influence of divergent parental attachment styles on adolescent maturation: Implications for family counseling practitioners. *The Family Journal, 22*(1), 35–42. Copyright © 2014 by SAGE Publications. Reprinted by Permission of SAGE Publications.

4. For more information, I refer you to two wonderful resources that are dog-eared and worn on my bookshelf: Bromfield, R. (2005). *Teens in therapy: Making it their own*. New York, NY: Norton, and Perl, E. (2008). *Psychotherapy with adolescent girls and young women: Fostering autonomy through attachment*. New York, NY: Guilford Press.

5. North American Montessori Center (2007, August). Similarities between toddlers and adolescents: A Montessori look at growing up. Retrieved from http://montessoritraining.blogspot.com/2007/08/toddler-and-adolescent-similarities.html#.VMfpa0uzDwI.

6. Back to the importance of genuineness, this is how I handle situations in my personal life too, with a dose of gentle sarcasm, so it feels easy and comfortable for me to infuse it in therapy. If this isn't comfortable for you, there are other ways to convey your feelings.

7. This is slightly different than the way that Dr. Green explains it in his book.

8. With older adolescents who drive themselves to therapy, I aim to do check-ins and checkouts by phone with parents.

Chapter Three

The Two-Way Street

Communication and Confidentiality

"I want her to be able to tell you anything ... but then you'll tell me, right?" This is a sentiment I hear over and over from parents regarding their teen's treatment. In some ways this is understandable. In most cases, teens will wait to seek treatment until things become serious (Stouthamer-Loeber et al., 1995), and parents often believe that once their teen forms an alliance with you, you will "get to the bottom of the problem." Many parents assume that you will convince their teen to be completely honest, and that once you have uncovered the truth, you will share that information with them. It is hard for some parents to understand that it is not a therapist's job to convince their teenager to be more law-abiding or honest (Bromfield, 2005). Parents may also struggle to understand that you can keep them informed while still protecting their teen's privacy, as we discussed in chapter 2.

The parents of my clients are not unique in this regard. Studies show that while parents support confidentiality between their teen and providers, many of them still expect to be privy to the content of your discussions (Dempsey, Singer, Clark, & Davis, 2009) and worry about being excluded from important conversations (Duncan, Vandeleur, Derks, & Sawyer, 2011). Furthermore, in a study of parents who brought their teens to a medical clinic, the topics parents most hoped to be informed about included depression, eating disorders, substance abuse, and other mental health issues (Duncan et al., 2011). As an adolescent therapist, that list essentially summarizes my sessions on a daily basis!

So, how do we keep parents informed while protecting our minor clients' confidentiality? Confidentiality helps teens share sensitive information (Ford, Millstein, Halpern-Felsher, & Irwin, 1997); yet some parents worry that confidentiality will promote risky behavior (McKee, O'Sullivan, & Weber, 2006). Research suggests that the recognition of teens' need for autonomy may play a role in parents' acceptability of confidential services (Tebb, Pollack, Millstein, Otero-Sabogal, & Wibbelsman, 2014). To understand this aspect of adolescent treatment, it is important to first understand the role of privacy and disclosure in the parent–teen relationship outside of therapy. Therefore, in this chapter, we will tackle the "clinical paradox" (Tebb, 2011) of confidentiality with adolescents by examining (1) parenting knowledge and means of obtaining information, (2) parents' views of adolescent confidentiality in therapy, and (3) issues related to "conditional confidentiality" in your work with adolescents.

WHAT DO PARENTS KNOW, AND HOW DO THEY KNOW IT?

One of the core tasks of adolescence is to increase independence. As a result, relationships with parents change, becoming more equal (Smetana, Campione-Barr, & Daddis, 2004). Interestingly enough, this goal seems in direct contrast to the development of intimate relationships, another milestone in adolescent development. How do teens develop close relationships while simultaneously striving for autonomy and independence? And how can parents help facilitate this process? A majority of parents will struggle with the notion that their teen is keeping things from them, and they will seek your help to manage their own anxiety. Many parents will have a particularly difficult time tolerating the "not knowing," although some of them will awe you with their appreciation and understanding of their adolescents' needs. After working with adolescents in therapy, I have come to appreciate the importance of parents' knowledge and the means by which they obtain information. Parental monitoring and adolescent willingness to self-disclose are two variables that lead therapy in many ways. Moreover, parents' views of monitoring adolescent privacy, along with their willingness to adjust related aspects of their parenting, can largely propel or stymie the progress that you reasonably are able to make over the course of treatment.

Parental Monitoring, Solicitation, and Control

The term *parental monitoring* reflects parenting practices aimed at gathering and managing information about children's experiences, both internal and external (Dishion & McMahon, 1998). Parents use a variety of monitoring strategies to keep track of where their children are, what they are doing, and with whom they are doing it (Waizenhofer, Buchanan, & Jackson-Newsom, 2004, p. 352), including the following:

- *Active method:* Direct attempts to inquire about or participate in the child's day; examples include participating in an activity with the child, asking the child, asking other parents, or asking someone else.
- *Passive-child method:* Also known as child self-disclosure; child volunteers information without the parent asking for it.
- *Passive-spouse method:* Spouse (or other parent) volunteers information without the parent asking for it.
- *Passive-other method:* Parent receives information from someone other than the child or other parent, or knows about a child's routine activity.

This practice changes as children grow and their abilities and needs change. As a parent of a toddler, my monitoring method is primarily active, and I rarely rely on the passive-child method. I need to be aware of what my son is doing and where he is at all times in order to keep him safe. Parents of school-aged children, in contrast, may feel comfortable leaving their children to play in the backyard while they watch from inside but are likely to heavily monitor progress in school and homework completion. As school progresses, parents' involvement with schoolwork may also decrease; parents begin relying on their children and teachers' feedback (i.e., passive-child, passive-other) about the completion of assignments and cease checking homework.

In adolescence, teens spend less time at home and under the supervision of adults, so parents can no longer rely solely on active methods and passive-other methods of parental monitoring to gain access to information. Parents do continue asking their teens directly about their activities (i.e., *parental solicitation*), but a heightened reliance on adolescents' voluntary disclosures (i.e., passive-child) emerges in order for parents to stay "in the loop" (Darling & Dowdy, 2010). At the same time, adolescents begin controlling parents' access to their developing self and daily interactions by establishing boundaries about what their parents can and cannot know (Finkenauer, Engels, & Kubacka, 2008).

I want to point out here that active parental monitoring, despite its decrease in adolescence, is still incredibly important. Parents who are involved in their teens' lives—through active engagement in activities and conversations with their teens and others who know them—appear to know the most about their adolescents' daily experiences (Waizenhofer et al., 2004). Alternatively, inadequate supervision and neglect (i.e., lack of material care, interest in education, socialization, or emotional support) have been linked to deviant behavior (Waizenhofer et al., 2004) and deliberate self-harm (Bifulco et al., 2014; Kaess et al., 2013).

When parents acknowledge that their teen is maturing and in need of more autonomy, they can collaborate to create a more developmentally appropriate relationship. Parents may "loosen the reins," while still staying invested and involved in their teen's life. In these cases, *parental control*—parents' rules and restrictions for their children—declines, yet adolescent disclosure and parental solicitation remains (Keijsers, Frijns, Branje, & Meeus, 2009; Stattin & Kerr, 2000). Controlling parents, on the other hand, create climates where teens feel that their privacies are invaded (Hawk, Hale, Raaijmakers, & Meeus, 2008). These parents often have good intentions; they are trying to protect their teens and keep them from engaging in delinquent activities. But, research has suggested that the importance of parental control has been overstated, and highly controlling parenting may be developmentally inappropriate (Kerr & Stattin, 2000; Stattin & Kerr, 2000).

Adolescent Secrecy and Self-Disclosure

Self-disclosure, or information one person communicates about him/herself with another person, is a voluntary activity that relies heavily on both individual traits and relationship closeness. In line with self-determination theory (Ryan & Deci, 2000) adolescents' decisions to self-disclose to—or withhold information from—parents assists in the development of intimacy/relatedness, autonomy, and competence/individuation (Tokić & Pećnik, 2011). Self-disclosure is a complex process that takes into account traits of the discloser and the recipient of the information (Hargie & Dickson, 2004), and it has been identified as an important predictor of parental knowledge of adolescents' activities (Stattin & Kerr, 2000).

Related to self-disclosure, *secrets* are an interesting social phenomenon involving purpose and intent. Teens choose to share secrets with others to show their trust, perceived intimacy, or "specialness" of the relationship. On the other hand, they may withhold secrets to hide perceived flaws, avoid punishment, protect others, have power, or prevent others from spoiling a special memory (Caughlin, Afifi, Carpenter-Theune, & Miller, 2005; Finkenauer et al., 2008, p. 43). Secrets help adolescents with the seemingly contradictory goals of autonomy and social networking by allowing them to control information about themselves (Finkenauer et al., 2008). Frijns, Finkenauer, and Keijsers (2013) propose that adolescents balance the costs and benefits of secrets—and sharing those secrets—by strategically sharing them with parents and others. In this way, they can control how much of the secret they disclose, and prevent isolation because of rigid concealment (p. 56).

Adolescents who share information with their parents demonstrate less problem behavior, anxiety, and depression (Jacobson & Crockett, 2000; Smetana & Metzger, 2008). They also exhibit greater willingness to have parental involvement (Trost, Biesecker, Stattin, & Kerr, 2007) and experience higher well-being overall (Jacobson & Crockett, 2000). It could be that teens who disclose more to their parents get the benefit of parental support; their caregivers can then help meet their needs. Intrapersonal factors, such as a teen's open and engaging personality, and/or interpersonal factors, such as positive disclosure experiences in the past, could also contribute to adolescents' willingness to share with parents (Frijns, Keijsers, Branje, & Meeus, 2010). Whatever the reason, it is important for parents to understand the delicate balance between facilitating openness while respecting secrets and privacy.

Unfortunately, parents—and many people in general—often have a very black and white view when it comes to secrecy. Family beliefs, culture, and past experiences often play a role in this view. To them, secrets are unhealthy, dangerous, and contradictive of healthy relationships (Finkenauer et al., 2008). Indeed, there are some definite disadvantages to secret-keeping: keeping secrets can be stressful, can convey a sense of "getting away with" misconduct, and takes away parents' chances to redirect behavior (Frijns et al., 2010). On the other hand, *shared secrets*, or secrets that are shared with some but kept from others, are not necessarily negative. In fact, these types of secrets have been associated with being well adjusted and increased competence in interpersonal relationships (Frijns et al., 2013). *Secrets kept private*, or concealed from everyone and known only to the secret-keeper, on the other hand, are associated with higher internalizing and externalizing symptoms, loneliness, and poorer quality relationships (Finkenauer, Engels, & Meeus, 2002; Frijns et al., 2013; Frijns, Finkenauer, Vermulst, & Engels, 2005). Interestingly, Frijns and colleagues (2013) also found that for those adolescents who had shared secrets, private secrets had less of a negative effect on mental health.

Remember when I told you that at times, knowing the literature can help give credibility to your discussions with parents? Secrecy in adolescence is one of those times. Again, many parents have the misconception that their teen's secrecy is something to be worried about, but I can often put these anxieties at ease by sharing what we (the field of counseling) know about secret-keeping. Once parents understand this, they can refocus their energy on being a good candidate for the recipient of a shared secret.

On Attachment and Monitoring

When teens and parents have a securely attached relationship, they have set the stage for a successful, reciprocal partnership. In this partnership, teens feel safe to share information when their parents request it; this makes monitoring and supervision less of an issue in the relationship (Waters, Kondo-Ikemura, Posada, & Richters, 1991). Secure relationships are associated with check-ins initiated by both parents and teens and increased parental knowledge.

Check-ins demonstrate parental availability and interest to teens, which then further strengthen and maintain the secure relationship and increase the likelihood that teens will disclose in the future (Kerns & Aspelmeier, 2001; van der Vorst et al., 2006). On the other hand, parents and teens that do not have a strong relationship may be less likely to engage in regular conversation, leading to less disclosure and possibly more intrusive, less teen-centered monitoring and solicitation strategies.

Facilitating Adolescent Self-Disclosure

I am often trusted with my adolescent clients' secrets, a fact that is not very surprising for most parents. After all, many of them seek out treatment so that their teen has someone to talk to, and although some overestimate their awareness of their teens' risky behavior (Helitzer, Sussman, Urquieta de Hernandez, & Kong, 2011), most are pretty accepting of the fact that their teen is not telling them everything. If, however, my goal is to eventually "work myself out of a job" and terminate treatment, my clients will need someone to talk to once I am no longer there. Enter parents.

One of my goals in writing this book is to point out great things that parents do, as well as parenting behaviors that can be problematic. I think there is a danger in assuming that parents are *always* to blame when adolescents refuse to share things with them, and as I just said in the last section, I use the literature to normalize adolescent concealment to parents, much in the way I have tried to do in this chapter. That being said, some parents do need my help in developing a means of parental solicitation that feels comfortable for them and their teen. This process often includes assisting parents with active methods of monitoring such as getting to know their teen's friends, carving out time for discussion, and participating in activities that their teen values. In addition, I am *constantly* working with parents to improve their potential as a confidant. I help them understand the importance of being perceived by their teen as available, discreet, nonjudgmental, patient, calm, willing to take issues seriously, and able to provide new insights or offer advice (Keijsers et al., 2009; Kelly & McKillop, 1996; Tokić & Pećnik, 2011). Adolescents are less likely to self-disclose to their parents when they fear negative emotional or behavioral consequences (Darling, Cumsille, Caldwell, & Dowdy, 2006). Specifically, some teens view their parents as intrusive or distracted, or they think their parents will lecture, punish (including anger/yelling, and the "silent treatment"), interrupt, break confidentiality, or tease them (Tokić & Pećnik, 2011).

The last one, teasing, goes along with lack of understanding and is particularly important in terms of adolescents feeling supported by their parents. For example, many teens tell me that their parents "just don't understand," particularly when it comes to social issues such as arguments with friends or romantic partners. I frequently remind parents that although a high school romance may seem "silly" when compared to a committed, long-term, adult relationship, it is far from trivial in the eyes of a teenager. I often have to tell parents that their adolescent's experience of romantic love is all that she/he knows, and minimizing it only makes her/him feel misunderstood. On the other hand, parents who can empathize, take their teens seriously, and maybe even appropriately self-disclose can facilitate disclosure and a closer relationship with their teens. Allie, sixteen, was "shocked" when her mother was able to empathize and give a helpful suggestion after Allie's boyfriend unexpectedly broke up with her. Allie told me,

> It was late, and I knew [my best friend] wouldn't be able to answer my text, so I was kind of stuck with my mom. I was expecting her to tell me that high school relationships are silly and that I shouldn't be upset. That's what she always does. But I took a chance and told her anyway, more to get her to go away than anything else. She looked really sad to see me so upset, and she just gave me a hug and told me she was sorry and that she knew it hurt. Then she asked if I wanted to go to [the grocery store] and get some ice cream. I don't know why—it's so cliché to eat ice cream after a break-up—but it actually helped to get out of the house.

I could not have been prouder of Allie's mom for this exchange. Her mom was available, empathic, nonjudgmental, and helpful. She responded in a way that felt comfortable for both her and Allie. These "wins" are possible with all parents if they are willing to prioritize their teens' needs over the urge to immediately solve every problem or make every interaction a "teachable moment."

Ideally, I want parents and adolescents to share at least a few secrets together and to have positive self-disclosure experiences. There is an inherent closeness that occurs when two people share a secret, and parents and teens can never have too many opportunities to develop and redefine a healthy attachment to one another. In my individual work with teens, I often act as a "thermometer," letting them test out their disclosures on me or encouraging them to think about what it would be like to tell these secrets to their parents. Together, we explore the barriers and facilitators that factor into the teens' decisions. I then use this information to assist parents in becoming more appealing outlets for their teens' disclosures. Imagine Isaac tells me that he would *never* consider telling his dad that he failed his most recent math quiz because his dad would assume he was not completing his work or trying hard enough. In our check-out, or the next time I see his dad, I might mention, "Isaac and I have been working on sharing feelings and thoughts with people in his life. I think he worries that no one understands him. I'm really working with him to take some chances with the people in his life. From you and his mom, I need you to be as accepting as possible with the things he tells you. You don't have to agree with him, but I think it's important that he learns that he can trust other people not to put him down or criticize him."

A Word about Parental Trust

In relationships, predictability, dependability, and honesty seem to make up the foundation of trust (see Kerr, Stattin, & Trost, 1999, for review), and the parent–teen relationship is no exception. Issues surrounding *parental trust*—parents' beliefs that their teen generally follows rules and makes good decisions—are common (Kerr et al., 1999). Just the other day, during a check-in, Kevin's mom told him that he was "impossible" to trust. This hurt Kevin, thirteen, deeply. He told me, "She's the only one who doesn't trust me, and it sucks." He went on to tell me about close friends who confided in him about family problems and special responsibilities he was given by his soccer coach. It did seem that many individuals viewed him as trustworthy. Furthermore, he felt that he contributed greatly to the needs of their single-parent home. When I spoke to his mom at the end of the session, she shared that she could not trust Kevin because he lied about completing homework and chores around the house. She complained that he often "made excuses" when his responsibilities were not completed. For her, Kevin's actions were not trustworthy, so *he* was not trustworthy.

Kevin and his mom are a great example of just how complicated the issue of trust is in therapy. Much of the information you get about your teens, other than what they tell you themselves, is from parents, and there may be only a small association between adolescents' reports of their own trustworthiness and parents' trust beliefs. Although parents often have a knack for spotting lies, they also tend to err on the side of pessimism, assuming that their teen is lying to them (Darling & Dowdy, 2010). This tendency to assume untrustworthiness can have negative consequences, or what I call *the cycle of nondisclosure* (figure 3.1).

When parents believe their teens are concealing information, they are less accepting and confident in them (Finkenauer, Frijns, Engels, & Kerkhof, 2005). This, in turn, affects the parent–teen relationship, which lessens the degree to which teens trust that their parents will respond positively to a disclosure. Adolescents use the degree to which they trust their parents to determine their willingness to disclose (Darling & Dowdy, 2010). If they choose not to disclose or to lie, parents may see them as even less trustworthy.

It is important that parents understand the role that distrust plays in their relationships with their teens. Teens, like Kevin, may feel hurt and less close to their parents when they are falsely accused of deception and deemed

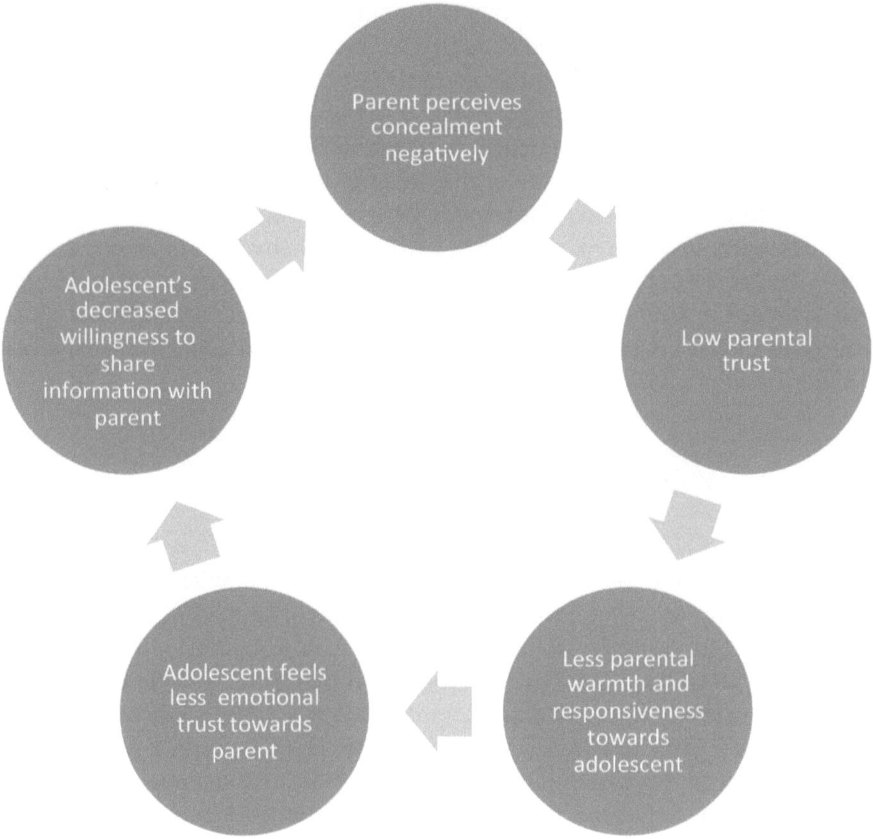

Figure 3.1 The Cycle of Non-Disclosure

untrustworthy (Feeney, 2005). This can also set the cycle of nondisclosure in motion. One of your objectives in cases where parental trust is an issue may be to assist parents in recognizing times when they are being pessimistic or evaluating their teen's overall trustworthiness using limited information.

Parental Knowledge and Adolescents' Confidentiality in Therapy

With so much pressure on parents to trust their teens and respect their privacy but also know what is going on, it is not surprising that the issue of confidentiality can be quite difficult for parents, teens, and their therapists. Consider, for example, the parent who struggles with excessive monitoring and control; the thought of "not knowing" is wrought with anxiety and fear. Alternatively, think about your own anxiety when you encounter a high-risk teen that lives with a low monitoring parent who is a poor listener. Only *you* can decide where your comfort lies when it comes to breaking confidentiality. For the rest of the chapter, I am going to summarize the literature on adolescent confidentiality, discuss how I approach the conversation with parents and teens, and demonstrate how I make decisions about breaking confidentiality in non-mandated situations.[1] They may or may not put you at ease, and ultimately, it is not up to me (or anyone else) to decide the situations in which you break confidentiality in high-risk situations. I would only stress that you do, in fact, make the decision, preferably before you are faced with a questionably high-risk behavior in your session with a teen. Once you have made that decision, you need only to explain it clearly to parents and teens, and then they can decide if you are the right fit for their family.

"CONDITIONAL CONFIDENTIALITY" IN ADOLESCENT TREATMENT

When it comes to confidentiality in therapy, many therapists do their teens a disservice by assuring them that their treatment is confidential. In fact, there is no legal basis for doing so (Fisher, 2013; Rae, 2001). Parents have the right to all of their teens' information, and therapists have an ethical and legal responsibility to break confidentiality when a client's behavior constitutes potential harm to himself or others (American Counseling Association, 2014; American Psychological Association, 2002). Thus, adolescents and parents must be informed that confidentiality is *conditional*, meaning that certain situations necessitate a break in confidentiality (Lothen-Kline, Howard, Hamburger, Worrell, & Boekeloo, 2003). Despite the fact that professional organizations recommend a clear discussion about confidentiality with clients, research suggests that some therapists avoid the discussion completely for fear of a reduction in trust, disclosure, or willingness to enter therapy (Crenshaw, Lichtenberg, & Bartell, 1993; Fisher, 2013; Haut & Muehleman, 1986).

There *are* possible negative implications to placing conditions on confidentiality, such as a decrease in clients' willingness to disclose difficult information (Ford et al., 1997; Lothen-Kline et al., 2003; Nowell & Spruill, 1993) or clients' discomfort in sharing information which may warrant a breach of confidentiality (Wallach, 1997). However, you place yourself in a precarious ethical situation if you fail to adequately explain confidentiality to your teens (Fisher, 2013). Studies have found that "no explanation" equates to "complete assurance of confidentiality" for many teens (Miller & Thelen, 1987), which we know is not the case. You may find yourself struggling with the best way to address teens' conditional confidentiality.[2] Therefore, I have included some teens' suggestions on how to explain confidentiality to themselves and their parents (Ford, Thomsen, & Compton, 2001, p. 158):

1. Emphasize the ways in which confidentiality can be protective.
2. Emphasize caring over legal obligation.
3. Be specific about what is and what is not protected by confidentiality.
4. Discuss how you will manage "gray areas" (Taffel, 2005).
5. Avoid the word "except" and the phrase "I promise."
6. Act trustworthy.

My sound bite about confidentiality to teens keeps each of these six recommendations in mind and ensures that teens understand exactly what confidentiality means:

> Many of the things we talk about in here will stay in here, like your thoughts and feelings (#3). But, there may be times that you tell me about something that makes me concerned for your safety (#2), and my number one job is to help you stay safe (#1). These times might include serious thoughts about taking your life or someone else's, or someone hurting you physically or sexually. Some teens struggle with substance use that is getting out of control, or they are making choices about sex that put them at risk. I work with some clients who are cutting themselves or involved in some dangerous eating habits. All of these things, depending on the circumstances, could be times that I decide that we need to get your parents involved. I call these "gray areas" because they can be tricky to figure out sometimes (#3). If I decide that your parents need to be informed, you and I will talk about how to do that (#4). I will never go behind your back or tell you that something will stay confidential if it won't (#6). Many times, my clients and I tell parents in a session, so that we can come up with some solutions together. These solutions might include some more sessions, some changes at home, or maybe hospitalization if things are serious. Do you have any questions about what would or would not be kept confidential, or how we would handle any potentially dangerous situations?

Parental Acceptability of Confidentiality

As a whole, the counseling field knows little about parental attitudes of confidential services for their adolescents (Tebb et al., 2014). However, a recently published study demonstrated that one-third of adult participants (47 percent of which were parents) believed that parents' authority should take priority in situations possibly warranting a break in confidentiality (Munoz Sastre, Olivari, Sorum, & Mullet, 2014). Additionally, other research suggests that demographic and sociocultural variables, such as cultural views about parents' role in teens' lives and changing expectations of involvement as teens age, may be involved (Tebb et al., 2012). Parental anxiety can also act as a barrier. Some parents worry that their teens' disclosures about the family will be unflattering or that their parenting practices will be viewed as abusive (Haut & Muehleman, 1986). Although a strong working alliance with parents may not completely eradicate their fears, it does help for parents to trust you and have confidence in your therapeutic skills (Tebb et al., 2012).

One step I take toward helping parents understand confidentiality in adolescent therapy involves a *child therapy contract*. This contract, seen in textbox 3.1, is used by many therapists around the country and was created

Textbox 3.1

Amie C. Myrick, MS, LCPC
Licensed Clinical Professional Counselor
1205 York Road, Suite 39B
Lutherville, MD 21093
443.220.7922 . amie.myrick@gmail.com

Child Therapy Contract

Prior to beginning treatment, it is important for you to understand my approach to child therapy and agree to some rules about your child's confidentiality during the course of his/her treatment. The information herein is in addition to the information contained in the Client–Therapist Agreement. Under HIPAA and the ACA Ethics Code, I am legally and ethical responsible to provide you with informed consent. As we go forward, I will try to remind you of important issues as they arise.

Therapy is most effective when a trusting relationship exists between the counselor and the patient. Privacy is especially important in securing and maintaining that trust. One goal of treatment is to promote a stronger and better relationship between children and their parents. However, it is often necessary for children to develop a "zone of privacy" whereby they feel free to discuss personal matters with greater freedom. This is particularly true for adolescents who are naturally developing a greater sense of independence and autonomy. By signing this agreement, you will be waiving your right of access to your child's treatment records.

It is my policy to provide you with general information about treatment status. I will raise issues that may impact your child either inside or outside the home. If it is necessary to refer your child to another mental health professional with more specialized skills, I will share that information with you. I will not share with you what your child has disclosed to me without your child's consent. I will tell you if your child does not attend sessions. At the end of your child's treatment, I will provide you with a treatment summary that will describe what issues were discussed, what progress was made, and what areas are likely to require intervention in the future.

If your child is an adolescent, it is possible that he/she will reveal sensitive information regarding sexual contact, alcohol and drug use, or other potentially problematic behaviors. Sometimes these behaviors are within the range of normal adolescent experimentation, but at other times they may require parental intervention. We must carefully and directly discuss your feelings and opinions regarding acceptable behavior. If I ever believe that your child is at serious risk of harming himself/herself or another, I will inform you.

One risk of child therapy involves disagreement among parents and/or disagreement between parents and therapist regarding the best interests of the child. If such disagreements occur, I will strive to listen carefully so that I can understand your perspectives and fully explain my perspective. We can resolve such disagreements or we can agree to disagree, so long as this enables your child's therapeutic progress. Ultimately, you will decide whether therapy will continue. If either of you decides that therapy should end, I will honor that decision, however I ask that you allow me the option of having a few closing sessions to appropriately end the treatment relationship.

____
Printed name of minor client

Printed name of parent or guardian	Signature of parent or guardian— Date
Printed name of parent or guardian	Signature of parent or guardian— Date

by the American Insurance Trust, the American Psychological Association's affiliated malpractice provider.[3]

For several reasons, this form has been a helpful addition to my intake packet. First, it highlights the importance of their teen's privacy from the very beginning of treatment. Parents are informed that the contract is not a legal document; rather, it acts as a mutual understanding of the importance of the therapeutic relationship. Second, although not legally binding, most parents do take it seriously. As a result, parents rarely demand to see their teen's records in their entirety, and in cases where they do request notes, most parents are content with a letter or summary rather than the entire chart. Finally, in cases where parents do refuse to sign the contract, I am aware immediately of their hesitation to relinquish access, and we can talk about it. I would much rather understand this mistrust or anxiety at the beginning of treatment than in the midst of a crisis.

After discussing the child therapy contract, I explain confidentiality with parents in a manner similar to my approach with teens:

> Many of the things [teen's name] and I talk about will stay between us. It is important that he feels safe in therapy to share any of his thoughts or feelings. However, my number one job is to help him stay safe. If he were to tell me about serious thoughts of killing himself or someone else, I would be legally required to intervene. If he were to tell me that someone was physically or sexually abusing him, I would be legally required to report it. But in working with teens, there are also some "gray areas" that often come up. Substance abuse, self-injury, eating disorders, and high-risk sexual behaviors are a few examples. In those cases, I would get some more information and

> decide whether or not you need to be informed. Usually, I look at the severity, frequency, and degree of risk. If I decide that you need to be informed, [teen's name] and I will talk about how to involve you. Many times, my clients and I tell parents in a session, so that we can come up with some solutions together. These solutions might include some more sessions, some changes at home, or maybe hospitalization if things are serious. Do you have any questions about what would or would not be kept confidential, or how we would handle any potentially dangerous situations?

It is at this time during the intake that I also introduce the check-ins and check-outs outlined in chapter 2 and welcome between-session contact. This helps parents understand the degree to which I plan to keep them regularly involved, which also assists with anxiety about being "kept in the dark."

THE DECISION TO BREAK CONFIDENTIALITY AND HANDLING "GRAY AREAS"

The question of when to break confidentiality is one that virtually *all* therapists struggle with, whether they see adults or minor clients. In fact, mental health professionals consider confidentiality dilemmas as the ones most frequently encountered in their work with clients (Pettifor & Sawchuck, 2006). Fears about clients completing suicide are high on the list of anxiety-provoking scenarios (Pope & Tabachnick, 1993), and therapists may experience feelings of anger, anxiety, and sadness when working with clients who engage in destructive behaviors (Fleet & Mintz, 2013). When I teach graduate level courses and the trainees find out how often I work with issues such as self-injury, substance abuse, and suicidality, many of them seem terrified at the prospect of high-risk clients, and understandably so. How do you help these individuals? How do you know when confidentiality should be broken? How do you manage the anxiety that must come with safety-related issues in therapy? We can all think of a clear example of a time when confidentiality needed to be broken. One of my colleagues once had an adult male take out a Swiss army knife during a session and begin self-harming. Although this situation was certainly scary, the seriousness of his intent and risk he posed to himself was clear. The times when I have to break confidentiality are usually less black or white and far more gray.

- Mary was a seventeen-year-old client who had been referred for obsessive compulsive disorder (OCD) related to cleanliness. Shortly after beginning treatment, she reported manic symptoms and was subsequently diagnosed with bipolar I disorder. Over the course of treatment (approximately one year), she and I worked through noncompliance with her medication,

unremitting OCD symptoms, and a significant life stressor—her parents' impending divorce. One week, she came into my office, tearful and depressed. Her father was unable to take her to her school dance, as he had a business dinner that evening, but he was unwilling to collaborate with Mary's mother to get Mary to the dance. Mary was crying and saying how unfair it was, when she mentioned that "maybe I should just kill myself … that would solve everyone's problems." She went on to say that even though she had thought about it sometimes, she "probably wouldn't act on it."
- Liam was fifteen years old when he first disclosed his drug and alcohol use. He was initially referred to treatment due to conflict with his parents over missed curfews and friends they considered "too old" for Liam. After three sessions, he admitted to social drinking and marijuana use with peers during weekend parties. He denied blackouts but did admit that sometimes he drank a little more than he had planned.

A tension exists when therapists consider breaking confidentiality. The negative nature of the behavior (i.e., frequency, intensity, duration, and risk) can push in favor of the break, whereas maintaining the therapeutic process (i.e., potential for behavior to stop without informing parents, seriousness of behavior, likelihood that treatment will continue after break, possible disruption of therapy) can cause a therapist to pull away from the break (Sullivan, Ramirez, Rae, Razo, & George, 2002). Taffel (2005) acknowledges, "[The risk of] irreparable rupture … is a key reason to push your client to start sharing more with parents before you'll be forced to" (p. 165). However, as we have been discussing, teens are not always in a hurry to disclose information, and it is often difficult to determine if an adolescent poses a *genuine* risk to himself or others (Sullivan et al., 2002). So many times, you are left with only your clinical judgment to guide you.

Out of all high-risk behaviors, I tend to break confidentiality for suicidal behavior the most quickly and frequently. This is in line with what Sullivan and colleagues (2002) found in their survey with psychologists: suicidal behavior was most likely to be reported to parents by therapists, followed by substance use, sexual behavior, alcohol use, and, finally, cigarette smoking. As a general rule, I do not discuss substance use or sexuality with parents unless the behaviors concern me. I determine how concerned I am by whether one (or more) of the following seems true:

1. The adolescent intends to continue engaging in the behavior and does not seem to understand the danger involved.
2. The behavior seems to be intensifying to a degree that the adolescent is in greater harm than before. I look to see if the behavior is increasing in

frequency (e.g., weekend use to weekday use) and severity (e.g., social drinking of beer to solitary drinking of liquor). This is especially true if I have prior knowledge of behavior, and it is continuing to worsen despite our discussions.
3. The teen has put himself/herself in a position of serious danger. Examples of this include self-harm that is infected or requires medical attention, frequent blackouts from substance use, or having unprotected sex with multiple partners.

With Liam, for example, I decided to work on the issue in therapy without informing his parents of the substance use. His substance use, as he described it to me, sounded social and mostly controlled. He denied blackouts, use during the week, or attempts to stop without success (#2, 3). In our weekly sessions, we discussed the progression of substance use (i.e., use, misuse, abuse, and addiction) and agreed on warning signs that his drug and alcohol use was becoming problematic. Liam identified drinking or smoking alone, buying his own marijuana, and blackouts from alcohol as concerning behaviors. We also continued working on his relationship with his parents so that he might eventually feel comfortable self-disclosing his experimentation with them.

Determining suicidal ideation, as in the case of Mary, typically involves a more in-depth assessment before I make any decisions about whether to break confidentiality.

ASSESSING SUICIDAL RISK

There is little agreement on the "best method" with which to assess suicidal ideation (Connor & Rueter, 2009), and some research suggests that clinicians tend to overdetect suicidal ideation when their teen clients mention thoughts about death (Holi et al., 2008). I would highly recommend the first six items of the Suicide Status Form (SSF; Jobes, 2006), a core piece of the Collaborative Assessment and Management of Suicidality method (CAMS; Jobes, 2006). The CAMS method fits seamlessly with the treatment approach I have been outlining so far because it emphasizes collaboration between the therapist and client,[4] and it considers six unique constructs from the suicide literature:

1. **Psychological pain:** hurt, anguish, and misery in your mind (*not* physical pain or stress)
2. **Stress:** general feeling of being pressured or overwhelmed
3. **Agitation:** emotional urgency, feeling that you need to take action (*not* irritation or annoyance)

These first three items are based on the cubic model of suicide (Shneidman, 1987) that highlights a suicidal person's subjective experience of unbearable suffering (psychache), overwhelming feelings due to internal and external stressors (press/stress), and "impulsive desire to do *something* to change or alter his or her unbearable situation" (Jobes, 2006, p. 12), referred to as perturbation/agitation. Shneidman theorized that the interaction of maximum levels of all three variables (i.e., the 5-5-5 conceptual corner) culminates in a suicide attempt (figure 3.2).

This is a particularly useful viewpoint in working with adolescents; low distress tolerance can be especially dangerous when combined

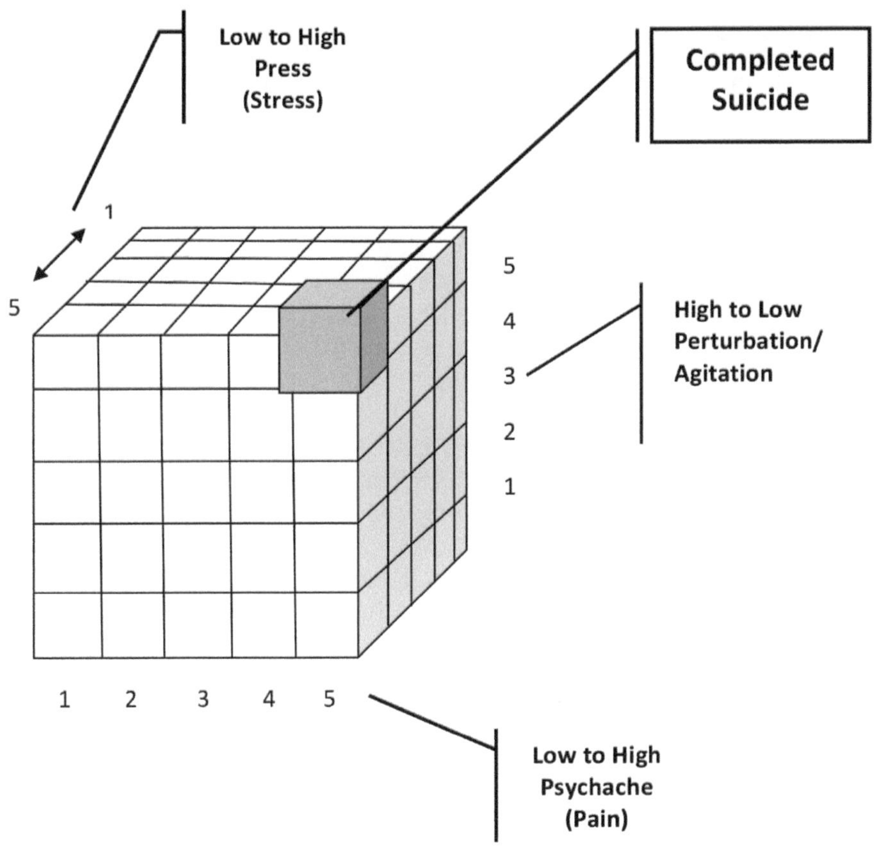

Figure 3.2 Shneidman's Cubic Model of Suicide. ***Source:*** **E. Shneidman. (1987). A psychological approach to suicide. In G. R. Vanden Box & B. K. Bryant (Eds.), *Cataclysms, crises, and catastrophies: Psychology in action* (pp. 147–183). Washington, DC: American Psychological Association. The use of APA information does not imply endorsement by APA. Reproduced with permission.**

with the impulsivity and poor judgment often associated with adolescence (Gibbs, 2011). Furthermore, adolescent psychache in particular has been shown to mediate the relationship between suicidality and a much-discussed variable in the suicide literature—hopelessness (Troister & Holden, 2010).

4. Hopelessness: an expectation that things will not get better

Hopelessness is a construct taken from the cognitive theory of depression. In this model, Beck asserted that when a person expects that a negative situation will never get better, it is difficult for them to develop hopeful thoughts about the future (Beck, Rush, Shaw, & Emery, 1979). Hopelessness is a relatively common feeling among adolescents (O'Connell, 2012) and has been linked to adolescent suicidality in studies (Hewitt, Caelian, Chen, & Flett, 2014; Zhang & Li, 2013), although the relationship between the two may be less salient than in research with adults (Rudd, Joiner, & Rajab, 2001).

5. Self-hate: general feelings of disliking yourself, poor self-esteem, low self-respect

This fifth variable incorporates the classic, psychodynamically minded conceptualization of suicide as a means to escape extreme, intolerable self-loathing and self-hatred (Baumeister, 1990). It is in line with research reports that one of the most commonly cited reasons for self-injury among teens is self-punishment related to a derogatory view of self (Glenn, 2013).

6. Behavioral assessment of suicidal risk: likelihood of killing self

Finally, the behavioral assessment of suicidal risk captures the question that needs to be asked: "Are you going to try and kill yourself?"

To assess these six items, I ask the teen to rate the degree of each on a scale of one (low) to five (high), and, if needed, I give them the brief descriptions provided above (Jobes, 2006). Then I combine these ratings with my clinical knowledge about the teen's current stressors, relationship with parents, past attempts, and so on, and consider their answers to the standard questions about the presence of a reasonable plan, means to obtain the plan, and future orientation. This approach helps me feel confident and comfortable—or as comfortable as I can be with a suicidal client—about the current status of the adolescent's safety. Once I know how I feel about my client's safety, I can decide whether to break confidentiality. As I see more and more teenagers, I continue to develop more and more trust in myself to make these decisions.

Textbox 3.2

Mary's Current Suicide Status

Measure	*Information*	*Risk Level*
Current Stressors	Missing school dance, discord within the family, ongoing OCD symptoms	Moderate
Relationship with Parents	Strained; low likelihood (in my opinion) that she would self-disclose suicidal ideation	Moderate
Past Attempts	None known	Low
Other High-Risk Behaviors	Denied	Low
Plan Details	Vague ("I just want to go to sleep and never wake up")	Low
Means to Harm Self	Access to psychiatric medications Access to sharp objects Access to car keys No firearms in home	Moderate
Future Orientation	Negative ("I just feel like it will never get better")	Moderate
Psychological Pain	4	Moderate
Stress	4	
Agitation	2	
Hopelessness	4	
Self-hatred	5	
Overall Risk	3	

After completing a brief assessment of Mary, I concluded that Mary was at moderate risk for a suicidal gesture (see textbox 3.2). This information, along with the fact that I was concerned at the suddenness of the symptoms and Mary herself did not feel safe, helped Mary and I decide to bring her mother into the room to discuss our options.

When the decision is made to break confidentiality, you have to decide exactly what information you will share with parents. I typically recommend the "less is more" approach in these cases; you only share the basic information you need to and encourage your adolescent clients to elaborate. You want to give parents enough information so that they know to take your concerns seriously, but not so much information that the teen feels any more exposed than absolutely necessary. You also need to come up with a plan that everyone—teen, parent, and yourself—is comfortable with and willing to follow; again this is done without disclosing too much about your clients' work and needs. To say that having conversations with parents about "tough stuff" is a delicate aspect of adolescent treatment would be an understatement. I have devoted all of chapter 5 to it, so fear not.

CONCLUSION

Adolescents make the conscious decision to share or withhold information from their parents every day as they work on developmental goals such as autonomy, decision-making, and meaningful relationships. During this process, many parents struggle to adapt to a new type of relationship with their teen. Communication between parents and adolescence presents a challenge for therapists tasked with assessing risk taking and potential safety concerns. Clear boundaries from the first appointment about confidentiality and its limitations are crucial. The assessment tools and strategies I have outlined in this chapter can guide you as you determine what can and cannot be kept confidential. Trusting your clinical judgment above all else will increase your confidence when gray areas appear.

NOTES

1. Each of the United States, District of Columbia, Guam, the Northern Marina Islands, Puerto Rico, and the Virgin Islands have identified mandated reporters of suspected child maltreatment. Thirty-two states also have institutional reporting laws, and fourteen of those states specifically state that providers are still obligated to make reports, despite any policies within the organization. Mandated reporting laws also exist in Canada, Australia, and much of Europe (Harries, 2002).
2. For the remainder of this chapter, conditional confidentiality will be referred to simply as "confidentiality."
3. The form shown here is modified slightly. The original form can be downloaded free of cost and in its entirety from http://www.trustinsurance.com. Reprinted here with permission.
4. This approach also stresses the importance of viewing suicidal ideation as a primary treatment goal. In this way, it is regularly assessed and examined in a collaborative fashion. This is a great approach to take with teens and their parents because it normalizes the discussion about suicide and models appropriate ways to approach the topic.

Chapter Four

ICYWW

Teens, Parents, and Therapists in the Digital Age

"I have never felt so old as when I am trying to read my daughter's texts," a mom told me recently. If you had to look up what the ICYWW in this chapter's title meant—In Case You Were Wondering—you are not alone. Working with today's digitalized teens not only involves staying current with trends, popular slang, and the endless stream of acronyms, but also making decisions such as whether to allow cell phone use during therapy, and supporting parents as they attempt to monitor social media. After the explosive growth of adolescents' social networking sites (SNS) approximately ten years ago, the market for parenting books followed suit, resulting in an overwhelming number of options for parents needing guidance to keep their teens safe online (Yan, 2008). For many parents, their teen's Internet usage is a source of great concern and anxiety, particularly as they attempt to balance these worries with developmentally appropriate decreases in parental monitoring, as we discussed in chapter 3. Because of this, working with teens will almost guarantee that parents struggling to determine and enforce effective digital limit-setting strategies will consult you. It is also likely that you, too, will have to make some decisions about the role of SNS and digital communication in your personal and professional worlds. But first, you need to have a clear picture of the functions that social media and digital communication serve in adolescents' lives.

THE ROLE OF SOCIAL MEDIA AND TECHNOLOGY IN ADOLESCENTS' LIVES

Adolescents have been called the "natives" of the digital world, meaning that their social world has always involved digital forms of communication such as text messaging, e-mail, and SNS (Kennedy, Judd, Dalgarno, & Waycott, 2010; Prensky, 2001). Although Facebook remains the most widely used SNS—nearly one billion users per month![1]—there are a number of other SNS that teens use, including, but not limited to, texting, microblogging, self-destructing, and chat applications, or *apps*.

IF YOU CAN'T BEAT 'EM . . .

Social Media and Technology for Parents

If adolescents are the natives of the digital world, that makes parents (and therapists) the "digital immigrants" (Kennedy et al., 2010; Prensky, 2001; Ransdell, Kent, Gaillard-Kenney, & Long, 2011). Older generations, in other words, remember what it was like to live in a world without the Internet. They formed their social identity without the use of SNS, so it is easy to see how they may not view and understand the use of technology in the same way as today's adolescents. Moreover, they may view technology as threats to "family time" (Ling & Yttri, 2006). Users of cell phones are in "perpetual contact" (Katz & Aakhus, 2002), so meals and vacations, previously designated for family, can now be permeated by texts, tweets, and ringtones (Ling & Yttri, 2006).

As we discussed in the last chapter, parents learn the most about their teens' lives by engaging in activities with them (Waizenhofer et al., 2004), so it makes sense that many parents attempt to connect with their adolescents through technology. Digital communication is a part of everyday communication between parents and their teens, with both positive and negative effects (Jordan, Hershey, McDevitt, & Heitzler, 2006; Padilla-Walker, Coyne, & Fraser, 2012; Pettigrew, 2009). Parents use cell phones to text and call their teens in an effort to check-in, and learn or confirm plans (Ling & Yttri, 2006; Padilla-Walker et al., 2012), and many believe that the ability to stay connected while physically apart is beneficial for their families (Kaiser Family Foundation, 2010). Similarly, teens report calling and texting their parents, although some teens do view the contact as encroachment on their emerging autonomy (Green, 2001; Ling, 2004) and many only text so that their parents know their whereabouts (Ling & Yttri, 2002). I have seen technology be a *wonderful* way for teens to connect with parents who are deployed, separated, or working night shifts.

Parents have also increased their SNS use (Madden, Cortesi, Gasser, Lenhart, & Duggan, 2012); a recent study revealed that almost 80 percent of adolescents' parents were on SNS (Doty & Dworkin, 2014). Studies estimate that about half of adolescents connect with their parents through SNS, although frequency of contact varies greatly (Coyne, Padilla-Walker, Day, Harper, & Stockdale,

2014). How comfortable teen clients are when social networking with parents is also largely variable and likely related to the overall quality of the parent–child relationship (Kanter, Afifi, & Robbins, 2012). Some teens struggle to get online distance from their parents, believing that SNS is for interacting with friends, and choosing alternative sites after their parents "invade Facebook" (Klein, 2012; Madge, Meek, Weelens, & Hooley, 2009; Wiederhold, 2012). Others actively choose to "friend" their parents and view the digital communication positively (Burke, 2012). Researchers suggest parent and teens' joint use of SNS can promote feelings of connectivity due to shared media interests, interactivity (e.g., games and shared videos), and online support (i.e., "liking" a picture, posting positive comments), particularly when parents can utilize SNS to better understand their teens (Coyne et al., 2014). Social networking, then, can act as "one of many 'tools' that parents can use to feel close to their [teens] and interact with them in meaningful ways" (Coyne et al., 2014, p. 11).

GUIDING AND SUPPORTING PARENTS IN THEIR DECISIONS ABOUT TEEN SOCIAL MEDIA USE

Although some parents may try to connect with their adolescents through SNS and may even consider themselves quite knowledgeable when it comes to social media, the reality is that adolescents are often more Internet savvy than the adults in their lives. This means that teens can engage in online activities that are unknown to parents, clinicians, and teachers, and understandably, this makes parents very nervous. Many of my clients' parents struggle with finding a balance between being overly intrusive and—as one mom put it—"stupidly unaware" of what their teens are doing on smartphones and computers, and they turn to me for guidance. Unfortunately, there is not a "one-size-fits-all" answer, and many approaches largely depend on teens' symptoms, parent–teen relationships, and parental monitoring styles. As a starting point, here are five basic guidelines I use with parents who are trying to promote safety in digital communication and social media.

1. Consider the role that digital communication and social media play in your teen's life.
2. Engage in Internet "spot checks."
3. Discuss rules for the Internet and SNS, clearly and objectively.
4. Identify consequences for breaking Internet rules clearly and objectively.
5. Talk openly about difficult Internet-related topics.
6. Set aside "unplugged time," and stick to it.

Let's look at each of these a little more closely.

Consider the Role that Digital Communication and Social Media Play in Your Teen's Life

It is important that parents keep in mind that social media serves as a place where teens can "explore, experiment, and engage" (Evans, 2014, p. 154), while texting and cell phone use assists them in maintaining relationships. Parents can connect with their teens by taking the time to learn about social media, showing the same level of interest that they would about a school play, sports game, or hobbies (Hannah, 2010; Weigle & Reid, 2014).

Engage in Internet "Spot Checks"

While I was in graduate school, I worked in an adult substance abuse clinic, and it was there that I first learned the power of random drug urinalysis. Conducting urine screens on a random schedule can deter drug use, discourage drug use after a screen (i.e., some clients will use immediately after because they know it will be a little while before they are screened again), and make it harder for clients to plan their drug use around testing. Furthermore, it allows therapists to see how clients are doing without relying on the client's self-report of drug use (see Vakili, Currie, & el-Guebaly, 2009, for review). Studies have suggested that such screens may be particularly useful in the treatment of adolescent substance use because teens may be less likely to willingly share the extent of their use and less intrinsically motivated to engage in treatment. Random drug testing, therefore, provides an external motivator to stay drug free until intrinsic motivation increases (Vakili et al., 2009).

In the same way, random "spot checks" of digital communication and SNS may act as a powerful deterrent for teens while also providing them with some space online. Barth (2014) cautions against exhibiting too much control over Internet and social media, as it can lead to teens feeling stifled or mistrusted. On the other hand, free reign on the Internet can lead to risk-taking and unsafe decision-making. For example, studies have linked a neglectful parenting style with higher rates of cyberbullying than more involved parenting styles (Dehue, Bolman, Vollink, & Pouwelse, 2012). Through spot checks, parents can allow their teen some freedom online, with the understanding that parents can and *will* check on their teen's usage from time to time.

Although some parents insist that they have their teens' passwords, I do not think this is absolutely necessary, and in some cases, it may do more harm than good. I can picture a few of my clients saying, "Well, then what's the point of a password?" or "How do I know you won't check what I'm doing more than you say you will?" I encourage parents to consider password knowledge as just one option to discuss with their teens. Another option might be to conduct the spot checks together, where teens sign in using their password and then look at their online histories with their parents. In this way, parents are allowing teens to see their own choices, and the shared experience can open up a discussion about such decisions. Parents might also give their teens the opportunity to let them know of anything that might be surprising beforehand. I once had a seventeen-year-old client who had been using the Internet to look up breast implants. Although this was not "against the rules," she worried about what her mom would think when she saw it in her browsing history. They were able to talk about it and decided to bring the body image issue into therapy.

Discuss Rules for the Internet and SNS Clearly and Objectively

One of the biggest strengths of parents who use an authoritative parenting style is their ability to establish *clear*, mutually agreed upon boundaries with their adolescents and then monitor those boundaries.[2] Teens of these parents are more socially responsible, independent, and cooperative than teens with permissive or authoritarian parents. They spend less time on the Internet than other teens, and they also have higher levels of trust and communication in their relationships with parents (Rosen, 2007).

Just as authoritative parents set limits on curfews, parties, and academic expectations, so too, can parents set clear, objective limits on Internet and social media use. Although most teens do not engage in "pathological computer use" (Weigle & Reid, 2014, p. 92), many do need parents' assistance on judging appropriate Internet behavior, ranging from the amount of time spent online and what is shared. With respect to time limits, Weigle and Reid (2014) suggest being clear about the start and stop time of Internet use. The use of timers or scheduling of Internet use around other activities (e.g., before dinner and before leaving for soccer practice) is less likely to result in a power struggle than a parent who arbitrarily decides when "enough is enough." In terms of setting limits on information sharing, parents need to be clear about information that is safe and unsafe to post online, whether GPS tracking or Location Services can be enabled on phones, what SNS are permitted, who (if anyone) can have the teens' login information, and specific times that parents do not want their teen posting their whereabouts or personal information (e.g., when parents leave teen home for the evening alone). Appropriate behavior, language, and discussions can also be topics upon which parents can set limits. Many people disclose more information online than they would in person (Christofides, Muise, & Desmarais, 2009), and this may be a good way for parents and teens to negotiate the sharing of information (i.e., "Is this something you would tell someone you just met?"). Although they may be challenging to enforce—and not welcomed by teens—such limits help teens make good choices online and balance technology use with other activities.

Limit-setting is an *ongoing conversation*, so remind parents to discuss limits anytime it seems appropriate. For example, one of my clients (Anya) went on vacation with her family to a Caribbean all-inclusive resort. While they were away, her sister (Cecile) got a terrible sunburn and posed for some pictures to document her experience. Anya's mother was horrified when she learned that Anya had posted a couple of these pictures—which featured Cecile wearing only a carefully placed towel to capture "burn-lines" along where her bathing suit had been—on Facebook. Anya and Cecile had not viewed these pictures as sexual in nature and found them funny, wanting to share them with friends. Anya's mother could have prevented Anya's post if she had set limits on the pictures' uses in the moment. This is in no way to blame Anya's mother for the post, or to suggest that parents must be able to read their teens' minds when it comes to posting on SNS. However, parents must be mindful of the fact that teens do sometimes post information that they later regret, either because they forgot certain people would see the information or because they did not realize how the post would be perceived (Child, Petronio, Agyeman-Budu, & Westermann, 2011).

Identify Clear Consequences for Breaking Rules, and Enforce Them

Along with clear rules, clear consequences must also be discussed and enforced. The simplest and most direct consequence, of course, is the removal of social media and technology. While this is a perfectly acceptable punishment, remind parents that they must *enforce* whatever amount of time they assign to the punishment, which can be a lot of work. Furthermore, removing the phone or Internet access may not address the problem. Many teens feel completely cut off from peers when their phones are taken away, and some may even view them as transitional, comforting objects akin to a young child's stuffed animal or beloved blanket (Barth, 2014; Erkolahti & Nyström, 2009; Ribak, 2009). There is a risk that teens will withdraw from their parents, or that they will fear that parents are violating their privacy by searching the phone (Marshall, 2014).

I really like an approach I read about in an article published this past summer (Marshall, 2014). One of the therapists interviewed suggests that parents first discuss the problematic behavior/decision with their teen and then limit phone privileges in a way that targets the problem. For example, a parent can delete an application that was used to engage in cyberbullying, or the phone can charge in the parent's room temporarily to help the teen focus on homework at night. This approach goes back to my first guideline—considering what social media and technology means for the teen—and focuses on correcting, not simply punishing behavior. Finally, it assists teens in setting limits when they are struggling to do so themselves. It would not be reasonable for many of us to go for long without access to the Internet or phone—I have logged countless hours online just in the writing of this book! Simply taking away teens' phones does not help them learn ways to manage social media and technology's daily presence in their lives.

Talk Openly about Difficult Internet-Related Topics

No parent particularly enjoys talking about sensitive topics such as sexting, online predators, and cyberbullying with their teens. Not only is it often uncomfortable for everyone involved, but parents also tell me that bringing up the issues makes them feel anxious when they think about the possibility of their teens being involved in some way. I often prepare parents for these discussions by giving them some basic information; this data helps offset the notion that "My son/daughter knows better than that," and it also gives parents information that they can actually use when they speak to their teens, if needed.

Textbox 4.1

Sexting

- Youth sexting is common, particularly when the definition includes both photographic and nonphotographic sexts (Strohmaier, Murphy, & DeMatteo, 2014).
- The majority of youths deny experiencing any negative social or legal consequences as a result of sexting (Strohmaier et al., 2014).
- Teens who sext are also more likely to engage in risky sexual behaviors such as unprotected sex (Drake, Price, Maziarz, & Ward, 2012), sex with multiple partners (Drake et al., 2012), and sexual activity while intoxicated (Temple et al., 2012).
- Many teens who sext have been bullied or cyberbullied (Drake et al., 2012).
- Peer pressure (Houck et al., 2014), perceived peer approval (Lee, Moak, & Walker, 2016), and the need for popularity (Vanden Abeele, Campbell, Eggermont, & Roe, 2014) are all reasons why teens sext.
- Teens may be prosecuted and convicted for their role in sexting. In some cases, teens and young adults have been placed on probation and required to register as a sexual offender (Strohmaier et al., 2014).
- Many teens are unaware that some states consider sexting among minors a crime.
- Teens who know the potential legal consequences of sexting engage in sexting significantly less than those who are unaware of the legal consequences (Strohmaier et al., 2014).

Online Predators

- Victims of online sexual offenders are often aware that they are conversing with adults, and offenders are often open about their sexual interest (Wolak, Finkelhor, Mitchell, & Ybarra, 2010).

- Nearly all victims of "Internet-initiated sex crimes" are between the ages of thirteen and seventeen (Wolak, Finkehlhor, & Mitchell, 2004).
- Interacting with strangers online and posting personal information online are two factors associated with proneness to risky Internet use (Ybarra, Mitchell, Finkelhor, & Wolak, 2007).

Cyberbullying

- Between 4 and 57 percent of teens admit being cyberbullied at some time (Dehue et al., 2012).
- Teen may not always define their behaviors as cyberbullying (Mishna, Saini, & Solomon, 2009; Vandenbosch & Cleemput, 2009).
- Some examples of cyberbullying behaviors include sending messages to frighten or threaten someone, spreading rumors on SNS, sending mean or insulting messages to someone, pretending to be someone else online for the purposes of hurting the victim (e.g., pretending to be the victim's crush) or getting the victim in trouble (e.g., pretending to be the victim), using vulgar or harsh language, excessive text messaging, and posting embarrassing pictures of the victim (NoBullying.com, 2015).
- Many teens fail to tell parents when they are being cyberbullied for fear that their parents will confiscate their phones or restrict their Internet use (Wolak et al., 2010; Weigle & Reid, 2014).

In order to have effective conversations about difficult Internet topics, I recommend that parents *specifically* talk about each issue, as opposed to engaging in general discussions about being "safe" or "smart." Returning to the notion of clear consequences for inappropriate or dangerous behavior, parents and teens can talk about appropriate courses of action if sexting or cyberbullying occur. In this discussion, parents can also assure teens that they will not be punished if they disclose that they are being cyberbullied.

Set Aside "Unplugged Time," and Stick to It

I will admit it: this is a tough one. I know it is tough because I have tried it and, on many occasions, failed miserably. However, I do truly think it is important, and I continue working on it in my own home so that my family can know and enjoy "unplugged time." Researchers are expressing more and more concern about the high levels of mobile phone and technology use among today's youth (Lopez-Fernandez, Honrubia-Serrano, Freixa-Blanxart, & Gibson, 2014), particularly in families where parents also report high rates of technology use (Bleakley, Jordan, & Hennessy, 2013). It is important for parents to remember that they are important role models when it comes to appropriate Internet and technology use (Weigle & Reid, 2014).

Whenever I am working with parents on implementation of new behaviors, I stress the importance of the change being attainable. For a family who spends the majority of their time on their computers, phones, gaming systems, or in front of the television, "unplugging" for the entire day on Sunday, for example, is completely unrealistic. For this family, we might discuss starting with *one hour* of unplugged time per week that gradually increases to one hour per day. To me, consistent quality is far more important than quantity. Just like any big change, limiting technology is hard, and parents and teens often struggle. One family was committed to unplugging after dinner. It was going great, until the father, a lawyer, had a conference call with clients in a different time zone. Evenings were the only time the call could occur. Giving parents permission to recover after a misstep or "relapse" is one of the most important things you can do as a therapist in their lives.

On Attachment in the Digital Age

Attachment is relevant when we consider how parents view and interact with teen Internet and phone use, as well as what digital communication means for teens. Parents who are struggling with their teen's emerging independence may experience great anxiety when it comes to Internet and phone use. These "helicopter parents" may try to keep teens from becoming too autonomous by instilling fear about the Internet or by using Facebook or texts to stay in constant contact with their teens (Cundy, 2015). As opposed to years past when, in order to talk to friends, teens needed to call their friends' houses and talk to their friends' parents, today, teens can largely communicate with friends without their parents even knowing, let alone giving permission. Anxious parents—and even securely attached parents—may worry about how adequately they are protecting their teens. Dismissive parents, on the other hand, may resent their teens for having constant access to them via phone or social media, and/or may not pay much attention to their teens' comings and goings in the digital world. These parents' teens may be the ones we talked about in chapter 2, who engage in risky behaviors in an unconscious attempt to get their parents' attention.

Insecurely attached teens may also rely intensely on social media and digital communication to connect with others. For some, it could be because the impersonal nature is easier to tolerate, while others may like it because it allows unlimited, constant contact with others. Indeed, Cundy (2015) suggests that cyberspace has "not just altered, but eroded, many boundaries" (p. 22). Securely attached teens, on the other hand, are more likely to develop and respect boundaries through digital communication. Their phones and access to others may provide some comfort and security but are not used excessively or in a way that challenges limits set by others.

SOCIAL MEDIA, TECHNOLOGY, AND THE THERAPIST

Many mental health professionals use technology every day, for both personal and professional reasons. This is not surprising; digital media is prevalent, accessible, and permanent (DeJong, 2014). Over time, professionals can expect that digital communication and social media will continue to play a greater role in counseling settings than ever before, and for therapists working with teenagers, it is not a matter of *if* they will need to address these issues in their practices, but rather *how* and *when* (Barth, 2014). Let's tackle some of the situations you may encounter in your work with teens and their parents, including, but not limited to, decisions about electronic communication and social media, cell phones in sessions, and using the Internet to look up information about clients. As you evaluate some of these decisions, you may also get a clearer sense of how you view technology in teens' lives, which can further inform the guidance you give to parents.

Google and Other Online Searches

Google has drastically changed the way we access information. I remember when the site first became popular and how exciting it was to simply "Google" the answer to a question or problem. So common is the usage today that "Google" was even added to the dictionary, defined as "to use the Google search engine to obtain information … on the World Wide Web" (Merriam Webster Online, n.d.). Because of the ease with which we can find information on places, people, and things, it makes sense that this practice has implications for the therapeutic relationship. Specifically, how frequently are clients Googling us? Should we Google clients? Should we search for them on SNS?

Client Searches

Online marketing is one of the most lucrative ways therapists are staying busy with new referrals. There are many articles and books that recommend having a positive online presence to reach prospective clients (Hanville & Snyder, 2012; Wallin, 2012). Therefore, it stands to reason that clients are searching for us online. One study found that 92 percent had found professional information about their therapists online (Kolmes & Taube, under review). What may surprise you, however, is that 70 percent of these participants also reported having found *personal* information about their therapist online. Most of the participants (87 percent) sought this information intentionally from sites such as Google, Facebook, and LinkedIn, and less than one-third discussed their findings with their therapists (Kolmes & Taube). Feelings of curiosity seemed to be the most common motivator to conduct a search (81 percent), followed by feelings of being in a one-sided relationship, interest in the therapist's daily life (i.e., married, children, in recovery), and wonderings about the therapist's political, religious, and sexual preferences.

I think I do a pretty good job of protecting my personal information online, but I am also very aware of the fact that I *do have personal information online*. I have a personal Facebook account, a personal blog where I write about crafts and cooking, and family members who use social media regularly. Because of this, and the knowledge that clients may search for me, I make sure that anything I post online would be okay for clients to see, should they ever stumble upon it. Since I know that a client may not ask me about something they find online, I want to make sure that the picture, the comment, or the statement is clear on its own.

I also do my best to share some small pieces of information with my clients so that they feel like they know something about me. If my teens and parents feel like they can ask me what my holiday plans are, for example, there is less of a chance of them searching for my Facebook page to catch a glimpse of my weekend. When my son was born, I chose a couple of pictures to share, and I did so with the few clients who asked. My pregnancy was not exactly something I could hide, after all, and after I returned to work, the pictures satiated any curiosity about this life event I had experienced. I also think it made some parents feel closer to me, as we now had a shared experience.

Therapist Searches

Now that you know that at least some of the parents and teens you see for therapy are searching for you online, let us consider your use of Google or SNS to gain information about clients. Although many therapists believe that clients should determine if and when they will share personal information, some professionals see little harm in conducting online searches for clients, reasoning that anything available on the Internet is public knowledge (DiLillo & Gale, 2011; Jent et al., 2011). In line with this viewpoint, many trainees—as many as 97 percent in one study (DiLillo & Gale, 2011)—admit that they have used the Internet to get information about clients, often out of curiosity or concern, or to establish the truthfulness of disclosures (DiLillo & Gale, 2011; Jent et al., 2011; Lehavot, Barnett, & Powers, 2010). Similarly, studies demonstrate that practicing therapists and other health professionals also conduct Internet searches on their clients (Kolmes & Taube, 2014) and would consider doing so to obtain additional information in the future (Jent et al., 2011).

There are serious ethical and alliance-related issues to consider if you conduct searches of your clients and their families online. First and foremost, doing online searches takes away clients' right to determine when and how personal information will be disclosed (DiLillo & Gale, 2011), which has potential consequences for your alliance with parents and clients. Adolescents and their parents may expect that their social media information will remain private unless they grant you permission to view their profile pages or sites. They may not have intended for you to see the information or be prepared to deal with the consequences once you do see it (Guseh, Brendel, & Brendel, 2009). Ethically, you need to decide what you will do with the information you find. In other words, is it appropriate to search without telling your clients? What should you do if you find information that suggests risk to self or others, or abuse? Could you ask your client for this information directly? In addition to these considerations, Clinton, Silverman, and Brendel (2010) suggest answering these questions prior to conducting an online search:

1. Why do I want to conduct this search?
2. Would my search advance or compromise the treatment?
3. Should I obtain informed consent from the client prior to searching?
4. Should I document the findings of my search in the client's record?
5. How do I monitor my motivations and the ongoing risk benefit profile of searching?

Personally, I do not search for my clients online, for several reasons. First, I worry about what I will find. One of my clients, Lindsey (age thirteen), was mortified after her mother found suggestive Facebook posts from a male Lindsey had been messaging privately. Through the conversation with Lindsey's mother, I learned that the male was an adult and that her mother had enough information to make a child abuse report. This situation would have been even more difficult if I had obtained that information myself, without Lindsey's or her mother's knowledge or consent. Similar issues can arise if you see suicidal statements or posts indicative of high-risk behavior (Cash, Thelwall, Peck, Ferrell, & Bridge, 2013). Because Lindsey and her mother shared the information with me, however, we were able to address it in therapy without anyone feeling as though their privacy had been violated. Second, I consider it a great step forward in our therapeutic relationship when teen clients show me their Instagram pictures, play their favorite music for me, or tell me about an embarrassing social media blunder. My genuine response to these disclosures would be lost if I already knew the information due to conducting online searches independently. By allowing those pieces of information to come into sessions as clients feel ready, I preserve the opportunities for those key relational moments in therapy. Finally, staying out of clients' Internet and social networking sets limits on what I am and am not willing to do for teens and their parents. Many of my referrals come from prior clients, and just as I set limits about my after-hours availability, so too has word "gotten around" that I stay out of my clients' social media.

Accepting Social Media Requests

Staying out of clients' social media means that I do not accept friend requests on any SNS, including LinkedIn, a site largely designed to promote professional networking and opportunities. This includes requests from parents, or situations in which a social media site tries to link me to a current or former client without my knowledge or permission (this has happened multiple times on LinkedIn). I utilize maximum privacy settings on Facebook, the social media site on which I am most active, and rarely post pictures. I never post about my day with clients because, despite the fact that it is unlikely that any client will ever see it, I do get referrals from many different places. It is entirely possible that a friend of a friend gets referred to me. How would I feel if I complained about my day, and that friend commented, making it possible for their friend (my client) to see it? I know this sounds a little paranoid, but I feel immense comfort in knowing that these types of issues will be prevented by my choices online. Furthermore, I worry enough about dual relationships and running into clients in uncomfortable settings (e.g., my son's pediatrician) without having the additional complication of having a client on a list of my "friends." In a profession full of grey areas, I, for one, like being able to simply say, "I do not participate in social media with my clients or their families."

E-mails and Texts between Sessions

Accepting e-mails and texts is another thing entirely, however. For one, I use e-mail with my clients from the beginning. As I shared in chapter 1, I typically send an e-mail to parents after our initial phone call and scheduling of the intake appointment. Personally, I prefer e-mails over phone calls from clients for day to day issues, and I often tell them that I can respond to e-mail more quickly than voicemails. The reasons for this are largely practical: in the ten minutes between sessions, I can read and respond to several e-mails, whereas I can probably only return one phone call. I am clear to state, however, that I do not conduct therapy over e-mail or text, so if there is an issue that we need to discuss, I insist we talk by phone or save the discussion for our next session. I try to reserve e-mail communication for appointment changes and quick things that parents want me to know before their teen's sessions.

Texts and e-mails can be "tone deaf," so my words are devoid of tone and therefore open to any interpretation by the client. I once had a client forget about an appointment. I called and left her a message, and she texted me back, apologizing and saying that she was overwhelmed. I started to respond to the text, planning to say, "Okay. Give me a call tomorrow and we can reschedule," but I accidentally hit send prematurely. The text she received said, "Ok." Given the high levels of anxiety and stress that this client was experiencing, she immediately called me, thinking I was angry because of my short text. This, of course, was relatively easy to rectify, but I can imagine it might not have been with another client, in a different situation.

A final reason that I limit the information discussed via e-mail or text is because of the very nature of e-mail and texting today. Thanks to smartphones, I have constant access to my messages, which means that I may see an e-mail while I am sitting on my couch watching television, or right before I step into a meeting. These situations are hardly ideal for responding to complex issues, as I may be distracted or wearing a different "hat" at the moment. Reserving more involved discussions for a time when I am completely engaged in a therapeutic space with the individual is a far more appropriate way for me to treat clients.

I do occasionally run into parents who struggle to respect the limits I have set for e-mail and text communication, and others have written about this issue as well (DeJong, 2014). I typically know that they are pushing limits when I began feeling pressured to respond therapeutically to e-mails, even though I know I am not comfortable doing so. These situations can be difficult because your options may be limited. I would encourage you to employ a model of limit-setting that feels comfortable to you, such as the A-C-T model of limit-setting that I use with children in my practice (Landreth, 2012). This model includes Acknowledging the feeling, Communicating the limit, and Targeting an alternative. In a situation involving excessive electronic communication, it may look like this:

A. Randy, I know you are really worried about your daughter and believe that e-mailing me several times a week "keeps me in the loop."
C. However, I cannot reasonably respond to this many e-mails. I also do not conduct therapy through e-mail.
T. You can send me an e-mail a week with a couple of the most important pieces of information, or you can choose to make a list for us to discuss during the check-ins before your daughter's appointment starts.

Texts during Sessions

Teenagers send hundreds of text messages per day in order to maintain relationships and have a feeling of "ever-present social support" (Dubus, 2014, p. 2). If you see teens, you *will* have the experience of a session being interrupted by a ring, ding, or other incoming text-message noise, and I would highly recommend making a proactive decision about how you would like to handle it. To consider your options, let us use the following example:

> Andie was a 15-year-old teen that just entered treatment for depression, self-injurious behavior, and family conflict. During the intake appointment, she told me that she was "interviewing" me because she had suffered through enough "terrible therapists who don't know the first thing about teenagers." After agreeing to see me again, she came to her first appointment, cell phone in her pocket. Approximately halfway through the session, her phone made an "oink oink" sound, signaling the incoming of a text. Breaking eye contact with me, she read the text message and quickly sent a response.

At this point in my session, I had a few options. I could (1) ask Andie to turn her phone off, (2) comment on the observation, or (3) ignore the text altogether. Admittedly, I did feel a little hurt and irritated, and I wanted to tell her to turn off the phone. Barth (2014) captured my experience perfectly in speaking of her own narcissistic injury when a client texted in her session; she shared that she wanted to feel appreciated and included and that she wanted her client to value their time together. Despite these countertransference feelings, I chose to ignore the text, and here is why: I consider that everything we do serves a purpose and that we only do things that make sense to our unconscious mind. Andie's texting in her session was no exception. I considered the possibility that Andie needed a "break" from our discussion, that her phone was a source of comfort, and that she may not want to explain the long time it took her to respond (i.e., not wanting peers to know she was in therapy). I also quickly considered the repercussions if I asked Andie to turn her phone off or tried to make a "therapisty"[3] observation, particularly in light of Andie's "warning" that I had better understand teenagers better than her last therapist. I thought this may be Andie's way of testing me to see how well I would be able to understand her world.

As time went on and our sessions continued, I began taking note of the times when Andie texted in our sessions. Indeed, those times did often coincide with difficult topics in the therapy room and when she seemed most distressed. Cell phones can act as a transitional object of sorts, providing comfort and constancy to teens, as well as connection to parents and peers (Barth, 2014; Erkolahti & Nyström, 2009; Ribak, 2009). In Andie's case, her phone also acted as a barometer of how tolerable she was finding her emotional experiences, a vitally important aspect of our work together to decrease self-injurious behavior. As sessions progressed and our alliance grew, I began gently pointing out times when I picked up on growing emotional discomfort. A telltale sign for this continued to be use of her cell phone to text or show me something, although this did become less frequent as our work continued. Over time, we were able to talk about what she felt when she texted with friends who really "got her" and ways in which she could seek this out from her parents and siblings. We also worked on affect regulation skills so that she could recognize her emotions and manage them without the immediate need for comfort from peers or self-injury. This included limit-setting within the session by actively telling me that she needed a break, rather than disconnecting passively via text messages. In looking back on the way Andie's treatment went, I cannot imagine her making the progress she did without initially being permitted to use the only coping skills she knew.

Of course, this is another decision that you must make for yourself and your practice. I certainly know therapists who insist that cell phones be turned off at the start of a session. For me, such a rule is not practical; because I have a small child, I am up front with my clients that I do keep my cell phone on and may occasionally need to interrupt a session if I get a call from his daycare.[4] Because of this, I do not necessarily think it is fair to mandate that my clients turn their cell phones off. I also know therapists who view their clients' cell phone use as an indicator of resistance or disrespect. I can certainly think of times when this might be the case, but again, I tend to think of this more in terms of *why* the client might be avoidant or resistant. Each therapist makes his/her own decisions regarding these issues, and my hope is that research will continue to work toward informing the reality of cell phones in therapy sessions.

Tips for Therapists' Responsible Social Media Use[5]

1. **Set clear boundaries** with parents and clients regarding your use of social media. Make decisions that you would be comfortable with across your caseload. Consider adapting a social media policy (see http://www.drk-kolmes.com/docs/socmed.pdf for a great example).
2. **Maximize privacy settings** and review your settings often. As SNS develop and grow, you may need to adjust your settings more than once.
3. **Show restraint** in your posts. Do not post anything you would not be comfortable with your clients seeing! Consider how your most sensitive or distressed client might respond (Kolmes & Taube, under review).
4. **Regularly check** your online presence (i.e., "Google" yourself).
5. Remember that you can and should **address any credible, threatening online behavior** from a client or client's family. More than half of the United States has laws against cyberbullying, which is a violation of privacy and safety (DeJong, 2014).

CONCLUSION

The role of today's technology is impossible to ignore in your therapeutic work, and your teen clients and their families, perhaps more than any other clients, will serve as a constant reminder of this fact. Assisting parents in understanding the role of technology and setting appropriate, feasible limits for their families can go a long way toward keeping your teen clients safe and keeping the lines of parent–teen communication open. Recognizing your place in a technological world and making choices with both your own and your clients' best interests in mind will not only protect you from possible liability but also model boundaries for your clients and assure you and your family of some privacy in an increasingly transparent world.

NOTES

1. According to March 2015 calculations of site traffic by eBizMBA Rank (http://www.ebizmba.com/articles/social-networking-websites).
2. I struggled to find the best place for a thorough discussion of parenting styles, mostly because it is a pervasive topic that applies to many of these chapters. It landed in chapter 7, since it is a big struggle that I encounter with parents, but absolutely applies when you are navigating guidelines for social media and technology.
3. This is an actual term that some adolescent clients have used when I say something they perceive to be analytical or "deep." As one male teen once asked me, "Do you *ever* think of things at face value, or do you always think about the 'hidden meaning'?" I love the term and have fully embraced my "therapisty-ness," sometimes even prefacing an observation or connection with a warning that I am about to sound "therapisty."
4. My phone is kept on "Do Not Disturb" mode, where my son's daycare is the only call that gets through; at the time of writing this book, I have only had to interrupt a session three times to take a call from them. Therefore, I feel comfortable telling clients about the small possibility that I may get a phone call. I have yet to work with a parent or teen who is adamantly opposed to this practice, although I recognize that other clients, depending on their symptoms and treatment needs, may feel differently.
5. Adapted from DeJong (2014).

Chapter Five

Inviting Parents into the Tough Stuff

"I had no idea ... what kind of parent does that make me?" Olivia's mother was asking after her daughter finally revealed months of self-harm. Giving parents an invitation to join you and their teen during the *tough stuff* is an interesting and valuable experience. It can also be terrifying, especially when you are not quite sure how they will respond and/or it is a very real possibility that they are contributing to the problem. Add to this uncertainty a grief experience that envelops many parents when they RSVP and learn what tough stuff their teen has been dealing with, and it is easy to see why some of my teens' former therapists have panicked right before their eyes.

In this chapter, we are going to discuss five topics that enter my office often: suicidality, non-suicidal self-injury (NSSI), substance abuse, teen dating violence (TDV), and sexual identity issues. I included sexual identity issues here because they reflect a different flavor of toughness. The first four topics reflect dangerous thoughts, feelings, or behaviors, and responses are largely centered on safety. In the case of sexual identity issues, the toughness comes less from imminent danger and more from parents' degree of acceptance and acknowledgment. This list is not intended to be all encompassing; I can easily think of at least five other topics that are the very definition of "tough stuff" (eating disorders, unexpected pregnancy, psychosis, religious issues, and criminal behavior, for starters). Instead, my hope is that I can help you take a deep breath and tackle the tough stuff one step at a time, beginning with knowing what exactly you are up against.

THE TOUGH STUFF

When I am sizing up a tough stuff situation and preparing to invite parents into it, I try to think of what I know about the topic on a basic level (the reality), parental issues that could be influencing or even driving the behavior, and possible parental responses. For those of you who work regularly with families involving teenagers, you may be interested in, but not altogether surprised by, some of the parental variables that factor into these difficult behaviors. The family therapy field has been identifying the power of family dynamics in the development of teen symptomatology for *years*. You may also be wondering about the individual factors that play a role in these issues. Like so many other things in this book, my decision to focus on parents is not meant to detract from teens' own personalities, cultures, mental health issues, and biology. Rather, it is simply my attempt to give you an overview of the role of the parents in your waiting room in these five throughly studied areas of adolescent mental health.

Suicidal Ideation and Attempts

Sherry, fifteen, was referred to me after a failed suicide attempt. Her mother reported that Sherry had been struggling with depressive symptoms for a couple of years, beginning shortly after her parents began embittered divorce proceedings. Sherry's relationship with her father was strained—she blamed him for the divorce—and her relationship with her mother was described as "insanely close" and slightly intrusive at times. She had never been in treatment before. During her hospitalization, she revealed to the staff that she had made two similar attempts that she had never revealed to anyone. Her father responded to this information by criticizing Sherry's mother ("See, Susan? You baby her, so she throws a temper tantrum whenever she doesn't get her way"), while her mother responded with depressive symptoms of her own ("I am a failure as a mother"). During our first session together, Sherry told me that she was looking forward to beginning treatment and believed it would be helpful. When I asked her what she had been thinking and feeling before her last attempt, she shared a desire to "get away from the drama" (in her family), prove to her dad that she was not "faking" her symptoms, and relieve her mother of having to "spend the little free time she has worrying."

The Reality

Approximately 15 percent of deaths in this age group are due to suicide, making suicide the third leading cause of death among adolescents aged fifteen to nineteen (Centers for Disease Control and Prevention [CDC], 2011; McIntosh

& Drapeau, 2012). An additional 15.8 percent of high school students seriously consider suicide, 12.8 percent make a plan, and 7.8 percent make an attempt (CDC, 2012). More than half of these teens attempt suicide at least once more (Géhin, Kabuth, Pichené, & Vidailhet, 2009). In many cases, adolescent suicide attempts are impulsive acts, occurring as little as a few minutes to one hour after the initial urge to act (Conner & Goldston, 2007; Swahn & Potter, 2001). For other teens, suicide attempts represent "a link in a chain of developmental non-successes … [youth] may 'work up' to such acts over time as they experience difficulties" (Conner & Goldston, 2007, p. 8). For teens who struggle with suicidal thoughts, many, if not most, will be able to tell you what the thoughts are, when they began, and what tends to trigger them (Bartimole, 2009).

Parental Factors

Parents have been discussed at length in the youth suicide literature, particularly with respect to the notion of the "expendable child" (Sabbath, 1969). As we discussed in chapter 2, some adolescents with insecure attachments perceive themselves to be expendable to their parents and families (Lyon et al., 2000), and Sabbath suggests that these parents may actually tell their teens—overtly or covertly—that they wish the teen did not exist. These parents may threaten to kick their teen out of the house (Lyon et al., 2000) or say and do other things to let their teens know they wish to be "rid of them." If you have ever had a parent tell you, "I just cannot deal with her anymore. She needs to go somewhere else; it would be better for both of us," you are likely treating an expendable child. Further, if a parent is willing to say this to you, you can almost guarantee that it has been said to the teen countless times. In terms of treatment for a suicidal adolescent, it is disastrous at best. Stone (1973) went so far as to say,

> Prognostic statements about suicidal adolescents, it would appear, are meaningless without inclusion of the parental factor … one needs to be familiar with the interaction between family and patient, both in the immediate past and in its vicissitudes over the years. (p. 190)

Research in recent years has substantiated this theory; high rates of parent–teen discord, parental hostility, neglect, overall family dysfunction and chaos, negative family events (e.g., deaths and abuse), and low levels of parental support have been linked to adolescent suicide attempts (Brent et al., 1998; Lyon et al., 2000; Meyer & Phillips, 1990; Noronha, 2000; Shepard, 1995; Tobin, 2000). Along the same lines, studies have supported the interpersonal theory of suicidal behavior, which suggests that adolescents attempt suicide following a failed sense of belonging and a feeling that they are a burden to their parents or others (Baumeister & Leary, 1995; Joiner et al., 2002), similar to what Sherry described above. Studies have found that those teens who experience low levels of belonging and high rates of emotional and/or physical separation from parents are at the highest risk for suicide (Timmons, Selby, Lewinsohn, & Joiner, 2011). Finally, parent's reactions following a suicide attempt have been associated with future attempts (Shamoo & Patras, 1990).

Parental Responses

The majority of individuals who complete suicide communicate their plans to another person, directly or indirectly (Barnes, Pazur, & Lester, 2014; Robins, Gassner, Kayes, WIlkinson, & Murphy, 1959), and teens often worry that their parents will be reassuring (e.g., "You have so much going for you!"), offended (e.g., "How could you do this to me?"), overprotective (e.g., asking multiple times a day about suicidality), over-reactive (e.g., "We're going to the hospital right now!"), or dismissive (e.g., "You are just doing this for attention").[1] Indeed, parents do sometimes discount their teen's suicidal thoughts or threats, particularly if the threats are recurrent, or if they believe they know their teens well enough that they would "never do that" (Barnes et al., 2014). Parents may also be reluctant to accept that their child could be at risk for suicide because they feel scared, helpless, uncomfortable, or guilty, do not understand the potential for a suicidal act, are overwhelmed or overburdened with home and work responsibilities, or are experiencing a range of other personal or cultural barriers (Barnes et al., 2014). All of this occurs despite research that suggests that parents are relatively knowledgeable about suicidal risk factors (Schwartz, Pyle, Dowd, & Sheehan, 2010).

Sometimes, parents do not even know when an attempt has occurred (Walker et al., 1990). I have worked with several teens, like Sherry, who told me about attempted overdoses that failed and ended with them waking up in their beds the next morning. Once parents learn of an attempt, they may experience emotions ranging from sympathy (James & Hawton, 1985) to outright hostility (Richman, 1986). They may deny the seriousness of the attempt, dismiss it as attention-seeking, or blame the adolescent for disrupting the family (Noronha, 2000). Parents may experience disappointment, humiliation, shame, or embarrassment, as well as anger, sadness, and other grief reactions (more on this below). They may feel hopeless, particularly if their teen has been in treatment and they perceive it as ineffective. As one parent once angrily told me, "It's *your* job to make sure she doesn't do this. What are you even *doing* in therapy?" (Of course, as a therapist, you know that suicide attempts are sadly inevitable when you work with depressed, anxious, traumatized, and otherwise impaired individuals, but more on countertransference in the next chapter.)

Non-Suicidal Self-Injury

Jennifer, sixteen, arrived on time for her second session with me and shared that she had been cutting for several months. She had told her previous therapist, who "freaked out" and promptly insisted that Jennifer's mother be brought into the session and told immediately. Blindsided, Jennifer's mother responded with panic, horror, and sadness, and Jennifer felt "like a terrible person." She refused to go back to see this therapist again.

Two years later, Jennifer came in for her weekly appointment with me and mentioned that a friend had disclosed his own self-harm. For Jennifer, who had not self-harmed in nearly one year, her friend's disclosure led her to consider her own experiences. She and I revisited the day she shared her self-harm with me, and Jennifer smiled and admitted that her disclosure had been a "test." She told me:

> I didn't want to waste my time with someone who was going to do more harm than good … the *only* reason my mom was even able to listen to and understand my need to self-harm was because you were willing to hear about it. That made me feel less ashamed and made my mom feel less panicked … like I wasn't a lost cause.

The Reality

As I mentioned briefly in chapter 1, NSSI is common among adolescents, like Jennifer and her friend. NSSI is the intentional and direct injuring of one's own body without suicidal intent (Nock & Favazza, 2009). Published prevalence rates range somewhere between 13 and 39 percent (Jacobson & Gould, 2007; Lloyd-Richardson, Perrine, Dierker, & Kelley, 2007; Muehlenkamp, Claes, Havertape, & Plener, 2012; Zoroglu et al., 2003).

I frequently hear parents and other adults refer to teens' NSSI as "attention-seeking," but it is so much more complicated than that. NSSI is also more complicated than teens simply trying to show their pain, and it is different from a suicide attempt, although Ougrin (2012) posits that NSSI is likely to be associated with a "spectrum of suicidal intent with purely suicidal and purely non-suicidal groups at each end of the spectrum and the majority of adolescents reporting mixed or unstable intent" (p. 1220). The research suggests that NSSI serves both automatic and social functions, such as:

- to suppress intense, negative emotions (automatic);
- to punish or reject aspects of themselves that are hated or feared (automatic);
- to express the pain and fear associated with growing up (automatic);
- to alert others to their distress, often by displaying scars for someone to "accidentally" see (social); and

- to demonstrate their increasing autonomy and power; no matter how desperately parents may beg, plead, threaten, or demand, teens have the power to self-harm or refrain from self-harming (Plante, 2006).

I also work with some clients who self-harm to "feel something" (automatic) and eliminate terrifying emotional numbness. Indeed, many individuals with trauma histories and complex post-traumatic symptomatology commonly engage in NSSI for this reason (see Smith, Kouros, & Meuret, 2014, for a review), and experiencing any form of abuse is a risk factor for engaging in self-harming behaviors (Fliege, Grimm, Grimm, & Klapp, 2009).

Parental Factors

The degree to which families are having difficulties can greatly impact NSSI. Multiple negative life-events are significantly related to NSSI (Baetens, Claes, Muehlenkamp, Grietens, & Onghena, 2011; Horesh, Nachshoni, Wolmer, & Toren, 2009), as are more specific experiences such as parental divorce and family losses (Nixon & Heath, 2009; Sourander et al., 2006). In general, research has found that teens are more likely to self-harm in single-parent households (Bifulco et al., 2014; Nixon, Cloutier, & Jansson, 2008; Whitlock, Eckenrode, & Silverman, 2006), when parents are struggling to meet basic needs (Brown, 2004; Bureau et al., 2010), or when a family member has health problems (Muehlenkamp, Hoff, Licht, Azure, & Hasenzahl, 2008). Interestingly, however, there is another pocket of research that has linked teen NSSI risk with membership in upper-class, white-collar professional families (DeChello, 2008; Yates, Tracy, & Luthar, 2008). One possible explanation for these findings is the presence of perfectionism and pressure to achieve within this demographic (Luthar & Becker, 2002; Lyman & Luthar, 2014).

In addition to demographic risk factors, there are, of course, relational risk factors for teen NSSI. Poor parent–teen attachment, as well as emotional neglect and abuse, has been implicated in the development of self-injurious behaviors (Bifulco et al., 2014; Gratz, 2006; Gratz, Conrad, & Roemer, 2002). High levels of emotional expression (EE), or the extent to which family members are critical or hostile toward and/or emotionally overinvolved with one another (Hooley, 1985, 2007), is associated with NSSI, particularly when adolescents' self-criticism is high (Wedig & Nock, 2007). Similarly, perceived parental control and over-involvement may contribute to increased rates of NSSI (Baetens et al., 2014; Bureau et al., 2010; Gratz, 2006). This all makes sense based on what we know about parents' role in their children's development of emotional regulation skills. Parents are responsible for providing an emotional climate that is accepting, tolerant, and validating of children's affective experiences. Therefore, families that are rejecting, punishing, dismissive, neglectful, or intrusive interfere with children's ability to develop, understand, endure, and express their emotions. NSSI enables teens to avoid the negative emotions that they are ill-equipped to handle.[2]

Parental Responses

Like parents of suicidal teens, parents of teens who self-injure experience a range of emotional responses. After learning that their teen is engaged in NSSI, many parents feel confused, hurt, shocked, distressed, guilty, helpless, and depressed (Raphael, Clarke, & Kumar, 2006). They may view the NSSI as an act of rebellion or "for attention" (Barrowclough & Hooley, 2003). Many transition quickly into what I call "mama bear mode" where they experience intense emotions and an unparalleled protective instinct that is only awakened when they perceive their child to be in danger. In this state, many parents will demand (to either the teen or the therapist) that the behavior stop—immediately—and they may express anger when this does not occur. I have seen this backfire in a big way, and sometimes parents' reactions and responses will actually exacerbate the NSSI (Hollander, 2008; Yip, 2005). In the days, weeks, and months after the disclosure, parents may feel uncertain about how to best discipline their teen and manage their households (Plante, 2006; Raphael et al., 2006). They may also express a want or need to work on their responses to their teens and feelings about the NSSI (Byrne et al., 2008).

Substance Abuse

Peter was sixteen years old and had been seeing me for about six months when he was caught with marijuana at school. Prior to this, our treatment had largely centered on feelings identification and expression. Peter downplayed his drug use, calling it "social" and "not a big deal at all." He confided in me that he had no plans to stop using just because it got him into trouble at school. He compared his own use to his father's longstanding struggles with alcohol and told me, "As long as I don't look like him [when I'm using], I'm good to go." His father was not a large part of Peter's life. Peter's mother was involved in Peter's life and treatment but admitted that she gave him "probably more space than I should." She spoke negatively of Peter's father and, after the school called to inform her that Peter was being suspended for possession on campus, told Peter that he was "turning out just like [his] father."

The Reality

Rates of alcohol and drug use are particularly high during adolescence, with approximately one third of teens reporting illicit drug use (Johnston, O'Malley, Bachman, & Schulenberg, 2011) and half reporting binge drinking over the last year (Epstein, Hill, Bailey, & Hawkins, 2013). Three-quarters of teens report having at least tried alcohol (Moore, Rothwell, & Segrott, 2010) and for many teens, marijuana is described as the drug of choice (White, Godley, & Passetti, 2004). Alcohol, marijuana, prescription medication, over-the-counter medication, ecstasy, spice, and inhalant use is down from recent years, but experimentation and use remains a public health concern (National Institute on Drug Abuse [NIDA], 2014; Skiba, Monroe, & Wodarski, 2004).

Adolescents generally report that they use substances because it is fun, enjoyable, and social (McIntosh, MacDonald, & McKeganey, 2005). Some adolescents occasionally experiment with drugs and alcohol, whereas others progress toward substance abuse. For those in the latter group, researchers have written about the tendency for some substances to serve as a "gateway" to other substances. The most commonly reported progression is (1) alcohol and cigarette use, followed by (2) marijuana use, which is then followed by (3) other illicit substances (Kandel, Hu, & Griesler, 2013; Kandel & Yamaguchi, 2002). Others have suggested that early substance use may not necessarily be a predictor of later substance abuse; rather, early use may act as a warning sign that adolescents have personality traits and coping styles that may leave them vulnerable to later abuse (Bobova, Finn, Rickert, & Lucas, 2009).

How should Peter's use be characterized? When does use become abuse? One of my biggest challenges in working with substance using teens is determining when recreational use or experimentation becomes misuse and abuse. While I was working as a substance abuse counselor, I taught a psychoeducation class for all new clients. In one of the sessions, we talked about the progression of substance use to misuse, abuse, and dependence. I discussed this continuum in a straightforward and simple way (see figure 5.1), and I have used the same method ever since. In fact, the guidelines I use when deciding whether or not to break confidentiality (chapter 3) are really another way to consider where someone falls on this continuum.

Parental Factors

Remember our discussion on parental monitoring in chapter 3? It plays an important role when considering adolescent substance abuse. Poor parental supervision and lack of knowledge about their teen's whereabouts contributes to drug use (Piko & Kovács, 2010), as does parental permissiveness (Deković, 1999; Li, Feigelman, & Stanton, 2000; Schinke, Fang, & Cole, 2008; Tolou-Shams, Hadley, Conrad, & Brown, 2012). Parental modeling—that is, their own alcohol and drug use—and attitudes about substance use also increase adolescents' risk of substance abuse (Andrews, Hops, Ary, Tildesley, & Harris, 1993; Highet, 2005; Kilpatrick et al., 2000; Wills, Sandy, Yaeger, & Shinar, 2001). Parents who set clear rules about drug and alcohol nonuse, voice clear

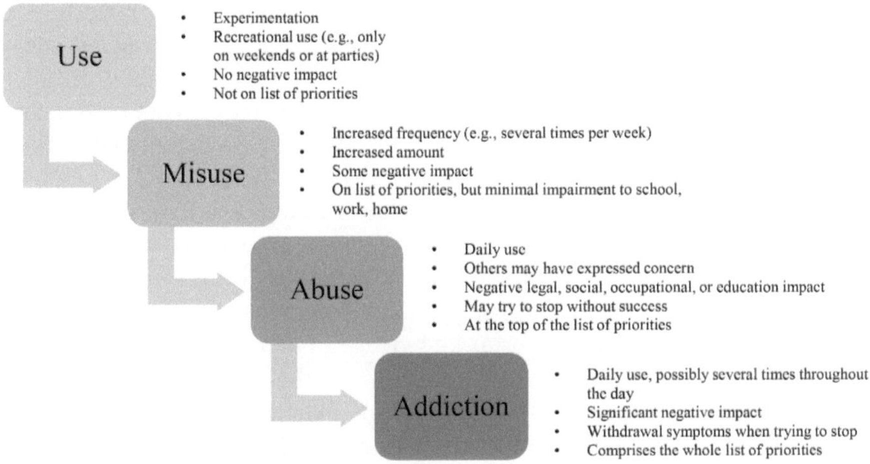

Figure 5.1 Progression of Substance Use

expectations, and speak often to their teens about abstaining from substance use are less likely to have teen who use these substances (Andrews et al., 1993; de Leeuw, Scholte, Vermulst, & Engels, 2013; Schinke et al., 2008).

Parent–adolescent attachment relationships have also been discussed at length in the adolescent substance abuse literature. Teens who feel supported by their parents as they make decisions and take steps toward independence are more likely to talk to their parents about problems instead of using substances to manage difficulties (Brook et al., 1998; Hair, Moore, Garrett, Ling, & Cleveland, 2008; Schinke et al., 2008). Additionally, strength of communication and cohesion within the family are both related to lower rates of substance use (Epstein et al., 2013; Piko & Kovács, 2010; Tolou-Shams et al., 2012). Emotional responsiveness within families is associated with the way in which teens manage their emotions, which in turn, is associated with teens' substance use (Tolou-Shams et al., 2012). Adolescents who do not learn, for example, that it is okay to cry when sad, show/express love, or experience anger, may turn to substances as a way to regulate difficult affective experiences (Hessler & Katz, 2010). Finally, the experience of child abuse and witnessing of domestic violence is associated with substance abuse (Begle et al., 2011; Hamburger, Leeb, & Swahn, 2008; Kilpatrick et al., 2000; Wright, Fagan, & Pinchevsky, 2013).

Parental Responses

In my experience, parents' responses to teens' substance abuse are a little different than their responses to suicidality or NSSI. As we just discussed, parental approval or disapproval of substance use can be quite impactful for adolescents, and attitudes toward underage drinking and illicit drug use seem to play a large role in parents' reactions. Many parents disapprove of other parents who permit adolescents to use substances, and they do not realize that their teens are accessing or using substances in their own home (Peterson, 2010). Some parents deny that their teens have ever tried alcohol, while others know about occasions on which their teens were drunk (Yoast, Fleming, & Balch, 2007). A lot of parents that I work with know (or assume) that their teens are using drugs or alcohol, but it is not until they "catch" them in the act that they respond. Highet (2005) suggests, "Parents 'catching' their children seems to be an event that transforms knowledge of their [drug] use into something that is impossible to ignore" (p. 119). Once their teens are "found out," parents engage in responses ranging from the extreme—panicky doling out of punishments (e.g., groundings, removal of privileges, and limited social engagement) and anxiety about legal problems, substance use disorders, reputations, and their teens' futures—to the other extreme of welcoming their teen to the "club" and grabbing them a glass, lighter, and so on. In less extreme cases, parents may handle learning about their teen's use by openly discussing the issue and communicating their expectations of abstinence. Parents may also take a harm reduction approach, negotiating boundaries with their teens and permitting them to use substances on special occasions and/or only under parental supervision (Highet, 2005).

Teen Dating Violence and Peer Sexual Victimization

Seventeen-year-old Katelyn told me in our first session that her boyfriend was "the best thing that ever happened to [her]." She described Jim as kind, caring, and someone with whom she could share anything. They had many things in common and spent the majority of their free time together. As our treatment progressed, however, Katelyn began sharing some of their arguments with me, largely surrounding Jim's mistrust of her. There had been some issues in the beginning of their relationship, and Katelyn had lied about drinking and occasionally smoking marijuana. When Jim found out, he had abruptly broken up with Katelyn, and although they had reunited, his mistrust of Katelyn remained.

Over time, I learned that Jim insisted on bringing Katelyn to her appointments with me so that he knew she was "really in therapy." He did not like her participating in social media and was only amenable if he had all of her passwords. Katelyn told me she did not mind giving him the passwords; she had nothing to hide. Once, Katelyn had told Jim that she was going to the mall to quickly pick up a gift and would arrive at his house within the hour. There was an accident outside of the mall, and it took Katelyn a long time to get in and out of the parking lot. When she arrived at Jim's house a half an hour later than planned, he accused her of lying and told Katelyn, "This is why I can't ever trust you. You started out as a liar and nothing has changed."

Zoe, eighteen, was relaying the weekend's events to me, and she shared that she had a "sort of scary" experience at a party. She told me that she had been drinking and flirting with a guy and that they had decided to go upstairs for some privacy. Once they were alone, Zoe said that they were kissing and "fooling around." She was having fun but then changed her mind about having sex. To her surprise, the guy became angry with her and told her that if she was going to be a "tease," the least she could do was perform oral sex. In recounting the story to me, Zoe shared that she had not been sure what to do but that she felt bad if she was, in fact, being a "tease." She performed oral sex and then went back downstairs to the party. They did not speak the rest of the night, and Zoe was a little worried that peers would find out what happened.

The Reality

Many teens would be surprised to learn that Jim's behaviors qualify as psychologically abusive and that Zoe was sexually assaulted. In fact, TDV refers to any behavior that inflicts pain or control on one partner, and it includes physical, psychological, and sexual victimization. Teens are at high risk for TDV due to immaturity, lack of life experience, misinterpretation of abusive acts as part of all typical relationships, and inaccurate perceptions of what constitutes love (Callahan, Tolman, & Saunders, 2003; Foshee et al., 2000; Silverman, Raj, Mucci, & Hathaway, 2001; Smith & Donnelly, 2001; Wolf, Ly, Hobart, & Kemic, 2003). Individuals in violent teen dating relationships often report similar levels of love, intimate self-disclosure, and perceived caring from partners (Giordano, Soto, Manning, & Longmore, 2010). However, high levels of verbal conflict, jealousy, time spent together, sexual activity, and power imbalances also characterize these relationships, and mutual violence (e.g., both partners are victims and perpetrators) is common (Giordano et al., 2010). TDV occurs in heterosexual and LGBTQI relationships (Dank, Lachman, Zweig, & Yahner, 2014), as well as relationships with adolescents and older partners. In fact, the wider the age gap between adolescents and their partners, the greater the risk for physical, psychological, and sexual victimization (Oudekerk, Guarnera, & Reppucci, 2014). For a victim of TDV, the experience can be one filled with varying degrees of fear: for self, for others, and for what may happen in the future (Burton, Halpern-Felsher, Rehm, Rankin, & Humphreys, 2013).

Physical victimization (PV) affects approximately 10 percent (CDC, 2007; Halpern, Oslak, Young, Martin, & Kupper, 2001; Halpern, Spriggs, Martin, &

Kupper, 2009) and includes a continuum of behaviors aimed at inflicting bodily harm ranging from scratching, pushing, and shoving to use of weapon or physical restraint (Saltzman, Fanslow, McMahon, & Shelley, 2002).

Psychological victimization (PsyV) is the most common form of TDV (Sears, Byers, & Price, 2007); in one nationally representative study, nearly one-third of adolescents had experienced some form of psychological abuse over the past eighteen months (Halpern et al., 2001). PsyV perpetration rates are also high (18–46 percent; Korchmaros, Ybarra, Langhinrichsen-Rohling, Boyd, & Lenhart, 2013; Renner & Whitney, 2010), and research has demonstrated that teens are using social media as a way to control, degrade, or invoke jealousy in their significant others (Korchmaros et al., 2013). In my experience, this is the hardest form of TDV to work with and possibly the most important. Teens tend to minimize the impact of PsyV, and more than once I have heard, "It's not like he hits me." However, studies have found unique relationships between adult PsyV, and subsequent symptoms and functioning (Norwood & Murphy, 2012), so it cannot be overlooked.

Sexual victimization (SV) can include harassment (e.g., being stared at in a sexual way and sexual/obscene calls or messages) and assault (e.g., kissing, touching, attempted rape, completed rape, and oral sex). Adolescents experience a great deal of sexual harassment throughout middle school and high school, around 40 percent for males, and between 50 and 75 percent of females, according to one study (Young, Grey, & Boyd, 2009). Rates vary depending on the definition of assault, with lower rates when only sexual intercourse is assessed (Bramsen, Lasgaard, Koss, Elklit, & Banner, 2012; Howard, Wang, & Yan, 2007). In Young et al. (2009), 26–28 percent of males and 40–53 percent of females experienced sexual assaults. A friend perpetrated approximately half of the assaults, while 15 percent of assaults were perpetrated by boyfriends/girlfriends.

Researchers have noted that the rate of SV by boyfriends/girlfriends has decreased over the years, and some have suggested that the changing nature of teen sexual relationships may be the cause. Less teens are committing to one another as boyfriends and girlfriends, and more are "hooking up," or engaging in sexual activity without any expectation of emotional investment or a romantic relationship (Paul, McManus, & Hayes, 2000). Studies have found that as many as 28 percent of adolescents have hooked up at least once (Fortunato, Young, Boyd, & Fons, 2010; Manning, Giordano, & Longmore, 2006), and the majority of the hook-ups are with friends or fellow students. Thus, some of the sexual assaults experienced by adolescents could be hook-ups that transformed into negative, coercive experiences (Kahn et al., 2000, as cited in Fortunato et al., 2010).

Parental Factors

As with some of the other "tough stuff" discussed in this chapter, parents and family environments have received a lot of attention in the TDV literature. For example, harsh parenting and witnessing parental intimate partner violence (IPV) predicts TDV perpetration (Foshee, Benefield, Ennett, Bauman, & Suchindran, 2004; Jouriles, Mueller, Rosenfield, McDonald, & Dodson, 2012; Wood & Sommers, 2011). Theorists suggest that through these hostile and potentially dangerous interactions, teens learn to respond quickly and aggressively to negative behavior or to ambiguous behavior that could be interpreted negatively (Wekerle et al., 2001). Conversely, a positive relationship between mothers and their teen daughters acts as a protective factor against dating violence (Cleveland, Herrera, & Stuewig, 2003). Childhood maltreatment is associated with TDV (Cyr, McDuff, & Wright, 2006; Herrenkohl et al., 2007; Kelly, Owen, Peralez-Dieckmann, & Martinez, 2007; Wekerle et al., 2009) and other risk factors (e.g., substance abuse, early sexual experiences, multiple sexual partners) that also increase teens' likelihood of victimization (Eaton, Davis, Barrios, Brener, & Noonan, 2007). Finally, living in an environment with high rates of crime and poverty (Foshee et al., 2004; Spriggs, Halpern, & Martin, 2009), and weak parental monitoring, particularly in high crime areas, greatly increases the risk for TDV victimization (Chapple, 2003; East, Chien, Adams, Hokoda, & Maier, 2010; Simons, Lin, & Gordon, 1998).

Parental Responses

In general, few adolescents report TDV (Ashley & Foshee, 2005). Many want to keep the victimization private, perceive it as too minor to warrant attention, or feel ashamed or embarrassed (Sabina, Cuevas, & Rodriguez, 2014). When help is sought, peers are usually told first, with parents and other adults as secondary options (Ashley & Foshee; Jackson, 2002; Ocampo, Shelley, & Jaycox, 2007). Teens share with parents more often than formal helpers such as therapists, but in general, adults are only told about 13 percent of the time (Weisz, Tolman, Callahan, Saunders, & Black, 2007). When victims seek help for dating violence, they are hoping for a nonblaming attitude, understanding, listening, and freedom to make their own decisions (Mahlstedt & Kenny, 1993). However, teens worry that their parents will make the situation worse, interrogate them, blame them, make them feel guilty, view them as weak, or not believe them (Black, Weisz, Preble, & Sharma, 2015; Gallopin & Leigh, 2009). Many also believe that their parents will force them to end the relationship or deny requests to date in the future (Liz Claiborne Inc., 2007).

Many parents do not know how they would respond if approached by teens about TDV (Rothman, MIller, Terpeluk, Glauber, & Randel, 2011), and Black and colleagues (2015) found that some parents' responses suggest that they would not recognize the seriousness of TDV and maybe even encourage the continuation of a potentially dangerous situation. This response matches some teens' tendency to minimize TDV (Rayburn et al., 2007). Parents may also respond in a way that is perceived by teens as intrusive, such as demanding that the relationship end rather than respecting teens' ambivalence in abusive situations, or in a way that further isolates the teen and helps the abuser (Miles, 2005; Tishby et al., 2000). However, Black and colleagues' (2015) findings also suggest that not all parents feel helpless and ill-equipped to handle TDV disclosures. Many participants respond in nurturing, supportive ways; few parents were likely to ground their teens after a TDV disclosure and many said that they would take their teens' disclosures seriously, encourage their teen to talk to them and end the relationship, and seek some form of counseling.

Sexual Identity Issues

Luke, fourteen, had endured a sexual assault by a male peer at a postchampionship game sleepover. He experienced a range of post-traumatic symptoms and feelings, including shame and powerlessness, and he worked hard in therapy to process his experience. In addition, he told me that for the last year or so, he had been thinking a lot about his sexuality. Prior to the assault, he had begun wondering if he was gay and had done some reading online. As more time passed, Luke was becoming more and more confident that he was gay or bisexual, but he worried that if he came out, those who knew about his assault would blame him or think that he had consented. Luke thought his mom would be supportive but said his dad would never understand. He expressed a lot of anger at the fact that his father still made comments about how Luke could have "fought off" the peer who raped him and told me, "Me saying I'm gay? That will add to the ammunition he needs to blame the whole thing on me."

The Reality

Rates of adolescents who identify as lesbian, bisexual, gay, transgender, queer, questioning, and intersex (LGBTQI) range, with many studies reporting that between 1 and 5 percent of teens identify as LGBTQI or report having same-sex experiences (Duncan & Hatzenbuehler, 2014; Reis & Saewyc, 1999). There are a number of psychosocial stressors and distress associated with being LGBTQI including suicidality (Kitts, 2005; Massachusetts

Department of Education, 2009), homelessness (Federal Policy Brief, 2012; Zavis, 2010), and harsher punishments at school and within the criminal system (Himmelstein & Bruckner, 2011). Clients like Luke also worry tremendously about what would happen if anyone at their school found out. They have good reason: some form of physical and verbal abuse and/or bullying at school is a reality for the majority of LGBTQI teens (Gay Lesbian and Straight Education Network [GLSEN], 2010).

Parental Factors

The current view of sexual orientation is that it is shaped through a combination of genetic (Langstrom, Rahman, Carlstrom, & Lichtenstein, 2010), hormonal (Hines, Brook, & Conway, 2004), and environmental factors (Goldberg, 2010; Golombok, 2000). One of the environmental factors that has been examined in the literature is growing up in a same-sex parent household. Like adolescents raised in heterosexual-parent homes, most of the teens raised by same-sex parents grow up to identify as heterosexual (Gartrell, Bos, & Goldberg, 2011; Wainright, Russell, & Patterson, 2004), although one study found that girls may be more likely to identify as bisexual when they were raised by lesbian mothers (Gartrell et al.). Studies have also suggested that teens of same-sex parents may simply be accepting of gender nonconformity (see Herek, 2014, for references) and be more open to the idea of same-sex relationships than teens raised in heterosexual-parent households (Bos & Sandfort, 2010; Gartrell et al., 2011; Stacey & Biblarz, 2001).

Parental Responses

A teen's decision to "come out" is an important step in identity integration. It implies the teen's acceptance of his/her own sexuality and represents an active willingness to share this identity with others (Baiocco et al., 2014). Although parents may not always be the first to know about their teen's sexual orientation and some have suggested that coming out to parents may not be the best course of action for some teens (Green, 2000), most parents *do* know (LaSala, 2000; Schope, 2002). It seems that the quality of the parent–teen relationship factors into teens' decisions about whether or not to come out to their parents (Carnelley, Hepper, Hicks, & Turner, 2011; Holtzen, Kenny, & Mahalik, 1995; Mohr & Fassinger, 2003; Willoughby, Malik, & Lindahl, 2006). Furthermore, perceived supportiveness and positivity from family members is associated with low levels of depression, suicidality, and high levels of self-esteem (see Baiocco et al., 2014, for references).

Unfortunately, as many as 52 percent of parents initially respond negatively following their teen's coming out (D'Augelli, Grossman, & Starks, 2008), making the process a stressful one for many adolescents

(Savin-Williams, 2005). Willoughby, Doty, and Malik (2008) have proposed parental reactions to coming out are related to family members' relational competences, beliefs about meanings of stressful events, and family stability. Other researchers have pointed to variables such as older parental age (Savin-Williams, 2001), younger adolescent age (LaSala, 2000), lower levels of parental education (Conley, 2011), traditional religious views and values related to marriage, family, and sex roles (Baiocco et al., 2014; Cramer & Roach, 1988; Newman & Muzzonigro, 1993), and high levels of concern for their teen (Conley, 2011) when trying to understand parents' negative reactions to their teen's coming out. Regardless of the reasons, however, the literature is quite clear: negative reactions can lead to many negative outcomes for teens, including negative views of self, substance abuse, unprotected sex, depression, and suicidality (Rothman, Sullivan, Keyes, & Boehmer, 2012; Ryan, Huebner, Diaz, & Sanchez, 2009). Fortunately, studies have found that, often, parents' initial negative reactions eventually transform into new ways of viewing their teens' sexual orientation, different behaviors, and renewed bonds with their teens, and, upon reflection, many parents appreciate the experience (Goodrich, 2009; LaSala, 2010; Phillips & Ancis, 2008).

On Attachment and Tough Stuff

NSSI and Suicidality

NSSI and suicidality have been conceptualized as "extreme attachment behavior[s]" (Adam, Sheldon-Keller, & West, 1996, p. 265) that teens utilize as a way to signal distress. When teens are securely attached, their parents are more likely to recognize the teens' emotional needs, meet them appropriately, and strive to create a safe environment in which their teens can learn more adaptive ways to cope with their distress (Glazebrook, Townsend, & Sayal, 2015; Yip, Ngan, & Lam, 2003). Secure attachment, then, can act as a protective factor against future suicide attempts and incidents of NSSI (Maimon, Browning, & Brooks-Gunn, 2010). When insecurely attached teens signal their distress, however, parents' responses may not demonstrate understanding and safety. Instead, teens may experience increased parental expectations, overreactions, parent–teen conflict, or intense parental emotions such as guilt, frustration, and anxiety (Yip et al., 2003).

As a result, insecure attachment in childhood has been linked with adolescent suicidality (Adam et al., 1996; Maimon et al., 2010; Violato & Arato, 2004; Zyrek, Gencoz, Bergman, & Lester, 2009) and NSSI (Adam et al., 1996; Hallab & Covic, 2010; Salzinger, Rosario, Feldman, & Ng-Mak, 2007).

Substance Abuse

Despite studies suggesting that family structure (i.e., who lives in the home) predicts substance use, more recent research is looking to parental attachment instead (Barfield-Cottledge, 2015). Schindler and Bröning (2015), in their recent review of the relationship between substance abuse and attachment, suggest that insecure attachment invariably has the potential to lead to substance abuse, albeit for different reasons. They suggest that anxiously attached teens may look to maximize their attachment needs, thereby using substances for self-medication. Alternatively, avoidant teens may try to impulsively distance themselves from others through the use of substances. Finally, disorganized teens may utilize substances as a means to control trauma-related symptoms. Understanding teens' attachment relationships with their parents may assist you in identifying their substance use goals, which you can then address in individual therapy, in work with parents, or through a referral to family therapy.

TDV

When parent–teen relationships are insecure, teens who have not experienced unconditional acceptance or security may enter dating relationships that, in many ways, look and feel similar. As opposed to securely attached teens whose relationships include feelings of safety, comfort with closeness, trust in partners, clear expectations, and the ability to cope with stress in healthy ways (Ulloa, Martinez-Arango, & Hokoda, 2014), insecure teens' dating relationships are characterized by low levels of connectedness and perceived support, and high levels of conflict (Li & Chan, 2012). Of all attachment styles, teens with an anxious attachment style are at the highest risk for TDV. Because they often become overly dependent on others and fear abandonment, they are the most likely attachment group to overlook and/or downplay warning signs and use sexual activity as a means of securing closeness (Mikulincer & Shaver, 2007; Sandberg, Suess, & Heaton, 2010; Yarkovsky & Timmons Fritz, 2014). Such teens may also demonstrate aggression, extreme feelings of jealousy, controlling behaviors, and poor problem-solving skills (see Ulloa et al., 2014, for a review).

Sexual Identity Issues

When considering attachment for teens who have recently come out or are questioning their sexual identity, the limited research that exists has considered the impact of parents' suspicions that their teen may be LGBTQI and/or their reactions to their teen's coming out. Studies have found that, in the coming out process for families with an LGBTQI teen, there is at least a brief disruption in the parent–teen attachment relationship (Ridge & Feeney, 1998). In a recently published study, higher rates of perceived alienation from attachment figures after coming out was associated with current attachment insecurity (Rejiester, 2015), and other studies have found that family rejection can have a tremendously negative influence on the well-being of gay and lesbian teens (Ryan et al., 2009). Further compounding the problem is reactions from those inside and outside of the family, which may also put increased pressure on an already stressed attachment system. It is important to have a good handle on the parent–teen attachment relationship as your teen clients explore their sexual identities and potentially prepare to come out to loved ones. Insecure attachment may make it difficult for teens to fully explore their sexuality and has been linked to fear about being LGBTQI, as well as nondisclosure of sexual orientation (Elizur & Mintzer, 2001; Mohr & Fassinger, 2003).

ACCOMPANYING PARENTS THROUGH THE TOUGH STUFF

Sharing with Parents: Sometimes It Can Wait, and Sometimes It Can't

When you learn about one of the tough situations we have discussed (and the ones we have not), your first parent-related decision is whether or not they need to know immediately. We spent some time talking about how to make the decision to break confidentiality in chapter 3, and I do a "triage" of sorts when it comes to difficult situations (see figure 5.2).

The pyramid helps me categorize behaviors quickly, while also serving as a visual reminder that in outpatient treatment, the majority of situations are *not* ones in which parents need to be informed immediately. Black Zone behaviors, for me, are often relatively easy to identify and address, and I rely heavily on my knowledge of teens, their histories, and their families to triage tough situations. Remember to consider teens' intentions of continuing the behavior(s), increasing frequency and/or severity, and any immediate danger (see chapter 3) for behaviors that fall in the Gray Zone. Pay attention to small signals that behaviors may be entering the Gray Zone; do not just look for glaring red flags (Taffel, 2005). Be clear with your teens about the reasoning behind your decision to break confidentiality or maintain it.

For behaviors in the Light (white) Zone, make a mental note to continue assessing the behaviors, and also consider whether it might be therapeutically appropriate for parents to know about the issue(s) at some point. I usually talk it over with my clients, and if they are interested in telling their parents in the

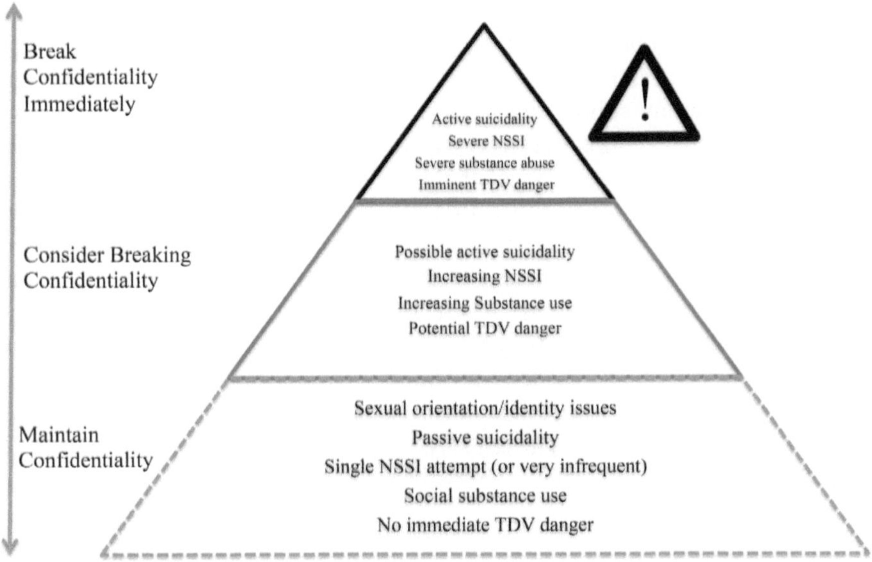

Figure 5.2 Triage Pyramid

future, we set it as a goal to work toward, and I consider ways to support this goal in my interactions with parents. For example, Willoughby et al. (2008) suggest that therapists treating LGBTQI teens work with family members to strengthen communication and problem-solving prior to teens' coming out.

Managing Expectations and Emotions

I feel proud to say that a large majority of the time, tough stuff disclosures go well with the parents of my teens. Like any other therapist, I definitely have those clients with whom it does not go so well, but over time, I have come to recognize and accept that I cannot control the way all of my teens' disclosures play out, just as I cannot always determine the way therapy goes. I would like to think that the working alliance I spend time building with parents early in treatment helps with this, and I also believe that my approach to these tough stuff disclosures has become fine-tuned over time. This approach is pretty simple: stay calm, psychoeducate, acknowledge parents' feelings, and then stay calm some more.

Stay Calm

You must, *must* be able to exude calmness in situations where parents are about to learn something new and potentially scary about their adolescents.

Calmness prevents parents from doing something rash in the moments after they learn about their teen's tough stuff, such as throwing teens out of their homes, filing criminal charges against abusive teen partners, terminating outpatient treatment, calling the school, cancelling their senior week, and so on. All of these reactions may be reasonable, or even necessary, given the particulars of the case, but none of these decisions can be made rationally and for the right reasons in those first minutes after a disclosure. It is critically important that you are able to remain focused, positive, supportive, and hopeful for your teens and their parents after a disclosure has been made. Remember that they are in the eye of the tough stuff storm. *You* know that they will survive it, but they may not.

Let me be clear that this does not mean that you cannot, should not, or will not have feelings. I have been brought to tears more than once in these tough sessions. When I am particularly worried, I am open with parents and their teens about it, and I strive to express this worry to them in a way that conveys hopefulness, comfort, and support. In other words, *no*, your teen is not beyond help; *yes*, I have worked with this type of issue before; and *yes*, I am here for both you and your teen. A perfect example occurred just a week ago, while I was in the middle of writing this chapter. Gavin, thirteen, reported suicidal ideation that I assessed to be in the Black Zone. His mood had suffered a rapid decline since our last session and his plan was specific, involving a somewhat accessible firearm. Although I am usually able to stay pretty calm, Gavin's words and intention scared me, and I knew they would terrify his mother, Joan. I invited her into the session and told her,

> So Gavin and I have been talking, and I am *very* worried about him. He's told me that he has been having some pretty serious thoughts about taking his life, and based on his plan, I think there is a good chance he will act on it. [By the look on Joan's face, I could tell she was horrified.] I know this is scary to hear, and to be honest, it's a little scary to say. I never want one of my clients to be in this much pain. The good news is that Gavin trusted me enough to tell me what he was feeling and now we can do something about it. I think you should take him to the [nearby] walk-in clinic right now. I can call and give them a heads up that you are on your way. Gavin and I have talked about this, and we both think this is a good plan. [Joan nodded.] Okay, great. I really think this will help Gavin. Now what questions do you have? How can I be most helpful?

We talked for a little while longer, Gavin and his mom left shortly after, and Gavin was (not surprisingly) admitted almost immediately. I called to check in with Joan a few hours later, and she sounded mentally and physically exhausted.[3] She was feeling scared, angry, and guilty. She told me, "Thank God he told you. I know it must be a horrible job to hear kids tell you they want to kill themselves all the time, but I'm so glad you knew what to do."

The way in which I handled Gavin's suicidal ideation is not unlike the way I handle most tough stuff conversations. I usually offer for the teen to start the conversation, but most of the time, they ask me to do it. I am okay with that, as long as the teen is prepared to participate in the conversation and provide some information that I have not. It matters not to me what the information is, just that the conversation between teen and parent has begun. From there, I can start working on psychoeducation so that the parent can understand what is going on with their teen. In most cases, the information I share is similar to that which teens and I have discussed in previous sessions, so that the parents and teens are now (somewhat) on the same page.

Psychoeducate

Psychoeducation is an important part of helping parents manage their expectations and emotions during and after a disclosure. *Protection motivation theory* (PMT) can assist you in deciding on what psychoeducational material to share with parents. According to PMT, when a potentially threatening situation occurs, we appraise the severity of the situation, the likelihood of its occurrence, our options for protecting ourselves from the threat, and how effective we think we are at carrying out the necessary steps to protect ourselves (Foshee et al., 2012; Rogers, 1975). For parents dealing with their teens' tough stuff, we want them to first recognize the seriousness of the issue in terms of safety, identity development, and the family's future and, second, feel competent in their abilities to effectively respond to their teens and the situation.

Providing parents with knowledge about the process that teens go through when determining their sexuality, for example, may help them refrain from calling their teen's sexual orientation "a phase" or from presuming "he doesn't know what he wants." It can also be helpful to use research to demonstrate how well adjusted many LGBTQI teens are; a lot of parents get caught up in the stereotype that all gay and lesbian teens are bullied, unhappy, and lonely. Parents may also be comforted to learn that this information will help them respond more effectively to their teens.

Psychoeducation can be particularly useful when dealing with the high-risk behaviors we have talked about. It is critical that parents realize that while behaviors such as substance abuse and NSSI are dangerous, they serve an important function for the teens that utilize them as a coping mechanism. Both are *extremely* effective in quelling emotional distress, which is why many teens are reluctant to give them up (Briere & Gil, 1998; Hollander, 2008).[4] I often liken these behaviors to crying when sad; I cry easily, and I find it incredibly cathartic at times. If someone told me that I could no longer cry when I was sad, I would feel helpless and completely uninterested in giving the behavior up. It would not be until that person helped me identify other ways to manage my sadness that I would *maybe* be willing to let go of crying as a coping mechanism. Such is also the case with NSSI, substance abuse, and other maladaptive coping mechanisms. Helping parents understand this may prevent them from telling their teen just to "stop it" and may also help prepare them to manage the long-term work that can accompany such behaviors.

Some parents can understand that it is not easy just to "stop it," but they ask some version of "So what do we do to make this problem go away?" It can be difficult to explain to parents why teens may not stop self-destructive behaviors even after learning other, more adaptive coping skills. Parents perceive these new coping skills as more effective, healthier, and better in every way. Why wouldn't their teen use those instead? It is a valid question, and I use a pie chart (see figure 5.3) to simply explain a somewhat complicated dynamic of treatment and recovery.

Using the pie chart design, I explain that, in the beginning, NSSI (or any other maladaptive behavior) is a tried-and-true, effective coping mechanism. It is often the only one that the teen is even willing to utilize, so it is employed 100 percent of the time (circle 1). Once we do some work in therapy and the teen feels competent in using another skill, NSSI may only be used 50 percent of

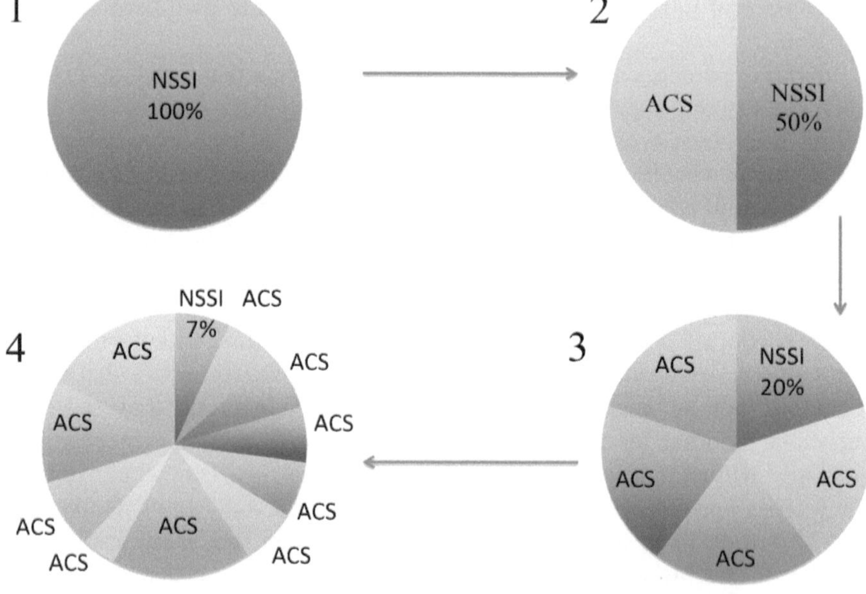

Figure 5.3 The Process of Adding Adaptive Coping Skills (ACS) to Tool Kit

the time (circle 2). With each new coping skill, the need for and use of NSSI will ideally go down (circles 3 and 4), but NSSI will *always* be an option. Physically drawing this out gives parents an idea of how unreasonable it is to ask their teens to give up their coping mechanism when there is nothing else in the tool kit (circle 1) and helps them conceptualize and begin coming to terms with the fact that there is nothing any of us can do to completely eradicate the possibility of the dangerous behavior in their teen's life (circle 4). If parents can accept this, they are less likely to panic when their teen mentions urges to self-harm or when a relapse has occurred.[5] The examples I have presented here tackle both aspects of PMT: they help parents take the issue seriously and provide them with enough knowledge to remain hopeful and feel equipped to continue their roles as parents while therapy goes on.

Acknowledge Their Feelings

As I have been highlighting throughout this chapter, anything goes when it comes to parents' reactions to tough stuff disclosures. This is because all people respond differently when faced with threatening, scary information. Remember that parents, for any number of individual and interpersonal reasons, may respond differently from what you or their teen are expecting. The only time I ever set limits on parents' responses is when the behavior threatens the emotional or physical safety of anyone in the room. I typically use the A-C-T model we discussed previously:

> John, it seems that you are feeling angry and blindsided by Manny's news that he is using cocaine. I understand, and it is okay to be feeling whatever you are (A). It is *not* okay, though, to stand over him, cursing and screaming (C). We can take a break if you need it, or you can take a seat and we can keep talking (T). If you choose to keep screaming and cursing at him, we will have to end the session.[6]

Many of the reactions you encounter in the moments immediately following the disclosure (and likely several sessions after), if not most, will be some form of a grief reaction.

THE GRIEF PROCESS

As we have been discussing, parents are likely to experience a multitude of feelings, many related to grief and loss, following their teens' disclosures of tough stuff. These feelings often begin in the immediate aftermath of a disclosure and can be quite prolonged, as new challenges present themselves and symptoms wax and wane (Godress, Ozgul, Owen, & Foley-Evans, 2005).

Parents must come to terms with the fact that their teen's life is different from the ones they had planned for him/her, and, depending on the issue, parents must also deal with the impact the issue has on the family (Godress et al., 2005). They may experience emotional distress, preoccupation with their teen's mental health issues, difficulties adjusting to changes related to the disclosure, and/or avoid discussing their feelings all together. Although the source of the grief will differ in each situation, a majority of parents report grief on a continuum. These responses can be compounded by the reality of tough stuff disclosures. Inpatient hospitalizations, detoxification and rehab, legal actions, and future relationships can all act as triggers or roadblocks, delaying or changing the course of parents' path toward acceptance and understanding. Kübler-Ross' well-known grief model—denial, bargaining, anger, sadness, and acceptance (Kübler-Ross & Kessler, 2005)—can be a useful way to conceptualize parents' reactions after a teen's disclosure (see figure 5.4). Although progression through these stages is described as a linear process, it is rarely so simple, and I frequently see parents skip stages or cycle through them more than once over time.

Some parents will *deny* that there is a problem or that the behavior is real and not just for attention. Emotional distress is low in this first phase because the parent is not willing to admit that there is anything to be emotional about. In the case of sexual identity, parents may view their teen's coming out as a phase or experiment. Parents may refuse to believe that their teen's partner is abusive because "(s)he is such a good kid." A suicide attempt may be termed an "accident." One of your jobs is to ground parents in the reality of

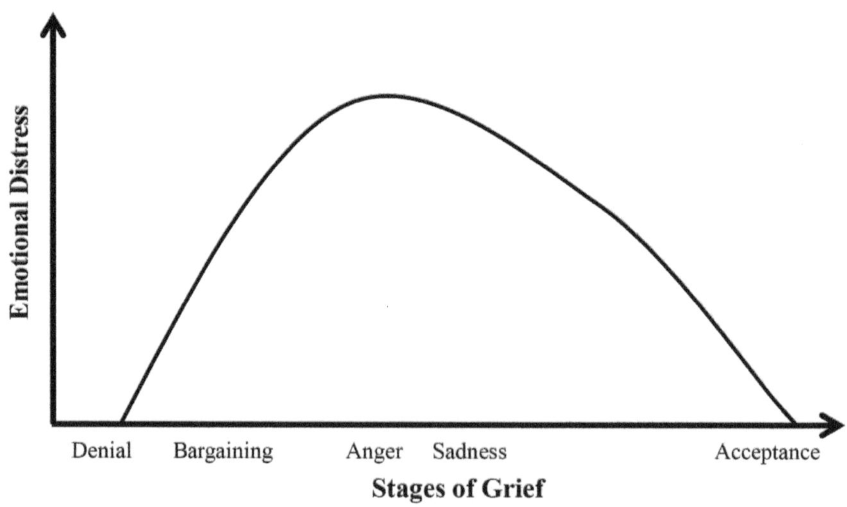

Figure 5.4 Level of Distress across Parents' Stages of Grief

the situation. One way to do this is through decisive words (e.g., "when," not "if") and by labeling experiences clearly (Hunter & Gerber, 1990). A father responded to his son's coming out by saying, "So you have been experimenting with a few of the guys; lots of people do that. It doesn't mean that you are definitely that way. If it turns out that you are … we'll deal with it then." I rephrased this by saying, "I think Brandon is trying to tell you that he is gay, not that he is just experimenting." Terms such as "suicidal," "self-injurious," "substance abuse," "abusive," and "gay" can help parents who are attempting to minimize or deny the issue by using unthreatening terminology (e.g., "a little problem," "a tough time," "attention-seeking"). Minimization is commonly seen in the *bargaining* phase, which occurs when an issue can no longer be denied. For example, after seeing the controlling texts that Jane's boyfriend sent her repeatedly throughout the day, Jane's mother told her, "He just likes to know where you are so that he knows you are safe." Emotional distress may begin to build, but it is still relatively low.

Anger is the third stage of Kübler-Ross' model, and one commonly encountered after tough stuff is disclosed. Emotions are now running high. As we discussed in the first section, parents often respond with anger to their teen's disclosures. This anger may be directed toward the teen, a perpetrator, peers, other adults, and the therapist. You can probably think of plenty of angry responses, but here are a few more:

- "You are just throwing your life away!"
- "What are you thinking?"
- "You must not care about me at all if you would be willing to put me through this."
- "I'm calling the police."
- "That is disgusting."
- "No wonder he thinks he can treat you that way—you let him!"

Let's not forget about passive aggressive responses. Refusal to attend future sessions, rejection of plans put in place during therapy, leaving the teen out of future events, or saying things like "Oops, is that going to make you go cut yourself?" all fall under this category. Rosenbaum and Richman (1970) discuss similar messages that parents give their suicidal children that go far beyond insensitivity to triggers.

Sadness occurs when parents are able to recognize and share the feelings of loss that accompany a difficult disclosure. Emotional distress is still high but beginning to stabilize and possibly decline. Much has been written about this in the LGBTQI literature, with parents grieving the loss of futures they had planned for their children. These futures might have included weddings, grandchildren, and a place in religious communities (Martin, Hutson,

Kazyak, & Scherrer, 2010). In terms of mental health issues, parents express sadness over several losses: the illusion of a "happy kid," the perception of themselves as "good parents," their sense of invulnerability in the relationship they thought they had with their teen, and possibly the futures they had planned for their children (Godress et al., 2005; Lowes, Gregory, & Lyne, 2005; Milliken, 2001; Oreo & Ozgul, 2007). They may worry about how people will treat their teen. Parents may also have to come to terms with feelings of loneliness or social isolation, sometimes self-inflicted and other times imposed upon the family (Kovarsky, 1989).

Ideally, parents' denial, bargaining, anger, and sadness gets resolved into *acceptance* of both their losses and their teen as someone dealing with safety issues, substance abuse, or an LGBTQI lifestyle. The same parent who grieved the loss of a child who would marry and have children may come to accept that many gay and lesbian couples decide to marry and build a family. A parent who envisioned a future full of hospitalizations and medications may see that in some ways, life can return to "normal" after a suicide attempt. Acceptance occurs on many levels and at different paces, with some parents able to accept only their losses (Broad, 2011). Some parents may choose to seek out their own therapy to help them cope. It is important to remember that in most cases, parents will not reach acceptance in that first session to talk about the tough stuff. It is important to normalize this for both parents and teens so that no one feels as though they have failed or that the situation is "hopeless." If you choose to use the grief model to explain the process to parents, I have found that it really depathologizes the different levels of responses and helps with guilt down the road.

CONCLUSION

Learning that your adolescent client has tough stuff going on can be difficult, and the thought of telling parents can be even more so. The realities of these issues, coupled with risk assessment, the role of parental factors, and the multitude of possible responses awaiting you oftentimes feel overwhelming. Once parents hear what their teen needs to tell them, their own feelings of being overwhelmed factor in, and your job expands to include managing your emotions and reactions in order to help parents and teens manage theirs. Through staying calm, teaching parents, and acknowledging their feelings, you can help parents recognize their grief and help them through it. If all goes according to plan, you and the teen can continue making progress in individual therapy. These treatment stories often have happy endings. But what happens when parents' own tough stuff gets in the way? What can you do when parental resistance and/or psychopathology becomes a piece of the treatment puzzle? If you have been reading this book and wondering how any of what I have been saying applies when you have an abusive, personality disordered, impaired, or destructive parent in your waiting room, the time has finally arrived! Chapter 6, here we come.

NOTES

1. Retrieved from http://www.speakingofsuicide.com/2013/05/29/parents-and-teens/.
2. For an eloquent review of this literature, I would highly recommend Sim, Adrian, Zeman, Cassano, and Friedrich's (2009) article titled "Adolescent Deliberate Self-Harm: Linkages to Emotion Regulation and Family Emotional Climate" (full citation available in the References section).
3. Parents frequently report feeling physically exhausted, mentally drained, and overwhelmed in situations where they receive difficult information about their child (Mulligan, MacCullough, Good, & Nicholas, 2012).
4. In fact, in line with Plante's (2006) assertion, I tend to believe that treatment for NSSI and substance abuse cannot truly begin until teens (and their parents) can acknowledge how much relief the behaviors provide; it is important that both understand that maladaptive coping skills can be difficult to let go of, especially if there are no other options in place.
5. There are also some other great psychoeducation materials out there about the topics we have discussed in this chapter, as well as other topics I could not get to here.
6. In the rare cases when parents have not been able to calm themselves, I have insisted that another adult come and pick the teen up to maintain safety. In the even rarer cases that I have felt that either my safety or the safety of the teen was in jeopardy, I have requested the assistance of one of the police officers who work with the crisis response unit housed within my office building.

Chapter Six

Parental Interference

"I'm not the client here." I feel like a football analogy is the best one I can give when trying to describe what it feels like to have parental interference in your treatment of an adolescent client. When everything is going smoothly, passes are completed and touchdowns are scored; parents transfer the therapeutic work to real life situations, teens are succeeding, and everyone is cheering. When things are not going smoothly, however, you will often feel like someone is perpetually hitting you from your blind spot, tackling you from behind, and seemingly coming out of nowhere to intercept, interfere with, and ultimately thwart your attempts to get the ball in the end zone.

There are some overarching issues, such as parent personalities and parenting styles, that factor into adolescents' treatment in potentially big ways. There are also matters such as parental mental health diagnoses, life stressors, and child abuse that may find their way into your office on more than one occasion. As in chapter 5, this chapter is by no means exhaustive. For example, there are a number of life stressors other than divorce that can affect parents in the therapy room, and parental mental health issues extend far beyond anxiety. My biggest challenge in writing this chapter was separating out such integrative concepts, so please read with the following in mind: *all* of the parents you encounter have a personality and a parenting style that you will learn and to which you will adapt. You may also encounter parent mental health and life stressor issues, which have a bidirectional relationship with personality and parenting style; these issues affect one another. Finally, child abuse is a difficult situation all around, one in which personality, parenting styles, mental health issues, and life stressors all play a role. These factors are crucial to understand if you are going to successfully work with teens and their parents.

PARENT PERSONALITIES AND PERSONALITY DISORDERS

Nick, thirteen, had been in therapy for over a year when he finally told me that he did not like his father, whom he visited every weekend. Nick perceived his father as demanding, inflexible, and sometimes verbally aggressive. He admitted that he was often afraid to express his opinions when he was at his father's house. Nick's mother tried to mediate the relationship by helping Nick express himself, but his father only viewed this as an attempt for his mother to "turn Nick against [him]." After a couple of failed attempts at scheduling phone or in-person sessions with Nick's father, I suggested a parent–teen session where they could talk together. The session went reasonably well, with both identifying things they could work on to improve their relationship, but Nick's father was defensive and unable to see the ways in which his responses hurt Nick.

We scheduled another session for a few weeks later, but Nick's father called me shortly afterward to cancel it. During this phone call, he also berated me for letting Nick's mother "manipulate" me, for failing him and his son, and he alluded to the fact that I was too young to be a therapist. He indicated that he would seek therapy for Nick and himself elsewhere—which I fully supported—and hung up on me. Although he never withdrew consent for Nick to see me for individual therapy, he never responded to any of my attempts to keep him engaged in Nick's work.

Many clinicians will tell you that, when it comes to diagnosing personality disorders (PD), they "know it when they see it" (Freeman, Breitmeyer, & Flint, 2013). There has been a lot of debate about the current conceptualization of PD, and it is quite possible that the field will soon move away from rigid categorical model and toward a dimensional model that considers patterns and severity of symptoms (American Psychiatric Association, 2013a, 2013b). The good news is that when it comes to working with parents of your teen clients, it is usually less important to know if a parent has a formal PD diagnosis than it is to understand traits as they pertain to parenting and building a working alliance with their teens' therapies.

When working with parents with PD or disordered personality traits, it is important to identify whether you are viewed as an ally or an enemy. Edward Budd (2012) eloquently describes this situation:

> Many people with personality disorders treat allies and adversaries quite differently. They are "circle the wagon" folks. Anyone inside the circle gets grub and a pat on the back. Those outside the circle get shot off their horses. (p. 36)

Indeed, if you are lucky enough to be inside the circle, PD parents will interact cooperatively with you, provided that you continue to endorse a narcissistic or paranoid parent's views and prevent a borderline parent from feeling abandoned. If you are doing your job well, however, you *will* challenge them eventually, at which point you begin getting treated in the same way as other adversaries (Budd, 2012). Although there are certainly parents who struggle with Cluster A and C personalities, I find that many of my parents have some traits common in Cluster B PD.[1] So let us focus this section on Cluster B parents.

Borderline Personality Disorder

Research on mothers with *borderline personality disorder* (BPD) suggests that these mothers[2] struggle to balance their desire to be a good parent and their own needs (Aidane, Wendland, Rabain, & Marie, 2009). They tend to feel less satisfied, less competent, and more distressed in fulfilling their parenting roles than non-BPD mothers (Newman, Stevenson, Bergman, & Boyce, 2007). Parents with BPD are often inconsistent in their parenting approach, sometimes demonstrating overinvolvement with their teen and other times ignoring teens' needs in order to meet their own affective needs (Aidane et al., 2009; Macfie & Swan, 2009; Reinelt et al., 2013). They are also at a heightened risk for abusive parenting (Bogacki & Weiss, 2007; Fontaine & Nolin, 2012).

Parents with BPD may especially struggle with adolescent youth. They are less accepting of their teens' increasing autonomy and may view teens' attempts at separation as threatening and withdraw love as a means of protection from the abandonment they fear (Aidane et al., 2009; Zalewski et al., 2014). Parents with BPD may also feel jealous and competitive toward their teens, leading to harsh criticism, mean-spirited teasing, and unrealistic expectations (Amianto, Daga, Bertorello, & Fassino, 2013).

BPD Parents in Therapy

There is a reason why professionals caution against having too many BPD clients on your caseload at one time. They can be exhausting. The same is true with parents, and may be even more exhausting since you are not directly working on the issues in therapy with them. Having a release to talk to parents' individual therapists (assuming they have one, which many will not) is sometimes helpful.

Boundary violations are probably the issues I come across the most with BPD parents of my teen clients. Parents may try to push boundaries related to sessions, out of session contact, your role in working with the teen. In the beginning, their requests may seem innocuous, but be careful. Parents with BPD may take a small, appropriate boundary crossing and interpret it as proof that they are special (Budd, 2012). A perfect example of this was a parent who had a conflict and had to bring her other child to the appointment. The child was young, maybe only four or five, so she could not stay in the waiting room while my client and her mom "checked out." The sibling was incredibly disruptive, but I did not say anything because it was a one-time occurrence. Or so I thought. Before I knew it, the sibling was disrupting our check-out every week.

Idealization is another issue that you may experience. After enough time working with BPD parents and clients, someone telling me how wonderful I am sets off warning bells in my head. I liken the experience of working with BPD to being on a really, really high platform overlooking a beautiful landscape. When you are at the top, you feel great. But when someone pushes you off that platform, the fall is unexpected, it happens quickly, and it hurts. The first time I ever experienced this plummet, I was working with a young adult female named Alexis. She had been in therapy with me for over a year and had presented as anxious, depressed, and immature. As time went on, I saw abandonment fears and interpersonal issues that were characteristic of BPD. One day, I said something that Alexis took offense to (I cannot even remember what now). I reflected her feelings, apologized, and expected that we would continue our session. But she blew up and began yelling and crying. She told me, "I guess you just aren't as good of a therapist as I thought you were." My descent had begun.

How to Handle It

A rule of thumb for me is that I am only willing to do for one parent what I am willing to do for all. Over time, this rule has helped me establish clear boundaries that I feel comfortable with, but it has also acted as a guide for when I may be dealing with a BPD parent. Most parents, even if they are anxious, can eventually respect limits I set with them regarding phone calls, e-mails, and session content. BPD parents will have a much harder time. I have had parents terminate their teen's therapy after I repeatedly set limits about after-hours phone calls; I suspected BPD in several of the cases. I am clear with parents that my role as a therapist for their teen does *not* include completing objective evaluations for court, discussing treatment for other members of the family (including other children in the home), or determining placement in cases involving Department of Social Services. To counteract the notion that I am doing parents a "favor," I am clear that they will be billed for any appearances I am asked to make at court, school, or other treatment settings.

Back to my example above, with the parent who was bringing her younger child to therapy, I empathized with balancing multiple schedules and child care but ultimately told the parent that I thought it would help everyone maintain focus if the younger child no longer attended our sessions. The parent told me, in a nasty tone, that it must be nice not to have to worry about child care. Though untrue, this statement hit a nerve for me because the week before, I had to work from home and cancel appointments because my son's daycare was closed. Effective supervision and consultation with colleagues over the years enabled me to maintain my composure, remain disengaged from her attack on me, and reiterate that I would be happy to work with her to schedule appointments she could attend without the younger child present.

When it comes to idealization, remember that you are not black and white, as the BPD parent may be trying to make you. You are not perfect, nor are you pure evil. I may try to reflect these parents' feelings back to them, but that is about all I do when they are trying to kick me off of an idealized platform that I never agreed to be on in the first place. In later sessions, Alexis and I talked about the tendency for me to be put on the platform and how unrealistic it was to think that I would never disappoint her. With parents, I have similar conversations. A father was furious at me for cancelling an appointment due to a family emergency, and he told me that he had "expected better" from me. I empathized with his frustration but gently reminded him that we all have emergencies and that I do not cancel appointments lightly. Finally, document any of these situations.[3]

Antisocial Personality Disorder

Parental *antisocial personality disorder* (ASPD) has been cited among the highest predictors of negative parent–teen interactions (Johnson, Cohen, Kasen, & Brook, 2008). This may not surprise you; parents with traits of ASPD, or *psychopathy*, often lack many of the behaviors that we expect to come naturally to parents, such as genuinely caring for and comforting their children (Moss, Lynch, Hardie, & Baron, 2002). Because these parents lack empathy and are emotionally unavailable, their parenting style often fails to protect their children from emotional injuries or teach children that they can depend on others to meet their emotional needs (Torry & Billick, 2011). Interestingly, not all antisocial parents are "cold"; rather, many mix loving and abusive parenting behaviors together (Leedom, Bass, & Almas, 2013). As Leedom and colleagues (2013) explain,

> These "loving behaviors" paradoxically also serve their parasitic and predatory goals … We believe that the "affection" that psychopathic individuals display is at times a genuine reflection of their pleasure with social contact (social reward). When a psychopathic individual says, "I love you," the meaning is likely, "I enjoy you when you do what I want." (p. 176)

In addition to conditional, limited parental affection, teens of ASPD parents often experience chaos and instability at home—particularly if their parent has been involved in criminal activity—as well as isolation and limited stimulation or engagement (i.e., neglect). While ASPD parents may take an interest in children in the family—even fighting for custody in some cases—these parents rarely see the value in engaging with their teens or supervising them and, when they do, may enjoy inducing fear. Particularly as children enter adolescence, ASPD parents often begin engaging their teens in antisocial behavior, by talking to them about it, manipulating them into covering for the parent, and/or directly involving the teen (Leedom et al., 2013). Do not be surprised to see ASPD choose "favorites" among their children or practice differential parenting. Also be alert to the fact that "noncompliant" or struggling teens (like the ones you may see for therapy) may have a particularly difficult time with ASPD parents (Beaver et al., 2014).

Abusive parenting is common among ASPD parents, in part due to the lack of remorse or insight that might prevent violence against others (Bogacki & Weiss, 2007; Fontaine & Nolin, 2012). Adolescence seems to be a time of escalating violence for children of ASPD parents (Leedom et al., 2013). In their review of adult children's recollections of childhood with ASPD parents, Leedom and colleagues discuss a specific type of abuse seen in these families:

> This abuse, which involves manipulation of the subject's perceptions of reality, caused the [children] to doubt their own perceptions of reality. These parents asserted their emotional attachments and efforts to support the child financially to the point of sacrifice. Typically the psychopathic parent would make a statement to the effect of, "I do it all for you (the children of the family)." The assertion of extreme devotion on the part of psychopathic parents is a form of "gaslighting" as its purpose is to invalidate perceptions of neglect and abuse. (p. 166)

ASPD Parents in Therapy

Parents with ASPD may be deceitful, manipulative, mistrustful, impulsive, uncooperative, cynical, and unconcerned with the needs or rights of their teens or you (McWilliams, 1994; R. C. Schwartz, 2000). They are so masterful at externalizing blame that nothing is ever their fault. You may also notice grandiosity and inflated sense of self-esteem. While some are incredibly unlikeable, many have a convincing, superficial charm. Psychopathic individuals are highly motivated to connect socially and to establish control over people in their lives, and they can actually be pleasant to engage with when they do not feel threatened or when they believe they are effectively manipulating you.

When this control is threatened, however, you may see a completely different side of them, as I often did when I worked as the coordinator of a supervised visitation center. During intake, parents were on their best behavior and did everything they could to convince me of the wrongdoing of their exes or of the Department of Social Services. Once they were expected to abide by the rules and learned that I would not bend them, no matter how charming the requestor was, I often witnessed the switch before my very eyes. Subtle (and not so subtle) threats; further attempts at flattery; attacks on me, the center, and the courts; and victimization ("I *want* to see my children, but you won't allow me to") were just some of the ways that I became certain of antisocial traits in the room.

Unfortunately, working with ASPD parents also means enduring blatant disregard or disrespect for their teens and you. These are the parents who will not show for appointments and not care. In the past, I had a suspected ASPD parent repeatedly strand his teen at my office; this is one of the reasons I have developed a rule that parents must remain in the waiting room during sessions. A parent with ASPD may make ill-intentioned, inappropriate jokes in the therapy session, to either you or their teen. I would not set your sights too high on parental engagement, unless, of course, the parent believes that it will help them personally in some way (e.g., in custody proceedings). Pain and anxiety are cited by clients of all ages as a motivator for change, but those with ASPD do not experience discomfort, pain, guilt, or anxiety. Their motivation to engage in therapy designed to enact change will be mortally low (Reid & Gacono, 2000).

How to Handle It

I tend to keep my interactions with ASPD parents to a minimum and as fact-focused as possible. This often means setting *a lot* of limits, which ASPD parents will repeatedly violate, and resisting the urge to enter into conflict when parents become adversarial. Supervision and/or consultation in these cases is key, as is documentation and planning. In truth, one of the most important ways that I try to protect myself against ASPD parents is by obtaining useful information in early encounters. Then I can set those necessary boundaries early on in a proactive, rather than reactive, way. A parent's extensive criminal background or abuse allegations often act as warning signs for me. What teens tell me about their relationships can also be useful; I might hear about repeated guilt trips, exploitation of weaknesses, and examples of cruelty. The degree to which parents try to manipulate me into being "on their side" is another. In the first ten minutes of my first phone call with one noncustodial parent, I was blasted with stories about his cheating ex-wife, the "screwed-up legal system," and several of the ways he had been mistreated throughout their divorce process. In the next breath, he was remarkably charming, thanking me profusely for taking the case and being willing to see his perspective. Other authors have discussed similar experiences (Richmond, 1992).

Narcissistic Personality Disorder

Parents with *narcissistic personality disorder* (NPD) generally struggle to meet their teen's needs because of their own self-absorption. Roles are often flipped in these parent–teen relationships; the parents are affectively unavailable to their teens while their teens must fulfill parents' needs, which may include admiration and recognition. Horne (1998) cautions that these teens are at risk for developing behaviors aimed at excessively pleasing others. While they seem empathic, they are actually based in fear. Others have termed this *co-narcissism*; after failing to break through their parents' self-absorption, teens become obsessed with pleasing others (Rappoport, 2005).

When parents struggle with narcissistic tendencies, they attempt to sustain and enhance self-esteem, achieve perfection, and avoid feelings of shame or embarrassment in any way possible. This comes at a tremendous cost to their children. As Shaw (2010) explains,

> Although each narcissist parent/child couple has its own uniquely complex story, one bottom line is that these patients … have been brought up to believe that they are always wrong and cannot win, by a parent or parents who claim unyielding infallibility. The justice system in such families has become rotten, corrupt. Any opposition from the child is characterized by the parent as signifying the child's moral failure, punishable by the withdrawal of the parent's love and administration of contempt. (p. 49)

This dynamic is particularly important to consider when working with adolescents. In order to remain compliant with the parent, a teen must remain the object of his/her parent's demands, requirements, and judgments (Shaw, 2010, p. 50). However, this goes directly against teens' developmentally appropriate task of figuring out who "I" or "me" is and threatens their ability to experience themselves as separate from their parents. With the risk that teens potentially pose to NPD parents' fragile sense of self, it makes sense that research has demonstrated a strong link between NPD parents and abuse perpetration (Bogacki & Weiss, 2007; Fontaine & Nolin, 2012).

NPD Parents in Therapy

Like ASPD and BPD parents, NPD parents may readily point out flaws in others, including their teens. They may struggle to control their anger, particularly when they believe they are being criticized, act insensitively toward their teens, and/or appear cold and arrogant (Adshead, 2003; American Psychiatric Association, 2013a). Parents with NPD can be guarded, hypervigilant, and reactive in therapy settings. They can be equally grandiose, exaggerating their accomplishments and abilities (Ronningstam, 2012).

Sometimes this grandiosity serves a defensive function (e.g., "Of course I know what my daughter needs; I'm the CEO of [insert corporation], I solve problems every day!"), while other times it is reactive (e.g., "We can afford to see any other therapist; I can fire you anytime I want to").

In some cases, the grandiosity is slightly annoying but manageable; I remember one father who bragged about his superior work ethic every time we met, no matter what the discussion. To that point, not all NPD parents are unmanageable or unlikeable, like Nick's dad above. Like ASPD parents, some can be quite charming, intriguing, and engaging, and you may have a hard time identifying NPD parents. Likeable or not, you can expect that parents with NPD will struggle to accept anything that they perceive as criticism. Undoubtedly, they will. You have shattered (or at least damaged) their fragile self-image. Some may respond to this vulnerability by criticizing you right back (e.g., "What do you know? You aren't even a doctor"). Other parents who are more skilled at managing their responses will try a different tactic, maybe choosing to exaggerate their concern for their teen. One mother told me, "Well, yes, I am far from perfect, but what we really need to focus on here is [my son]. I sincerely worry that he will never find anyone [to share his life with] because he is so mean and selfish." If the conversation then shifts to her son's selfishness and cruelty, the narcissistic parent has succeeded in quashing the criticism directed at her.

How to Handle It

Early in treatment, your work with NPD parents will center on alliance building, as with any other parents. With NPD parents, I try to remain especially accepting and task-oriented (as suggested by Ronningstam, 2012, and others). Interpretations of behaviors (parents or teens) and/or attempts at feedback may be perceived as intrusive, controlling, or condescending. Therefore, I try to keep the focus on one thing at a time, even when parents try to veer the conversation away from perceived criticism and cushion the perceived blows by highlighting their importance in the process. In the example above, I empathized with the mother: "I certainly understand why you would feel concerned about your son, and I promise that he and I are going to be working on lots of things in his individual sessions. But I also know that, as his mother, you are one of the most important people to his success. How do you think you might be able to help our work?"

Remember to balance your accepting stance and objectivity with effective guidance and gentle criticism. Despite your best work, it is quite possible that you will hit a nerve and get assigned the villain role, so pack your thickest skin. Calmness and an ability to keep your feelings contained will be your best armor against a narcissistic parent's attacks, but at times it will be difficult. Narcissistic parents can be accusatory and confrontational. One father was convinced that I disliked him and wanted him out of his daughter's (my client) life. He was so sure of this that he began acting in ways that in fact made it nearly impossible for me to like him. He would fail to show for sessions, accuse me of aligning with his ex-wife, and threaten to withdraw consent for his daughter to continue therapy. In truth, every time his name came up on my caller ID, I sighed. My only rebuttal against these accusations was a calm, engaging, pleasant demeanor. In each conversation, I encouraged him to attend sessions, I empathized with how difficult it can be to be the noncustodial parent after a divorce, and I acknowledged his right to terminate his daughter's therapy if he thought it was best. At the end of the day, I knew that I had done nothing to substantiate his allegations of unfair treatment.

Countertransference Issues

Parents who struggle with PD or disordered personality traits bring up all kinds of countertransference reactions in their teens' therapists. Betan, Heim, Zittel Conklin, and Westen (2005) identified eight countertransference patterns among therapists treating PD clients, outlined in table 6.1.

Results of Betan and colleagues' study revealed that Cluster B clients evoked overwhelmed/disorganized feelings, helplessness, hostility, disengagement, and sexual attraction. This was in contrast to reactions to Cluster A clients (i.e., criticized/mistreated feelings) and Cluster C clients (i.e., nurturant and warm feelings). Similarly, other researchers have found that Cluster B clients often elicit negative countertransference feelings (Colli, Tanzilli, Dimaggio, & Lingiardi, 2014; Rossberg, Karterud, Pedersen, & Friis, 2010). Colli and colleagues (2014) also found that special/overinvolved feelings were common among therapists working with BPD.

It may also be helpful to know that research has found that the more significant the symptoms, the more negative therapists' countertransference reactions (Lingiardi, Tanzilli, & Colli, 2015). I share this as a helpful "heads up" that the more difficult parents you encounter, the more likely you are to feel overwhelmed, angry, or disengaged, but also as a means of assessment. If you encounter a parent who is evoking strong, negative countertransference reactions in you, take a step back, think about whether you may be dealing with a PD, and then proceed accordingly.

On Attachment and Parental Personality Disorders

Due to their character fragility, immaturity, and own insecure attachments (Brennan & Shaver, 1998), parents' PD can greatly complicate attachment relationships. Parents who struggle with impulse control, fickleness,

Table 6.1 Patterns Identified Through the Countertransference Questionnaire

Pattern	*Definition*	*Example*
Overwhelmed/Disorganized	A desire to avoid or flee the client and strong negative feelings, including dread, repulsion, and resentment	"I wish I had never taken him/her on as a client."
Helpless/Inadequate	Feelings of inadequacy, incompetence, hopelessness, and anxiety	"I feel anxious working with him/her."
Positive	The experience of a positive working alliance and close connection with the client	"If he/she was not my client, I could imagine being friends with him/her."
Special/Overinvolved	A sense of the client as special (relative to other clients) and problems maintaining boundaries, including self-disclosure, ending sessions on time, and feeling guilty, responsible, or overly concerned about the client	"I self-disclose with him/her more about my personal life with him/her more than my other clients."
Sexualized	Sexual feelings toward the client or experiences of sexual tension	"I find myself being flirtatious with him/her."
Disengaged	Feeling distracted, withdrawn, annoyed, or bored in sessions	"I feel annoyed in sessions with him/her."
Parental/Protective	A wish to protect and nurture the client in a parental way, above and beyond normal positive feelings toward the client	"I feel angry at people in his/her life."
Criticized/Mistreated	Feelings of being unappreciated, dismissed, or devalued by the client	"I have to stop myself from saying or doing something aggressive or critical."

Source: Betan, Heim, Zittel Conklin, and Westen (2005, pp. 892–893).

criticism, jealousy/competitiveness, or aggression are less likely to instill feelings of unconditional positive regard, stability, or predictability in their relationships. They often do not provide the empathy and interpersonal sensitivity teens need as they work through problems and toward identity development; parents may be relationally detached or overly intrusive (Amianto et al., 2013). Furthermore, PD parents may be experiencing lower feelings of mastery and self-acceptance and struggle with low resourcefulness, which makes it difficult for them to model and develop these feelings in their children. Amianto and colleagues suggest that parents suffer from a lack of *self-transcendence*, or "the ability to detach from himself and from concreteness and keep in touch with the deepest emotional and relational realty," which interferes with parents' ability to build deep, secure relationships with their teens (p. 808). These obstacles are important to consider as you assist teens in meeting their developmental and treatment goals, as they may get in the way of teens' abilities to make and/or sustain certain gains.

PARENTING PRACTICES

Tammy was sixteen when she first began treatment for anxiety and depression. Her mother came to all of her sessions, and Tammy considered her a close friend. Tammy did not get along well with her father, whom she perceived as mean and uncaring. Not long after beginning our work together, she began complaining about her home life. She viewed her parents as "inadequate" and gave examples of the ways in which her younger brother "walked all over them." Tammy was frustrated that she was the only one who did chores or attempted to keep the house clean, that no one noticed her unless she was "screwing up," and that, despite her trustworthiness, she was allowed less freedom than her older brother. She also complained that her older brother received much of the attention from their parents. Tammy reported that they were always setting goals for him and helping him, while she felt that she was alone in her hard work. She told me, "When I have kids, I won't have to worry about learning how to parent. I'll just take everything my mom and dad do, and I'll do the opposite."

Parenting Styles

Parenting style typically refers to the interplay between *parental responsiveness* and *parental demandingness*. Responsiveness represents supportiveness and attunement to the needs and wants of their teens, whereas demandingness

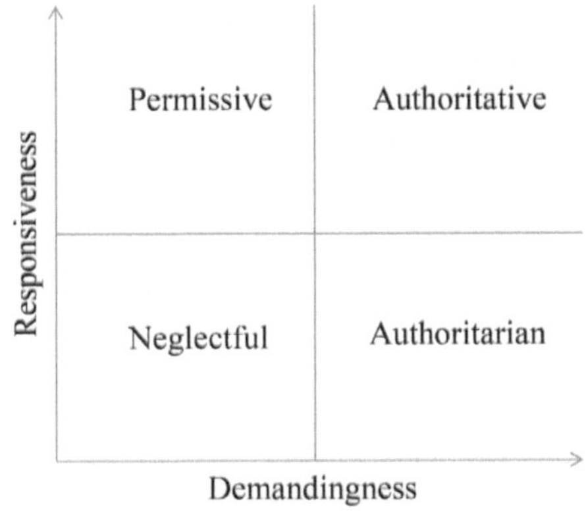

Figure 6.1 Parenting Styles Continuum. ***Source:*** **Based on Maccoby and Martin (1983).**

includes the ways that parents try to compel their teens to behave and follow certain rules (Baumrind, 1968, 1971, 1991; Steinberg, Lamborn, Darling, & Mounts, 1994). Where parents fall along the continuum of these two terms helps professionals identify what type of parenting style they use: permissive, authoritarian, neglectful, or authoritative (see figure 6.1; Maccoby & Martin, 1983).

Permissive parents tend to be high in responsiveness but low in demandingness. They parent in a nonpunitive, accepting way, include teens in decision-making, provide explanations for family rules, demand very little, and give their teens a lot of freedom to make their own decisions and "do their own thing." Tammy's description of her parents might fit into this category. There are no established standards by which these teens are expected to behave, and parents tend to have low expectations for maturity (Baumrind, 2003). For some teens, control over their own behaviors is okay; it promotes self-reliance and competence. For others, it can be problematic. Permissive parenting has been associated with substance abuse and delinquent behaviors.

Authoritative parents are high in both responsiveness and demandingness. Assertive, but more nurturing than punitive, authoritative parents establish rules and boundaries, and establish consequences when either is broken (Baumrind, 1991, 2003). However, these consequences are usually rational and discussed with the teen. There is an interesting balance in which parents exert firm control but do not overly restrict their teens. The parent is comfortable with the teen's emerging identity but also sets standards for future behavior, standards that may or may not line up with the teen's desires (Baumrind, 2003).

Authoritative parenting has long been thought of as the optimal parenting style, largely because studies have found that adolescents raised with this parenting style have positive self-esteem, adaptive coping skills (Aunola, Stattin, & Nurmi, 2000; Wolfradt, Hempel, & Miles, 2003), high life satisfaction, high rates of academic achievement (Im-Bolter, Zadeh, & Ling, 2013), and low levels of depression (Milevsky, Schlechter, Netter, & Keehn, 2007) and illicit drug use (Bahr & Hoffman, 2010). However, research suggests that this largely depends on context and that, in some cultures, authoritarian or indulgent parenting may be equal, if not preferable, to authoritative parenting (Darling & Steinberg, 1993; Dwairy, Achoui, Abouserie, & Farah, 2006; García & Gracia, 2009; Steinberg, 2001).

Neglectful parents are low in both responsiveness and demandingness. While they provide basic needs for their teens, they minimize contact and are indifferent to their teens' needs and wants (Baumrind, 2003). In these parent–teen dyads, parents' needs are always the top priority, similar to what we observe in the PD parents discussed above. Teens of these parents struggle with immaturity (Steinberg, Blatt-Eisengart, & Cauffman, 2006), low empathy, self-esteem, and competitiveness (Schaffer, Clark, & Jeglic, 2009). Vulnerable narcissism, in which teens feel unappreciated and angry when they are not noticed or given positive regard when they feel they have earned it, has been linked to the limited feedback and poor monitoring seen in neglectful parents (Mechanic & Barry, 2015). Teens of this parenting style also demonstrate high rates of self-destructive behavior, limited coping skills, and low academic achievement in comparison to other teens (Aunola et al., 2000; Calafat, García, Juan, Becoña, & Fernández-Hermida, 2014; Montgomery, Frisk, & Craig, 2008).

Authoritarian parents are low in responsiveness while high in demandingness. These parents can appear quite controlling as they attempt to shape and alter the teen and his/her behaviors to match a predetermined code of conduct. Their methods of obtaining obedience can be punitive, forceful, and restrictive; these are the "because I said so!" parents who are uninterested in engaging in verbal give and take. Rules are rules—there is no debating them. There is considerable overlap between authoritarian parenting and psychologically controlling behaviors such as guilt induction, anxiety induction, and love withdrawal (Barber & Harmon, 2002; Rudy, Awong, & Lambert, 2008).

As with permissive parenting, authoritarian parenting has been linked with positive outcomes such as success in school and limited involvement in delinquent behaviors. However, it has also been associated with conduct problems (Rodriguez & Eden, 2008), substance use (Calafat et al., 2014), high psychological distress (Wolfradt et al., 2003), poor peer relationships, low motivation, and limited internalization of values (Grolnick, 2003).

Parental Conditional Regard

Another important parenting practices involves the degree to which teens perceive their parents' affection and approval to be contingent on the teen's achievement of parentally valued outcomes or behaviors (Assor, Roth, & Deci, 2004). *Parental conditional regard* can be positive or negative. With *parental conditional positive regard* (PCPR), the teen perceives that he/she will receive more affection and attention when he/she meets parents' expectations; *parental conditional negative regard* (PCNR) involves a perception that parents provide less affection and attention when the teen fails to meet parents' expectations (Assor, Roth, Israeli, Freed, & Deci, 2007; Roth, Assor, Niemiec, Ryan, & Deci, 2009; Segrin, Givertz, Swaitkowski, & Montgomery, 2015). Both types of parental conditional regard refer to specific domains, such as sports or academic achievement. PCPR differs from positive feedback because it tends to focus on the product rather than the process (i.e., the outcome not the teen's effort). Similarly, PCNR is not the same as psychological control, which involves intrusiveness, manipulation of thoughts and feelings (Barber, 2002; Barber & Harmon, 2002), and psychological abuse (see chapter 8), although there may be love withdrawal in both cases.

Research has demonstrated that the use of parental conditional regard teaches teens to view achievement as vital to their self-worth (Assor, Vansteenkiste, & Kabuth, 2009). This can lead to tremendous anxiety, perfectionism, and even avoidance; after all, teens perceive these experiences as threatening to the love they receive from their parents. If they succeed, feelings of relief and temporary grandiosity follow, in tandem with praise and love from their parents (Assor & Tal, 2012). If they fail, feelings of shame and worthlessness await, and teens are alone, their distorted cognitions unchallenged—and possibly even reinforced—by their disappointed parents (Elliot & Thrash, 2004; MacGregor & Elliot, 2005).

As I continued my work with Tammy, I learned that she greatly craved positive regard from her parents. This drove many of her behaviors at home (e.g., doing chores without being asked) and was a driving force behind her perfectionism at school (i.e., doing well at school would get her some positive attention from parents). She also feared negative regard from her mother, whom she felt was the only person in the family who cared about her.

Helicopter Parents

If you ever have a parent who still e-mails coaches about playing time, solves social problems, and completes age-appropriate tasks for his/her teen (e.g., college applications), you have experienced a helicopter parent. *Helicopter parents* are "highly invested, extremely concerned for the well-being of their children, and well-intentioned albeit misdirected" (Padilla-Walker & Nelson, 2012, p. 1178). They are always hovering nearby. Despite good intentions, this type of parenting involves developmentally inappropriate involvement, including intrusive micromanagement and unsolicited affection (Rubin, Burgess, & Hastings, 2002; Segrin et al., 2015). These are the parents who unconsciously use the words "we" and "ours" when talking about their teens; as in "*We* just want to make sure that *we* get this anxiety under control so that it doesn't impair *our* goals." Of course, most parents just want the best for their children, but when you are dealing with helicopter parents, you will find an inordinate amount of unnecessary intervention (i.e., "swooping in") and a limited awareness of the impact this behavior could have in the long term (Coburn, 2006).

Helicopter parenting can be tricky, as many parents really do believe they are just engaging in "good parenting" (Padilla-Walker & Nelson, 2012), and it *has* been associated with positive types of parental involvement, including guidance and emotional support. However, it is also associated with low levels of parental autonomy granting and teens' limited proactive engagement with activities (Padilla-Walker & Nelson, 2012). Both the academic community (Padilla-Walker & Nelson, 2012; Segrin et al., 2015) and general public (Gabriel, 2010; Gottlieb, 2011; Marano, 2010) are beginning to recognize that overprotective, oversolicitious, helicopter parents, despite their best intentions, may be limiting their teen's opportunities to practice autonomy, problem solving, and decision-making, skills that are essential to teens success in adulthood. Padilla-Walker and Nelson (2012) considered, "While it may not be directly *destructive*, helicopter parenting may not be *conducive* to growth during emerging adulthood" (p. 1187).

Differential Parenting

Differential parenting, or differences in parental behavior toward each child, is a reality in many families. Some differential parenting is unavoidable, particularly as parents recognize different needs and abilities in their children, a teen is influenced both by the way parents treat all of the youth in the home and the way parents treat the teen him/herself (Feinberg & Hetherington, 2001). Parents may not realize their behaviors are different with each child, may believe they are acting fairly, or may have a rationale for the differential treatment that the teen does not know (Kowal, Kramer, Krull, & Crick, 2002).

Studies have emphasized the importance of the teens' *perception* of fairness when it comes to parents' differential practices. When teens view the practices as generally fair or can form attributions to explain the discrepancies, differential parenting seems to have less of an impact on sibling relationships and problem behaviors (Kowal & Kramer, 1997; McHale, Updegraff,

Jackson-Newsom, Tucker, & Crouter, 2000). Differential parental behavior that is perceived as unfair, on the other hand, has been associated with poorer sibling relationships and adolescent problem behaviors, particularly if teens believe they receive less parental warmth or more parental control than their siblings (Hetherington et al., 1999). These findings are even more pronounced in blended families (Henderson, Hetherington, Mekos, & Reiss, 1996; Mekos, Hetherington, & Reiss, 1996).

As I mentioned, Tammy complained a lot about the differential treatment she received at home. Knowing now what I have learned about differential parenting, her complaints are not surprising. Her parents, who insisted that they were parenting each child exactly the same, did not share her perception of the unfairness. Tammy, on the other hand, was highly sensitive to the differences she observed in their parenting strategies, as is the case with many adolescents who have younger siblings (Tamrouti-Makkink, Dubas, Gerris, & van Aken, 2004).

Parenting Practices in Therapy

It probably will not take long for you to see these parenting styles play out in therapy. For the most part, authoritative and permissive parents will be the ones who seem the most supportive of their teens and accepting of their feelings. You will recognize emotional attunement between teens and both types of parents. The differentiation will come when you learn more about the demands placed on the teens. Sometimes this does not happen until I start assigning tasks in between sessions; other times I learn which type I am dealing with when I hear about school expectations and rules at home.

Neglectful parents will likely be the ones who drop their teen off, are quick to end their involvement in the session, appear uninterested in participating, or participate but do not follow through on any of the things you discuss during check-ins or check-outs, whereas helicopter parents will be the ones who take intense notes and come back having accomplished every goal, whether they were supposed to be a part of the goal or not. They may or may not have included the child—think of the parents who complete their children's science fair projects for them. Remember to be on the lookout for the use of "we" when speaking about the teen's thoughts, feelings, experiences, and goals. Helicopter parents may also struggle to leave the check-ins on time; most would gladly sit through the whole session if you did not ask them to leave.

Similarly, authoritarian parents and those who utilize PCR are overly intrusive and, like helicopter parents, may also be quite demanding of your time and have high expectations of you. Unlike helicopter parents, however, authoritarian and PCR parents are critical and demanding of their teens as well. Their goals for therapy may be high and unrealistic, and they are unlikely to support the teen in his/her struggle through the process (Segrin et al., 2015). Such an intrusive, demanding style may result in their teen feeling like they cannot—or do not want to—disclose personal experiences.

Differential parenting can come out at any point in the therapy and can be difficult to pinpoint. You may start hearing clients complain that their parents treat them differently from siblings, or parents may tell you about times that they handled things differently than they would have with older children. Remember that this issue is not necessarily problematic; it only becomes therapeutically relevant when it is distressing for the client.

How to Handle it

When it comes to tackling parenting practices in therapy, I would encourage you to be *realistic*. After spending some time observing parent and teens' interactions with one another and getting to know the family, focus parents' efforts on things that they think they can change. You will encounter parents who, due to cultural beliefs, personality styles, or family dynamics, are unwilling to change anything. We will talk a little bit about that resistance at the end of the chapter, but in my experience, most parents can find *something* that they are willing to work on, even if it is very small. I frequently tell parents that I would rather them choose something small that feels manageable than something bigger that is unreasonable. I often have parents tell me they would like to improve their communication with their teens. Great! I work with them to objectify this goal, maybe by deciding to do one check-in daily where both the parent and the teen share a funny moment from their day. Many times, parents struggle the most to transfer their goals into tangible steps. Here are a few other examples:

- "I am willing to let him be a little more independent."—Parent and son agree that for the next week, parent will allow son to do his homework with parent checking for completion.
- "I want to be more involved in her life."—Parent and daughter make a date to get lunch together one time before next session.
- "It would be nice if the kids pitched in at home more."—Parent agrees to have a family meeting before next session where possible chores are discussed.

Psychoeducation can go a long way when it comes to working with parental styles. I would highly recommend using what you know about the parent and his/her style to dictate the way in which you give them information. For example, you may choose to share data with an authoritarian parent whose style is black-and-white. Emphasize studies that demonstrate benefits to setting goals for oneself, show the utility of granting autonomy to teens, or highlight the role of parent–teen attachment in future academic, occupational, and social success (Gunnoe, Hetherington, & Reiss, 2006; Myrick et al., 2013). Similarly, with a helicopter parent, discuss the importance of limits within the therapeutic relationship and the ways in which it positively impacts therapy outcomes. For these parents, who act inappropriately out of good intentions, they may be more likely to respect their teens' privacy or allow the teen to work on some goals independently if they believe it will be useful to their teen's future success (Asano et al., 2013). We will discuss the anxiety helicopter parents may feel (and what to do about it) in the next section. Encourage parents who are engaging in differential parenting to discuss their reasoning with their teens. Many parents have reasons why they parent one child differently from another, but few consider sharing it with their children (Kowal, Krull, & Kramer, 2004).

Finally, you may also meet with some success if you can assist highly demanding parents in *lowering the bar* when it comes to expectations, particularly when teens are struggling with depressive symptoms that make them feel as though they cannot complete even the smallest of tasks effectively (Wells & Albano, 2005). These same parents can often benefit from some guidance on ways to *catch their teen being good*; that is, they can provide more positive feedback when they notice efforts and positive progress toward goals (Wells & Albano, 2005). I find that I am most successful in helping parents lower demandingness and increase warmth when I am able to frame it within the context of the teens' symptoms and refrain from blaming the parents. For example, despite the fact that I know that the parent's demands regarding schoolwork are a large contributor to my client's depression, I might tell his authoritative or conditionally regarding parent, "One thing we know about depression is that it makes people feel like they are incapable of doing anything and fail anytime they try. I wonder if it might be helpful to fight against these depressive thoughts and feelings by setting Tim up for success. What is something you think we could 'lower the bar' on, to help him experience some success?" and then, "How can you let him know that you notice the work he is putting in?"[4]

Countertransference Issues

Every therapist was once a child; thus, every therapist holds thoughts and feelings about parenting styles (Freedman, Rosenberg, Gettman-Feizien, & Van Scoyk, 1993). You may believe that your parents' style was the "best way," or you may be averse to any style that mirrors your upbringing. Your reactions to parents of your teen clients will reflect these thoughts and feelings. If you are a parent yourself, you will also have reactions based on how closely the parents' style matches the one you have chosen to employ with your child(ren). Do your best, and utilize supervision and consultation, to observe your teens' parents as objectively as possible. Know your own blind spots. Remember that there is no one way to parent effectively, and while the research does support some behaviors over others, there is no such thing as a "perfect parent," and no one needs one anyway.

On Attachment and Parenting Practices

When considering attachment and parenting styles, I mostly think about how different parenting practices impact the parent–teen relationship. Helicopter parents and authoritarian parents who grant little to no autonomy often sacrifice a quality relationship with their teens, and some teens may even disengage from their family as soon as they get the chance (Mayseless & Scharf, 2009). One of my clients frequently tells me, "I can't wait to go to college and just *get away*." Surely no parent wants to hear that from his/her child, and many parents' fear of this very thing often becomes a self-fulfilling prophecy, leading them to over-controlling behaviors that then push their children away. On the other hand, parents who make compromises and concessions regarding their teen's increasing autonomy while appropriately supervising and expressing warmth and affection are able to maintain and strengthen a secure attachment through their parenting practices (Karavasilis, Doyle, & Markiewicz, 2003; Zimmer-Gembeck, Ducat, & Collins, 2011). Be sure to give parents who are successfully striking this balance a lot of credit—it is *not* easy!

Differential parenting also has an interesting connection to attachment. Research has shown that it is not just important to consider what type of warmth and affection teens receive from parents but also what they receive relative to their siblings. Preferred siblings may receive more sensitive caregiving than nonpreferred children in the home. This leads to strong, more stable attachments that are typically rewarding to parents. Parents then continue to pay closer attention to these attachment relationships, to the detriment of the other relationships in the home (see Sheehan & Noller, 2002, for a review). Assuming your client is the disfavored child, you may need to work with parents to help them understand the ways in which their differential treatment plays a role in presenting problems. For example, Sheehan and Noller (2002) found that those who received less warmth and support from parents typically reported more controlling, coercive parenting. These teens were less confident or comfortable with closeness in relationships than their other siblings.

STRESS AND PARENTING[5]

Bradley was initially referred for treatment at age thirteen for anxious symptoms stemming from a bullying incident that occurred in the months before. After a brief time in therapy, Bradley's symptoms improved, and he and I mutually agreed on termination. I was surprised, then, to receive a call from his father a few months later, indicating that "something else had come up." He explained that Bradley had begun refusing to see his mother, who had divorced from his father the year before. No one was entirely sure what had changed in their relationship, which had previously appeared loving and strong.

When Bradley entered treatment he told me that he "couldn't take it anymore." He talked about his mother's mental health issues, her dependence on him to be a listening ear, her negative comments about his father and his new girlfriend, and his feelings of being the "man of the house" who was responsible for taking care of anything she could not. Since he was only there twice a month, he told me, he was usually able to tolerate his mother's issues and behaviors. However, as he was starting to get involved in more extracurricular activities, he reported that his mother was giving him "a hard time" and "trying to guilt trip [him] all the time." His mother's own issues, it seemed, were not only interfering with Bradley's well-being but also threatening the parent–teen relationship in a big way. Rather than hear these complaints, Bradley admitted, it was easier to tell his mother he was busy and could not come over for his weekend visits.

Mental Health Issues: Spotlight on Parental Anxiety

I hear elements of Bradley's story repeatedly in my work with teenagers, and I see the impact that parents' own mental health issues can have on parenting style, teens' mental health, and teen's treatment outcomes. Many parents have a lower level of psychological well-being than their teens (Evenson & Simon, 2005), and research suggests that is especially true when the difficulties of parenting outweigh the rewarding aspects of their role (Pace & Shafer, 2015).

Parental anxiety has received a lot of attention in literature, as it is related to inflexible, restrictive, and non-nurturing parenting styles (Lindhout et al., 2006) and strategies that often lead to unproductive interactions with their teens (Woodruff-Borden, Morrow, Bourland, & Cambron, 2002). They may manage their own anxiety by controlling, limiting, or even ignoring teens' experiences (Ballash, Leyfer, Buckley, & Woodruff-Borden, 2006; Nanda, 2012; Woodruff-Borden et al., 2002) or becoming overly involved (Hudson & Rapee, 2004).

Anxious parents can be a notable risk factor for teens, particularly when the parents demonstrate separation anxiety. Some anxious parents struggle to relinquish control to their adolescents as they work toward autonomy or are unable to normalize teens' needs to separate and develop their identities (Hock, Eberly, Bartle-Haring, Ellwanger, & Widaman, 2001). Likewise, socially anxious parents struggle to show warmth toward their teens, are more likely to interpret their teens' actions negatively, and are more likely to correct or control behaviors that they fear will reflect poorly on them (Crosby Budinger, Drazdowski, & Ginsburg, 2013, p. 413). Self-criticism is a big part of social anxiety disorder (Cox, Fleet, & Stein, 2004), and parents struggling with these symptoms may view their teens' actions as a reflection of themselves.

Parents with anxiety may also present as perfectionistic, or with traits in line with an obsessive compulsive personality disorder (OCPD; Fairburn, Cooper, Doll, & Welch, 1999; Lilenfeld et al., 1998). When both parents and teens are anxious, it creates a dyad that communicates ineffectively and enhances frustration, fear, nervousness, and helplessness (Hudson et al., 2014).

Parental Anxiety in Therapy

While parents' mental health issues can certainly impact teens' treatment, the nature of the relationship can vary. Some parents experience a "spillover effect" from their teens' treatment and feel relief just from entering treatment in a peripheral way. Parents with their own mental health issues may recognize the importance of treatment and be more motivated to participate actively for the good of the teen and family (Schleider et al., 2015). In other cases, mental health issues contribute to parenting strain, which affects parents' ability to engage positively with their teens in and out of therapy (Crawford & Manassis, 2001). To this end, parental depression has been linked to low levels of satisfaction with treatment for youth (Furey & Basili, 1988), and both parental depression and anxiety have been associated with poorer youth treatment outcomes (Cobham, Dadds, & Spence, 1998; Southam-Gerow, Kendall, & Weersing, 2001).

Parents actively struggling with their own mental health issues are often significantly affected by their teens' emotional experiences, sometimes even more so than the teens themselves. These parents often have a low threshold for frustration (Neger & Prinz, 2015), and if they cannot tolerate teens' reactions, parents may use emotionally avoidant language or emotion suppression strategies (Coyne & Wilson, 2004; Murrell, Wilson, LaBorde, Drake, & Rogers, 2008). These approaches may become evident in therapy sessions. For example, I have heard parents tell their teens to "pull themselves together" when they are crying in my office. These parents give the message that negative emotions should be avoided, which can lead to teens' symptoms worsening almost before your eyes. Similar to the helicopter parenting we discussed above, anxious parenting may include overinvolvement and intrusiveness; these parents may have difficulty respecting limits of the therapy.

Separation anxious parents often experience jealousy and possessiveness over their teens or take their teens' attempts at individuation as rejection (Hock et al., 2001). They may attempt to pathologize their teen's desire for independence. They may be unable to enjoy events that highlight their teen's increasing autonomy (Soenens, Vansteenkiste, Duriez, & Goossens, 2006). One mother insisted that her daughter send her texts repeatedly throughout her senior prom. Her daughter later told me that she was unable to enjoy herself because she knew her mother would "freak out" if she did not respond. Parents may struggle to adapt to their changing roles as treatment progresses; oftentimes, teens rely less on their parents than before, especially when the teen presented with anxious symptoms themselves. This change can be extremely distressing for a separation anxious parent, who subsequently becomes less satisfied with their parental role (Esbjørn et al., 2014). Socially anxious parents may be critical, doubtful of your assessment of their teen's performance (e.g., "I don't think she is doing it right"), and cold toward their teens (Crosby Budinger et al., 2013).

You may witness a spike in anxiety among parents, particularly as their teens' symptoms begin improving. Lindsey, thirteen, struggled with perfectionism and anxiety that was characterized by ruminative, obsessive thoughts. She confided in me that she could not even paint her own nails for fear of "messing them up." We designed an exposure at home where she could paint her nails, identified a number of coping strategies to help her, and solicited the help of her mother, who was also quite anxious but supportive of treatment. Her mother's immediate response to the planned exposure was "But what if she spills nail polish on the table?" In that moment I became painfully aware of the ways in which Lindsey's mother's own anxiety was interfering with (if not sabotaging) Lindsey's efforts in therapy.

How to Handle It

Anxious parents often need reassurance, and a lot of it. This may involve normalization of parents' feelings that they miss their adolescents' dependence on them while also normalizing teens' increasing autonomy and need for a secure base in their parents (Hock et al., 2001). Everyday parenting struggles may seem insurmountable, so they may need some extra time or support to make changes in their parenting. They may be particularly susceptible to the feelings of stigma, self-blame, and shame that we discussed in chapter 1, so remember to take a kind, nonblaming stance. I often tell anxious parents about similar cases that I have worked on to remind them that they are not the only families with mental health needs and concerns.

Research demonstrates that parents' own improved mental health trickles down to their teens (Cuijpers, Weitz, Karyotaki, Garber, & Andersson, 2015), so I use this to support my statement that parents must take care of themselves in order to be the parents they can be. Parents must be reminded to "put on their own oxygen masks before assisting others," just as we are reminded before every airplane ascent. You may need to do this around the time that your teen client starts making some changes in his/her life or trying new things. Jason was a preadolescent with severe social anxiety and some aggressive behavior; peer rejection had been a longstanding issue that was both a cause and effect of behaviors. He was excited but nervous, then, when he was invited to a peer's birthday party, but not nearly as nervous as his parents, who actually considered telling him he could not go. They greatly feared that Jason might "have a tough time," and to say that they were catastrophizing would be an understatement.[6] Jason and I worked tirelessly in the weeks leading up to the party, engaging in exposures and identifying a coping plan, and I also scheduled a session with his parents to help them manage the anxiety they were feeling about this new terrain.

To combat the inflexibility linked with many flavors of parental anxiety, focus some of your interactions on increasing psychological flexibility. *Psychological flexibility* involves openness to thoughts, feelings, and experiences and the ability to choose and engage in behaviors consistent with values (Moyer & Sandoz, 2015). Help parents tolerate distress caused by seeing their teens struggle with difficult experiences. Empathize with how helpless or distraught they may feel. Provide psychoeducation as to why it is important for teens to learn coping skills. I often work with parents to "let themselves off the hook" when it comes to rescuing their teens. Finally, be patient; anxious parents may only be able to tolerate distress for short periods of time.

Finally, Budd (2012) suggests protecting yourself from being an easy target of anxious, perfectionistic (possibly OCPD) parents by being on time, returning phone calls and e-mails promptly, setting limits, and meeting deadlines. For example, I require twenty-four hours to write a letter, and give a time frame in which I will communicate with other providers or look into resources (e.g., before the week is out).

Countertransference Issues

Anxious parents can evoke a variety of feelings in me. I genuinely like many of them, and some lead me to feel warm and nurturing countertransference feelings (Betan et al., 2005). This is particularly true with parents who focus a lot of their energy on developing a relationship with me and/or perceive me as knowledgeable, supportive, and protective (Disney, 2013). I sometimes find myself wanting to intervene in parents' mental health issues or considering taking them on as an individual client (Freedman et al., 1993).

However, as Bornstein (2012) points out, anxious parents can also invoke strong negative countertransference reactions in therapists, such as when they use self-deprecation to maintain care and support by the therapist. When this happens, I experience an "empathy meter on low." I find myself getting tired of empathizing with their feelings of self-deprecation and feeling irritated. I begin feeling exhausted by their endless streams of "What if?" I am well aware that these behaviors are ones for which I have less tolerance than others, so I am careful to use consultation, supervision, and self-care to prevent my feelings from negatively affecting the adolescent's therapy. As always, knowing *your* triggers is an important part of managing countertransference, particularly with parents affected by mental health issues.

Parental Divorce

Half of marriages end in divorce (Behrman, 1994), resulting in parental feelings of loss, grief, isolation, and failure (Cohen, 1998) and issues that negatively impact parenting abilities, such as financial stress (Ponnet et al., 2013), being forced to leave the home (Anthony, 1997), and abuse allegations (Penfold, 1995). Cohen (1998) explains,

> By its very nature, divorce constitutes a narcissistic threat. It raises questions about the individual's ability to love and be loved and embodies his or her failure to maintain an important relationship. The individual's shortcomings are, moreover, publicly exposed. (p. 200)

These feelings can be further compounded by infidelity and remarriage (Gunsberg, 2013; Shopper, 2013). Parents respond in a variety of ways intended to manage such a threat, and unfortunately, their teens often become involved. This is not to say that all parents intentionally triangulate their teen in the dissolution of their marriage. Shopper (2013) observes,

> Although many divorcing parents know or are told that they should not "involve" their children in their divorce, it is very difficult for parents to be abide by that advice even if it is their conscious wish to do so. (p. 120)

A vengeful, hurt, or distraught parent, then, may attempt to discredit the other parent, prevent or sabotage visitation, and otherwise damage the relationship between their teen and the other parent in an effort to exact revenge on their ex (Baker & Brassard, 2013; Shopper, 2013). Teens may get drawn into parental conflict, be expected to choose sides, or be asked to spy on a parent

(Baker & Ben Ami, 2011), causing great distress and conflict within the teen (Afifi & McManus, 2010).

Sometimes, parents end up allocating all of their emotional resources to management of the marital issues or divorce proceedings, and ineffective parenting strategies, including neglectful parenting and inconsistent discipline (i.e., less warmth and responsiveness) damage teens' perception of their parents as supportive or emotionally present (Krishnakumar & Buehler, 2000; Tritt & Pryor, 2005).

Parental Divorce in Therapy

Teens enter therapy at different phases in their parents' divorce, and research suggests that divorces that occur when teens are later in adolescence (i.e., between fifteen and nineteen years) do not seem to have the same negative impact as divorce occurring earlier (i.e., before age fifteen; Zeratsion et al., 2013). Siskind (2013) discusses four situations that you may encounter:

- Divorce is imminent; parents are requesting therapy for teen proactively.
- Parents wish for you to be a consultant to them as they navigate coparenting after divorce. They are not looking for a therapist to conduct individual therapy with their teen.
- Divorce proceedings have begun, and parents are noticing signs of stress in their teen.
- The teen begins treatment for an issue unrelated to divorce; divorce proceedings are initiated at some point during the treatment.

Aside from the chaos that a divorce can cause within the family, the issues I see most often in therapy revolve around parents' disclosures to their teens. Understandably, parents are distracted by their own grief, anger, loss, efforts to redefine their relationship with their former spouse, or their new role as a noncustodial parent (Cole & Cole, 1999; Wall & Levy, 1994). They do not always realize how their experiences affect what they tell their teens and the emotionality behind the disclosures (Afifi, 2003; Afifi, Afifi, & Coho, 2009; Afifi, McManus, Hutchinson, & Baker, 2007). Furthermore, research has shown that the more distress they feel because of the divorce, the more likely parents are to share negative information with their teens (Afifi et al., 2007).

Afifi and colleagues (2009) identified eleven types of disclosures that parents make to their adolescents, including *relationship-based* (e.g., asking the teen to serve as a mediator, discussing parents' relationship with the teen, or asking the teen to choose sides), *teen's relationship with parents* (e.g., commenting on teen's relationship with self or other parent), *partner-based* (e.g., commenting on other parent's personality or behaviors), *self-based* (e.g., commenting on own personality or behaviors), *teen-based* (e.g., commenting on teen's personality or behaviors and the ways in which they contribute to the divorce, family, or relationship with parents), *living/custody arrangements, finances, parenting practices* (e.g., expressing feelings about own or other parent's style of parenting), *role burden* (e.g., expressing feelings of being overwhelmed, of role within the family, and/or satisfaction with role), *general discussions about marriage and divorce*, including teen's feelings about own potential marriage one day, and questioning or commenting on either parent's *dating, remarriage, or new spouse* (p. 529–530).

Parents may—intentionally or unintentionally—speak negatively about the other parent, prod for information, treat teens as "messengers," or test the teen's loyalty, leading teens to feel caught in the middle. I have had many teen clients, like Bradley, complain about their parents' inability to act civilly toward each other, and other therapists sometimes miss that the parent is at fault when teens know more than they ought to. I once had a debate with a family therapist who insisted that my teen client, May, was "refusing to act her age" when she brought up financial issues that were occurring as a result of her parents' divorce. When I expressed my concerns about this teen's role in the parental conflict, I was told that May needed to be "put in her place." Fortunately, most of the family therapists I collaborate with take a much different stance in these types of situations, and they understand the complicated dynamics at play, but in this case, the parents got no feedback that their behaviors were inappropriate, the negative disclosures continued, and so did May's overinvolvement (and distress).

How to Handle It

In each possible situation Siskind outlines, she recommends setting firm limits and clearly stating that you will *not* take a position on divorce disputes, will *not* meet with attorneys, and will *not* provide documents that can be used in court proceedings. I, too, have to agree with Siskind; setting limits from the beginning will save you from the inevitable headache caused by an attorney's request and/or threat of subpoena. During the writing of this book, I received an e-mail from the attorney of a former client's parent, requesting that I testify on the parent's behalf. Because I had been clear with the parent back when her son began treatment with me, it should have come as no surprise when I refused, with my agency's support.

Furthermore, Siskind argues, "the therapist's best chance of safeguarding the continuity of treatment is to maintain the most rigorous professional stance, which includes the firm resolve to abstain from involvement in any divorce-related decisions" (p. 338). Since your primary responsibility is to the teen and not his/her parents, staying out of the mess caused by divorce strengthens the likelihood that the therapeutic relationship can continue and the teen will not be forced to endure yet another loss.

Once your role (and limits) is clear, you can encourage parents with decisions regarding what information and how much information to share with their teens about the divorce (Afifi, 2003; Afifi et al., 2007). Parents often ask me for help with this; they worry that they will share too much information or do so inappropriately. Some parents disclose information in emotionally charged or critical ways, transmitting their anxiety to the teen and/or putting the teen in a position where he/she feels responsible for the parent's well-being (Afifi, Hutchinson, & Krouse, 2006; Alexander, 2003; Lehman & Koerner, 2002; Wallerstein, 1985); more about parentification in the next section. Moreover, many parents experience arousal after they share something negative with their teen (Afifi et al., 2009). When consulting with parents, emphasize the importance of sharing at least some information with teens about the reasons for the divorce, answering questions about the parents' relationship now, and explaining what will happen next (Afifi & Schrodt, 2003). Remember that, like May's parents, many parents do not realize the effect that their comments have on their teens (Golish, 2003). Without your guidance, they may continue the maladaptive behavior.

Countertransference Issues

Intentionally or unintentionally, many parents tug at my heartstrings when they are in the midst of a divorce. Finances, time off work, moving, and custody battles are just a few of the issues that come with the dissolution of a marriage. There is also a redefinition of the parents' relationship from partners to coparents and a good deal of grief (Cole & Cole, 1999). I can empathize with parents' struggles to prioritize and juggle responsibilities while parenting effectively, and we *all* have stressors that affect multiple areas of our lives. None of us balance everything perfectly all the time. I might find myself wanting to extend leniency for lateness or missed appointments, for example. I may notice that parents are attempting to use me as their therapist as opposed to seeking their own treatment. I have to be extremely careful to maintain my boundaries and keep the focus of therapy on the teen when parents are experiencing significant life stressors. After all, the teen is experiencing grief too, along with whatever issues they are bringing to treatment.

Divorces, especially ugly ones, can also lead to your identification with one parent (Freedman et al., 1993). Whatever the reasoning for identifying with one parent over the other—it could literally be anything—once you do, you begin viewing that parent uncritically and compassionately while the other parent becomes the villain. Personality disordered parents may further complicate this issue. It can be hard to remember in the moment that divorces are complicated, and rarely are they fully one spouse's fault. These feelings are important to pay attention to; chances are that you are experiencing a struggle with allegiance similar to that of your adolescent client.

Finally, I try to remember that parents of divorcing families are greatly struggling to put aside their own feelings about the dissolution of the marriage to focus on their children's needs. This is likely to strain their empathic capacities and may, at any particular point in time, be more than either of them can reasonably handle. Although it may be obvious to you that the parents have to separate their opinions of each other as former partners from their opinions of each other as coparents, it is a complicated and overwhelming experience for many parents of your teen clients (Ehrenberg, Hunter, & Elterman, 1996).

The Parentified Teen

A final issue that Bradley's story highlights is parentification. Parentification is an interesting phenomenon that occurs when children recognize their parents' vulnerabilities and try to act in ways that either (1) causes the least trouble or (2) actively contributes to the well-being of the parent and family (Earley & Cushway, 2002; Peris, Goecke-Morey, Cummings, & Emery, 2008). Parentification can involve taking on instrumental tasks (e.g., household chores) or catering to the emotional needs of the family (e.g., being a peacekeeper, confidante, or decision-maker; Hooper, 2007), and it results in the roles of parent and child being flipped, with children assuming the role of caregiver (Byng-Hall, 2008; Rose & Cohen, 2010). Parentification, like so many other dynamics, operates on a continuum, with varying degrees of burdens and responsibilities placed on children, and some research has suggested that teens may learn resourcefulness and feel a sense of accomplishment (Mmari, Roche, Sudhinaraset, & Blum, 2009; Ungar, Theron, & Didkowsky, 2011), or that the parentification can be short-term in response to a family crisis (DiCaccavo, 2006). In other cases, however, teens feel overburdened by their responsibilities and the adult role they have taken on in the family (Mmari et al., 2009; Rose & Cohen, 2010) and view their parents as less close and warm than their parents themselves might report (Peris et al., 2008). These experiences are stable and associated with internalizing and externalizing adolescent problems (Peris et al., 2008).

Parentification can originate from parents who treat their teens as peers or who inappropriately seek support; it can also originate from children's efforts to comfort or relate to their parents (Peris et al., 2008). Regardless of who initiates the dynamic, however, parentified children come to worry about their parents incessantly, feel increased responsibility for their parents' well-being, and tend to bear the burden alone and in secret (Knutsson-Medin, Edlund, & Ramklint, 2007; Pölkki, Ervast, & Huupponen, 2004; Van Parys & Rober, 2013). Moreover, children become attuned to any behaviors that will provide clues regarding how their parents are doing at that moment. This dynamic has been observed among children of addicted (Kelley et al., 2007), depressed (Van Parys & Rober, 2013; Woolgar & Murray, 2010), divorced (Peris et al., 2008), and deployed (Harrison & Albanese, 2012) parents.

Parentification can occur at any age, but it is of particular concern for adolescents who are physically and psychologically more capable of taking on the responsibilities of caring for younger children, mediating conflict, completing chores around the house, and understanding their parents' stressors. One of my clients, whose mother struggled with substance abuse, was worried about her siblings after they were all placed in foster care. She told me, "I know they are just my brothers and sisters, but in some ways I feel like their mom. I made them dinner, took care of them, got them to bed at night. My mom made them, but I raised them."

Parentification in the Therapy Session

Much of the time, parents fail to notice that their teens have become parentified, and their viewpoint of the relationship may be very different from that of their teen (Peris et al., 2008). After all, if the teen steps in, there is nothing to alert parents to a problem; their needs are fulfilled. I do not mean this to villanize parents; instead, I mean it to demonstrate just how integral to the functioning of the family the teen's parentified role has become. However, there are a few parental "clues" to the possibility of parentification. Some examples include parents' descriptions of their parent–teen relationship as one upon which they can rely for advice, high expectations of the teen, difficulty allowing the teen to do age-appropriate activities that might interfere with family responsibilities, positive reinforcement for a teen taking over adult roles in the home, and references to the teen as "my good kid" or one who makes "herself invisible." One of my clients was denied a chance to play soccer for her high school because she needed to be home to retrieve her younger siblings from the bus stop. A recently divorced father also praised his daughter for "essentially keeping the house running smoothly."

When considering the types of parentification teens may be exposed to, Jurkovic, Morell, and Thirkield (1999) have developed profiles that encompass the roles assigned, levels of supportiveness, age appropriateness and extent of responsibilities, degree to which teens prioritize their parents' needs, and internalization of the caring role. Teens will describe feeling guilty when they are unable to meet their parents' needs, anxious about and overly responsible for their parents' well-being, and, often, being "the man (or woman) of the house," like Bradley. They may worry about "adult things" (e.g., the cost of sessions) or have difficulty acting their age in sessions. I have worked with teens who truly struggle to engage in play, expressive arts, or games. One preteen told me, after I asked her to draw a self-portrait, that she expected that we would be spending our time "more productively." As I got to know her better, I began to see many signs of parentification, including one disturbing interaction with her mother and two younger siblings in the waiting room. The younger siblings were being loud, and the mother was trying in vain to quiet them down. When we came out of my office to get the mother for a check-out, my client turned to her siblings and said, "Remember I told you that if you were good during my appointment, I would play a special game with you later," and promptly quieted them. Her mother, turning to me, declared, "She's so much better with them than I am."

Finally, parentified teens may be more likely than other clients to worry about you or defer to you in sessions, as they have become quite "adept at anticipating the needs of others as his or her primary way of relating" (DiCaccavo, 2006, p. 470). When I was pregnant, for example, a teen told me, "Just let me know if you need to stop because you are getting uncomfortable."

How to Handle It

In addition to any work you will do with the teen (see DiCaccavo, 2006, for suggestions), I would highly recommend discussing your concerns with the parents and, if they are open, guiding them toward some changes that will shift the caregiving back to the adults in the family. Simple ways to start this process might involve the parent reassuring the teen that he/she is okay, that it is the parent's job to take care of the house and siblings, and that he/she wants the teen to be a teen. Parents may need some support as they seek out appropriate outlets for their feelings (e.g., therapists, spiritual leaders, and adult friends). They may need help understanding why teens should not be referred to as heads of the household and/or assistance correcting others who refer to their teens in that way. For example, a simple response to someone's assertion that the teen is the "man (or woman) of the house" could be "He may be the oldest, but he is still a child. I have got it under control."

Countertransference Issues

There is a lot of convincing literature that warns counselors about the personal feelings and experiences that may be triggered by a parentified client. Commonly referred to as "wounded healers," some therapists do go into the helping profession to rework their own childhood hurts and disappointments.

In this way, they can care for themselves at a distance, through their clients, while also receiving validating feedback that may have been lacking from their own families (see DiCaccavo, 2002, for a review). In these cases, unresolved childhood issues can make it especially difficult to consider parents objectively or to refrain from permissiveness and gratification in the therapeutic relationship (Gabel & Bemporad, 1994). Regardless of whether you have a personal history of parentification, be aware of feeling overwhelmed by these vulnerable teens, falling into a caretaker role simply to alleviate your own anxiety, or shutting down to avoid the painful feelings that may be awakened (Byng-Hall, 2002; Lackie, 1999). Finally, be on the lookout for "rescue fantasies" in response to teens' ambivalence, disappointment, or grief over their real relationships with parents (Malawista, 2004).

On Attachment and Parenting Stress

Simply put, parents' stress spills over into parent–teen relationships. As parents' stress increases, they are less able to manage their own feelings and experiences, let alone those of their teens. Parents' supportiveness and availability—both physical and emotional—decreases (Almeida, Wethington, & Chandler, 1999; Nelson, O'Brien, Blankson, Calkins, & Keane, 2009; Repetti & Wood, 1997), and parents who do not usually value their teens' experiences may even further reduce their accessibility and responsiveness. Parents' stress, combined with decreased warmth and affection and negative views of teens' emotions, can lead teens to feel unstable and uncertain and seems to moderate the relationship between parental beliefs about teens' emotions and teens' attachment security (Stelter & Halberstadt, 2011).

The way in which parents manage stress and navigate their parent–teen relationships may be particularly important during highly stressful times, such as in the midst of a divorce. Parents who are just trying to get through their day and manage their own emotions related to the end of their marriage often have little left to offer their children. Teens are all too aware of this, and many will stop relying or going to their parents for support, even if the parent has never explicitly rejected them or significantly changed their caregiving. In addition, parental availability often literally changes as one parent moves out and often has less daily contact. Once secure attachments may become insecure as teens become avoidant to protect themselves from rejection and "keep the peace" at home by limiting conflict and demands (see Faber & Wittenborn, 2010, for a review). With parents, I try to normalize these possibilities without judgment so that they can actively work to maintain the secure attachment relationship by remaining available, warm, and consistent and, if needed, get into their own counseling so that they do not neglect their own needs during such a difficult time.

ALLEGATIONS OF CHILD PHYSICAL ABUSE[7]

I received a call one Monday afternoon from a school counselor about a client, Ella (fifteen). The school counselor had called Ella into her office because Ella was falling behind in her schoolwork, largely because she was not completing her homework. The counselor suggested that they call Ella's parents to discuss the issue and come up with a plan to ensure that homework was completed. Ella's parents were well known to the school; they were highly involved and had made numerous monetary donations throughout the year. Ella also had two younger sisters who attended the school.

At this point, Ella had burst into tears and begged the school counselor not to call her parents. She disclosed that, over the weekend, an argument between Ella and her father over incomplete chores had escalated into physical violence. Ella alleged that her father had pushed her to the ground and then grabbed her by the neck. She said that her father had been screaming at her the whole time and that she felt scared he would seriously hurt her. After she started crying, Ella's father had thrown her back down to the ground and left the room.

The school counselor was clearly upset by Ella's disclosure, and she asked me what I thought she should do. I suggested she let her administrator know so that they could follow protocol, but I also told her that, in my opinion, the allegations had to be reported to Child Protective Services (CPS). She balked but agreed, and I asked her to let me know once the report had been made. I also planned to follow up with Ella at our appointment later that week.

I received a call back from the school counselor a couple of hours later. She told me that after telling Ella that she was planning to report the allegations, Ella had recanted her story. She told the school counselor she just did not want to get in trouble and that she had "exaggerated" what happened with her father. The school counselor was calling to let me know that she no longer planned to make the report now that it was "clear that Ella had made the whole thing up to avoid getting in trouble."

Professionals' mandated reports make up a large percentage of substantiated abuse reports (67.3 percent in 2004; see US Department of Health and Human Services, A. o. C., Youth, and Families, 2006). Yet many, like Ella's school counselor, do not report the cases they encounter or inconsistently do so. Lack of obvious evidence, limited knowledge about abuse, views of mandated reports as confidentiality breaches, uncertainty about the correct way to file a report, and fear of adverse consequences are among the reasons cited for failing to fulfill mandatory reporting requirements (Flaherty et al., 2006; Levi, Brown, & Erb, 2006; Melton, 2005; Webster, O'Toole, O'Toole, & Lucal, 2005). Furthermore, many counselors experience conflict when they consider reporting alleged abusive behavior by parents with whom they have spent much time building a working alliance (Feng, Chen, Fetzer, Feng, & Lin, 2012).

This may even be truer for counselors who treat adolescents. Although studies suggest that adolescents experience similar, if not higher, rates of physical abuse, emotional abuse, and neglect than young and school-aged children, child protection agencies become involved far less often when teens are the victims (Finkelhor, Ormrod, Turner, & Hamby, 2005). Physical abuse and neglect allegations are also substantiated less when adolescents are the identified victims, possibly due to misconceptions that adolescents are more capable of caring for themselves than they actually are or that they are more deserving of physical punishment due to their oppositionality or breaking the rules (Powers & Eckenroade, 1988).

So what are the requirements for abuse reporting? No state mandates that a therapist be able to prove that abuse or neglect has occurred prior to making the report, so if you suspect abuse, you should make a report (Alvarez, Donohue, Kenny, Cavanagh, & Romero, 2005; Harper & Irvin, 1985). When a teen comes in with bruises or injuries, this decision is easy. I think most professionals would report those situations. It is the unclear cases, like Ella's, where there are no visible injuries, no *proof*, in which it can be hard to decide what to do. A supervisor once asked me, "Let's say you don't make the report. If you found out later that the abuse did happen, how would you feel?" I told her I thought I would feel like I should have reported it when I had the chance, and she told me, "Then you have your answer. You should report it." I have asked myself that question many times since, and if I am asking the question, I almost always end up making a report.

In the Therapy Session

Many times, hearing allegations against a parent will come as a shock (see textbox 6.1 for some risk factors), and telling a parent that his/her teen has made an abuse allegation against them can cause anxiety and distress. Nevertheless, it is an important and necessary part of the reporting process (Racusin & Felsman, 1986). At the very least, parents need to be informed of your decision to break their teen's confidentiality to file the report, but I have found that sharing the decision with parents before the report is made also serves a couple of other functions. I can explain my reasoning for the report, answer any questions about the report or process to come, encourage the parent to be a part of the reporting process, demonstrate respect by informing rather than blindsiding the parent, decrease the secrecy that may be allowing problematic behaviors to continue, assess parental anger and take any

Textbox 6.1 Parental Risk Factors for Physical Abuse

- High anger/hyperreactivity; difficulty considering alternative interpretations or solutions before responding
- High anxiety
- High psychopathology (e.g., depression, bipolar disorder, schizophrenia, and ASPD)
- High levels of personal stress
- Perception of the teen as a problem
- Inaccurate perceptions of the situation
- Poor empathy
- Alcohol and substance abuse
- Authoritarian and/or coercive parenting style
- More frequent use of physical aggression when disciplining
- Poor parent–teen relationship
- High family conflict
- Marital issues
- Low family cohesion
- Personal history of abuse and harsh discipline
- Poor attachment to own parents

See De Bellis et al. (2001); Haskett, Scott, Willoughby, Ahern, and Nears (2006); Mammen, Kolko, and Pilkonis (2003); Milner (2000); Rodriguez (2010, 2013); Schaeffer, Alexander, Bethke, and Kretz (2005); Rodriguez and Tucker (2011); Stith et al. (2009); and Walsh, MacMillan, and Jamieson (2002).

actions to defuse the situation and protect the teen. Although many therapists do worry that parents will abruptly terminate treatment or that clients will suffer worse abuse if their parents find out about their allegations, these worries are unfounded in the majority of cases (Alvarez, Kenny, Donohue, & Carpin, 2004; Harper & Irvin, 1985). Some parents and clients report feeling relief once a report has been made (Weinstein, Levine, Kogan, Harkavy-Friedman, & Miller, 2002). In fact, failing to share the information with parents can actually increase the teen's risk of physical harm (Racusin & Felsman, 1986).

I met with Ella the day after she made and recanted her story. I had already decided that I planned to make a report based on her initial statement to the school counselor, but I wanted to see what Ella would tell me about the argument with her father. Rather quickly, she admitted that the abusive incident had occurred as she had initially described it. She told me she had recanted because the school counselor looked "terrified" and like "she didn't know what to do next." Ella also told me that she was scared about what would happen if her parents found out she had told. I normalized all of these feelings and empathized with her fear after disclosing; however, I also reminded her of my duty to report. We talked about the anxiety she was feeling and what would happen next.

After our session, I called both her mother and father and let them know about Ella's allegations and my role as a mandated reporter. Both parents denied the argument and were, understandably, angry and scared. They both begged me not to make the report, promising to go to family therapy, a suggestion I had been making for many months. As with Ella, I empathized with their feelings but remained firm on my legal and ethical responsibility to report. I spent quite some time on the phone with them, discussing the reporting process and ensuring them that I was not firing Ella (or them) as clients. I gave them referrals for family therapy (again) and told them that I would be making the report as soon as we hung up the phone so that they knew when they might expect a call from CPS. In the weeks that followed, I remained available for the parents as they went through the investigation process and continued weekly therapy with Ella.

Guidelines for Informing Parents of Mandated Reporting

- *Highlight your care and concern* for the family as a whole. Draw on the relationships you have built with parents to express your desire to help everyone involved. I have never fired a client after learning of abuse, and parents are sometimes comforted by the fact that I do not view them as untreatable villains or terrible people. Feeling judged or bad about themselves is a common experience among parents who have abuse allegations made against them (Saint-Jacques, Drapeau, Lessard, & Beaudoin, 2006).
- *Remind parents of your legal and ethical responsibility* to report any allegations of abuse. As you covered the limitations of confidentiality with parents and teens in the beginning of treatment (and possibly throughout, depending on the issues that have arisen during therapy), this should not come as a surprise to parents. I often use this as a way to deflect parents' denials, blaming of teens, or insistence that they were simply using corporal punishment by reminding them that I am not accusing anyone of any wrongdoing, but merely following the reporting requirements of mental health professionals.
- *Explain the process of reporting.* I often use something like figure 6.2 to show parents that there are a number of steps that happen after a report is made, most of which do not include removal of the child from the home or criminal prosecution. Many parents (and sometimes therapists) have a negative view of CPS and do not realize that CPS's goal is to keep families intact, not tear them apart. Once a report is made, CPS accepts the report or does not. Reasons that they may not accept the referral include incomplete information or lack of details.[8] If the report is accepted, CPS begins an investigation typically involving interviews with the victim, alleged perpetrator, nonoffending parents, reporter (you), and witnesses. In cases

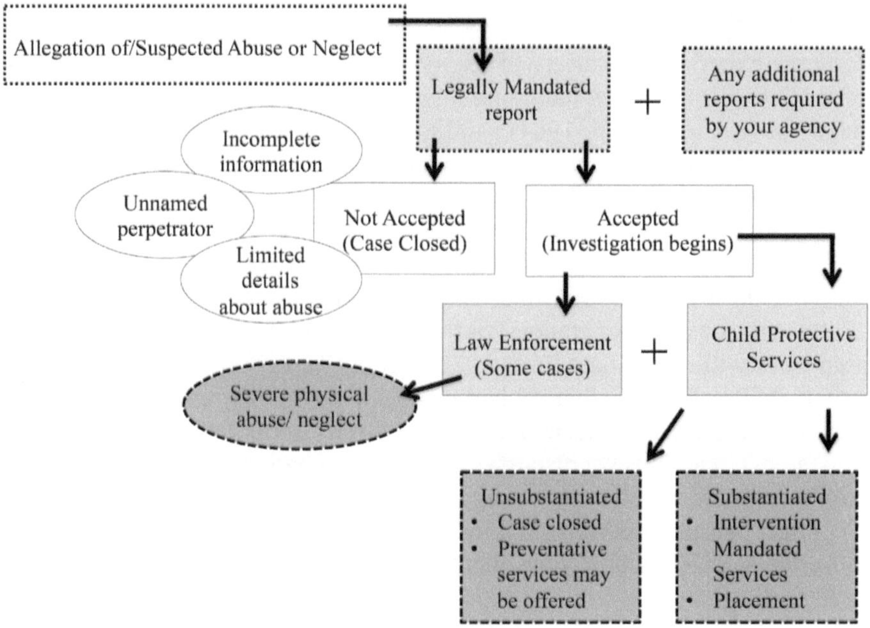

Figure 6.2 What Happens After a Mandated Report?

of severe physical abuse or neglect, a criminal investigation may also coincide with CPS's investigation. At the end of CPS's investigation, the report will be considered substantiated or unsubstantiated. In cases where it is unsubstantiated, the case is closed. Preventative services are sometimes offered and continued treatment is encouraged. In the case of substantiated reports, CPS will keep the case open in order to provide interventions, preventative services, and, in rare cases, placement services. Criminal charges may also result.[9]

- *Encourage the parent to be a part of the reporting process.* When parents agree to this, they demonstrate recognition of the problem, acknowledgment of the seriousness of the report, and ownership of their actions. Furthermore, parents may feel a little less powerless or helpless when they participate in making the report.
- *Demonstrate willingness to help* the teen and parent through the process. I think it is important that parents understand that once I have made the report, my obligation has ended, but the therapeutic work has just begun. In these situations, I try to help parents accept and tolerate their feelings of guilt (i.e., "I made a bad parenting decision") while working through feelings of shame (i.e., "I am a bad parent," or "I am a bad person"). Referrals to individual and family therapy may also be appropriate (more on this in chapter 8).

Countertransference Issues

You may experience a variety of reactions toward parents following allegations of abuse or neglect, including disgust, anger, sympathy, guilt, fear, and judgment (Krell & Okin, 1984). Additionally, many therapists feel anxious about the future of the treatment, overwhelmed, discouraged, depressed, punitive, or uncertain if they should have made the report (Krell & Okin, 1984; Pollak & Levy, 1989; Shuman, 2000). I know I have also experienced feelings of incompetence, particularly in cases where I have been working with families for a long time before learning about abuse. In my *head*, I know that I assess for trauma thoroughly and that I can only know what clients are willing to share with me, but in my *heart*, I often feel a sense of responsibility and think that if I had just been a better therapist, I might have been able to protect the teen and help the family sooner. All of the countertransference reactions we discussed early in the chapter can also factor in, as parents who are abusive may struggle with mental health issues and/or PD. It is important that you have a good support system, including supervisors, consultants, peers, and/or your own therapist to work through these complicated feelings.

On Attachment and Child Physical Abuse

Not surprisingly, physical abuse greatly affects attachment. Abused children must cope with frightening parenting behaviors and are more likely to develop negative views of their parents and themselves (Sternberg, Lamb, Guterman, Abbott, & Dawud-Noursi, 2005). Adolescents who have experienced physical abuse often experience ambivalence about their parents: on the one hand, they love their parents and rely on them for protection, but on the other, these parents are the ones who are making them feel unsafe. The literature on *betrayal trauma* is relevant here. Betrayal trauma occurs when someone relied on for survival significantly violates trust or well-being (Freyd, 2008). This theory suggests that teens are confused by abusive situations. Social norms dictate that they withdraw from someone who is hurting them, but in cases of physical abuse, it is not so easy. The abuser is also their caregiver and primary source for physical survival and emotional connection. This theory also suggests that in an effort to manage such opposing information between the "bad" and "good" parent, abused youth may try to disavow, ignore, or repress the abuse.

The theory and research on betrayal trauma coincides with attachment research findings that avoidant-insecure attachment is the most common type among physically abused children and adolescents. The theory of such findings has been well summarized by Finzi, Ram, Har-Even, Shnit, and Weizman (2001):

> For the abused child, the attachment figure is both a source of danger and the natural provider of protection … These children remain with the feeling of being unprotected and might beware of proximity which for them means being helpless and in danger … Confused by their contradictory feelings of love and hate, abused children might defensively exclude from the awareness the working model of the "bad" unloving parent and retain conscious access only to the loving model (the "good" parent) … In this case, the parents' violence evokes their rage, but they recoil from protest and cut off, repress, or falsify their anger to minimize the hurt … The avoidance could viewed as their way of suppressing the recognition and expression of their emotional vulnerability … and maintaining control over their own prospective reactions to their parents. (p. 779)

The good news is that these attachment relationships *can* be repaired. In their study of adolescents, Sternberg et al. (2005) found that abuse experienced five or six years earlier was not related to adolescents' current perceptions of their attachments with parents, even though more recent physical abuse was related to attachment with mothers. This suggests that teens' attachments with parents can improve, even after physical abuse allegations.

RECONSIDERING RESISTANT PARENTS

This chapter has focused on a range of parental variables that can be described as varied forms of *resistance* and which leave therapists inundated with countertransference feelings. If we were going to put teens' parents on a compliance–resistance continuum, there would be some parents who would fall at the compliant, "good parents" end. These parents are not barriers themselves; they have "done everything right" and still have a teen who will be on medication and in treatment for the rest of his or her life. These parents experience shame, grief, regret, and confusion. As one parent asked me, "Why me? Why us?" Andrew Solomon, in his *New York Times* bestseller, *Far from the Tree*, hits the nail on the head when he observes, "Parents whose kids do well take credit for it, and the obverse of self-congratulation is that parents whose kids do badly must have erred" (2012, p. 537). On the other end of the continuum, of course, are the parents who are destructive, uncooperative, and hostile, many of whom we have discussed throughout this chapter. They epitomize resistance. But even these parents, those who get most things wrong, manage to do a few things right (Robinson, 1990). The majority of parents fall somewhere in the middle, displaying varying degrees and forms of resistance.

Some therapists fall into the trap of assuming that any behavior that is not 100 percent compliant with their treatment approach should be framed as resistance. This can be especially true in dealings with parents; after all, why would they bring you their teen if they did not want to listen to your thoughts on the issues? They must be resistant to your approach, your style, or your interpretation of their family. Childress (1992) reflects,

> We overvalue the strength of the parent, crediting him or her with the power to cause psychopathology, and get angry at them for not parenting right … we may feel that they are using their black magic to interfere with our own potential to be omnipotent reflects curers ourselves. (p. 31)

When I first started working with adolescents, I found myself frustrated with the parents I encountered. Over time, however, I have come to expect resistance and view it less negatively, a sign that something is wrong. After all, do I really want my clients and their parents to agree blindly with everything I say? Do I really expect that my clients and their parents can make changes easily? Change is *hard*; if it were easy, parents would have made changes without ever including a therapist in the mix! A colleague once told me, "If your client is mad at you, you are probably doing something right." In that vein, I have begun to reframe resistance as a sign that change is occurring and to normalize it as a natural, sometimes facilitative, reaction to feeling a loss of control or predictability.

Additionally, VanFleet (2004) suggests that resistance is not an all-or-nothing phenomenon. In considering daily experiences, she proposes that compliance and resistance do, in fact, coexist much of the time. Here is an example from my own life: I would like to increase the amount of time I spend exercising; this is a long-term goal. Currently, I get to the gym approximately twice a week. Daycare schedules, work deadlines, family obligations, and succumbing to my comfortable bed in the morning result in resistance. It would be unfair, though, to overlook any of the progress I have made toward my goal, or to assume that my lack of fully achieving the goal is just because I do not want to change. Furthermore, anyone invested in helping me achieve my goal would first have to understand the reasons that exercise is pushed down on my priority list at times, recognize the limitations inherent in my schedule, and support me as I try to make this change. This, too, is our role as we help parents and families make changes.

The Role of Anger

It is so easy to dismiss angry, seemingly irrational parents as *resistant* when they enter our therapy offices, but the reality is that anger corresponds with many other emotions, such as shame and fear, and influences perceptions of condescension and criticism (Lobbestael, Arntz, & Wiers, 2008; Margolis, 1991; R. Schwartz, 2000). The angry parent who wants you to "fix things" but is unwilling to try any of your suggestions may be experiencing fear and helplessness. Research has also demonstrated that anger-invoking situations involving personal contact—like therapy—are more likely to prompt heightened physiological anger responses than those involving nonpersonal contact (Lobbestael et al., 2008). The parent sitting in your office may feel intruded upon or even threatened as you outline your concerns.

Angry parents often have inaccurate views of power in the therapy room. Although it can be argued that there is a power differential any time a person seeks out professional help, some parents have unrealistically high expectations of your power to make changes in their family. Simultaneously, they may have low estimates of their own power, leading to feelings of helplessness, shame, and even anger.

Finally, parents, like everyone, engage in dysfunctional thought patterns that distort situations. These may incorrectly lead to assumptions about your thoughts, feelings, or motivations. The mother who interprets my concerns about her son's behavior in class as a reflection on her failures as a parent may demonstrate anger that is confusing to me. It is important to remember that, in general, we do not engage in behaviors that do not make sense. Parents' angry behavior is, from their perspective, purposeful, rational, and justified (Margolis, 1991, p. 332).

Managing Resistance

One of the most effective ways that I have found to manage and diffuse situations in which parents appear angry and/or resistant is through *perception checking*. Perception checking includes describing your own perceptions of the parents' feelings, asking whether or not the perception is accurate, and managing your own feelings of judgment (Johnson, 1990). This might be as simple asking a mother of a suicidal teen, "I know that this is a lot of information to take in at once. It seems like you are maybe feeling some anger. What do you think? Is that how you would describe it?" If she says yes, I can take the opportunity to normalize the feelings and explore what she thinks is driving the anger. If she says no, I can explain my reasons for thinking she was angry and explore the feelings in the way she would describe them.

I also utilize aspects of *motivational interviewing* (MI). MI is conducted in such a way that parents are able to (1) identify their strengths, which will facilitate their teen's treatment and (2) take ownership of their difficulties, the variables that may act as barriers (Horwath & Morrison, 2010). This can be something that is done with teens in the room or during a separate, parents-only session. Facilitators and barriers can be psychological, material, environmental, or individual, and some parents are not aware of the useful skills they possess or the hurdles they are placing on the treatment track. The MI literature recommends a number of strategies to help parents with this process, including asking evocative questions (e.g., "What needs to change?"), encouraging parents to elaborate or give examples (e.g., "Tell me about a good day you had with Tommy recently"), exploring the costs and benefits of change (e.g., "What makes you want to see this change through?" "What makes you want to keep things as they are?"), and considering the future with this change (e.g., "How will things be different if this changes?"). Parents can also identify how ready they feel to engage in the steps necessary for change (e.g., use a 1–10 scale) while also rating the degree of resistance or internal struggle they feel (Iannos & Antcliff, 2013).

CONCLUSION

We have taken quite a journey in this chapter, through personality disorders, parenting styles, mental health issues, life stressors, and child physical abuse. Just as this chapter may have felt a little overwhelming at times, so, too, can be the experience of working with parents struggling with any of these issues. In many cases, you will be working with parents struggling with *several* of these issues, so early identification, when possible, is key. Keep a close eye on your countertransference in these situations, particularly when you feel tempted to oversimplify a parent as "resistant." Supervision, consultation, and personal awareness are key strategies for keeping feelings and reactions in check and getting the ball successfully in the mental health "end zone."

NOTES

1. Much of the research on Cluster C parents will be encompassed in the section on anxiety below.
2. Much of the research on BPD in parents has involved mothers.
3. I would recommend documenting any of the issues we are talking about with PD parents, in fact.
4. Because this approach puts the parent somewhat in control, I frequently use it when I am dealing with PD parents.
5. A big thank you to my RA, Lauren Gregory, who assisted me in writing this section.

6. One concern raised by Jason's mom: "What if he trips and falls off the deck where the party is, and everyone laughs, and he cannot deal with everyone laughing, so he starts hitting people?"

7. Allegations of childhood sexual abuse (CSA) will be discussed in chapter 7, and the presence of psychological abuse will discussed in chapter 8.

8. Approximately one-third of reports are not accepted for further investigation (US Department of Health and Human Services, 2003).

9. In 2003, approximately 27 percent of reports were substantiated following investigation (US Department of Health and Human Services).

Chapter Seven

When the World Implodes

Nonoffending Parents and Adolescent Trauma

"It's like my absolute worst nightmare has come true." When I was a freshman in college, I had the great fortune to land in a class taught by one of the most skilled trauma therapists in the field today. Amazingly, she saw something in me during that introductory course and offered me a small research assistant position. In offering me this position, she gave me access to a world that I knew very little about but would soon become entranced by: trauma. Eleven years later, we continue to do research together, and I consider her one of my closest colleagues and dearest friends. She taught me so much of what has made me the trauma therapist I am today. What she did not teach me, I have learned from my clients and the parents sitting right beside them, as they live through their worst nightmares before my eyes.

From the time I started conjuring up this book idea, I knew I wanted to focus an entire chapter on working with nonoffending parents of traumatized adolescents. Working with these parents is difficult, yet rewarding, and over time I have realized that I have a real passion for helping these secondary victims of trauma. Now that I am a parent myself, I feel even more drawn to them, men and women whose worlds have just imploded because of the harm others have intentionally inflicted upon their children. What I have heard, however, from the parents who come to see me, and in discussions with colleagues, is that not every therapist knows how to handle this delicate population. Parents' experiences may be minimized by professionals or the parents themselves in a misguided effort to meet the needs of the traumatized teen (Myrick & Green, 2013). There is no way to adequately address each of the unique trauma populations that exist, so I have chosen two that I encounter often in my work as a trauma therapist: parents of sexually abused teens and those affected by school violence. My hope is that, by the end of this chapter, you will have a clear idea of what these nonoffending parents go through, how their reactions impact their teens, how to support them as they witness their teen's journey through trauma treatment, and how to manage the feelings that trauma will inevitably bring up for you.[1]

NONOFFENDING PARENTS' REACTIONS TO SEXUAL ABUSE[2]

Like their teens, nonoffending parents range in their responses to trauma and may present with psychosocial difficulties (Tavkar & Hansen, 2011). These reactions typically include affect and cognitions directed toward the self, the child, and the offender. Additionally, parents may have complex thoughts and feelings related to the judicial system (Turner et al., 2012).

Parents' Feelings about Themselves

Nonoffending parents of child abuse survivors report significant emotional distress as well as post-traumatic and grief symptomatology (Elliott & Carnes, 2001; Manion et al., 1996) for an average of two years beyond disclosure (Stauffer & Deblinger, 1996). The most commonly reported feeling toward oneself is guilt. In other cases, parents may report deep shame (Kilroy, Egan, Maliszewska, & Sarma, 2014). To help you differentiate between guilt and shame, remember that guilt arises from actions (i.e., "I misjudged her safety") and shame results from feelings of being damaged or unworthy (i.e., "I am a bad parent"). When dealing with both guilt and shame, you may see parents holding themselves to unrealistic standards, believing they "should have known" that the perpetrator was dangerous. One parent shared that his daughter's new boyfriend failed to shake the parent's hand when they first met. The parent believed that this perceived lack of respect should have "tipped [him] off" that the boyfriend was "no good."

Following trauma, parents may have difficulty managing daily situations, further reinforcing guilt reactions. A qualitative study that examined effects of child abuse on nonoffending parents (McCourt & Peel, 1998) found that learning of the trauma affected parents' health, finances, housing, career, and marital relationships. Accruing debt after moving away from an abusive person, giving up jobs that limited parental monitoring, and impaired communication between spouses are among the stressors mentioned by parents (Kilroy et al., 2014; McCourt & Peel, 1998) and those that I frequently hear from parents. One father told me that he judged himself for even "wasting session time" mentioning these stressors. Reactions from others can also play a role in parents' guilt (Heflin, Deblinger, & Fisher, 2000; Regehr, 1990). Parents in McCourt and Peel's (1998) study reported that, in some cases, initially supportive individuals became critical over time, blaming either the parent or the child, and became frustrated when parents failed to return to previous levels of functioning quickly.

Alternatively, denial may occur in the wake of abuse disclosures (Manion et al., 1996). Parents may deny that the abuse happened or, as noted in incest literature, fail to take any responsibility for family dysfunction that may have contributed to abuse (DelPo & Koontz, 1991). In both scenarios, denial serves as an unconscious defense mechanism, aimed at protecting the parent from the overwhelming feelings associated with the teen's trauma. Refusal to participate in treatment also falls under this category. McCourt and Peel (1998) found that it was particularly difficult for protective males in traumatized children's lives to engage in treatment. Little exists in the literature for assisting these nonoffending fathers with treatment, largely because many opt not to partake in treatment or related research (Grosz, Kempe, & Kelly, 2000). More about denial and ambivalence below.

Parents' Feelings about Teen Victims

Parents experience a wide range of feelings toward traumatized youth, one of which is often anger. With younger children, parents are usually aware that their anger at the child for failing to prevent the abuse or tell them about it is inappropriate. Perhaps more challenging for parents, however, are the feelings of anger directed at teenagers, particularly when the breaking of a rule precipitated the abuse. Carolyn, the mother of a female high school student who was raped at an after-prom party, told her daughter, "I told you that you were too young to go to an after-prom sleepover." Research on blame attribution has found that individuals, especially males, are more likely to blame sexual abuse victims who do not physically resist an assault (Rogers, Davies, & Cottam, 2010). Parents may also wonder whether their adolescent consented to the sexual activity (Regehr, 1990) or experience a decrease in trust in the parent–teen relationship (Davies, 1995). We will talk more about blame below.

Finally, parents often experience anxiety, particularly surrounding fears that their teen will be permanently and psychologically changed. This is particularly true when teens demonstrate unfamiliar and sometimes frightening post-traumatic behaviors (Cohen, 2009). Lena was distraught to learn that her daughter had been engaging in sexualized conversations with strangers online. She wondered if her daughter would be able to move forward from her trauma and "see value in herself for things other than sex." These attributional fears may also mirror those of their teens; interpersonally traumatized youth often report that they feel different from their psychologically adjusted and nontraumatized peers (Mannarino, Cohen, & Berman, 1994), or they fear that they are beyond help and damaged (Meiser-Stedman et al., 2009).

Parents' Cognitions and Affect Regarding Offenders

Many parents feel malice toward the perpetrator that disrupted and adversely affected their teen's lives. Particularly in situations where the perpetrator was a trusted friend, partner, or other family member, parents feel betrayed and unable to trust their own judgment or relationships (Grosz et al., 2000). Five months after being sexually molested by a friend's father, one client reported that his mother, Jill, was unsupportive of his new friendships. Jill admitted that she had fears related to her son visiting a friend's house. She was also apprehensive of becoming involved at her son's school again, scared that she would misread another parent. Jill's anxieties over allowing her child to encounter positive life experiences, coupled with lack of interest in or avoidance of social activities, are typical affective reactions shared by many nonoffending parents (McCourt & Peel, 1998).

Parents of traumatized children also report fears about seeing the perpetrator again (Kilroy et al., 2014; McCourt & Peel, 1998). The notion that most perpetrators are known to their victims intensifies this fear for many parents and can result in parents' increased social withdrawal (Brestan & Payne, 2004). Gutner, Rizvi, Monson, and Resick (2006) found that social withdrawal was elevated in both primary and secondary victims who knew their perpetrator. Finally, parents may again struggle with guilt, as they realize that their children's disclosure has disrupted another family as well as their own. Jill stated, "No one wins here," when discussing the perpetrator's family and the impact of the upcoming trial on them.

Parents' Appraisal of "the System"

The same feelings that parents experience toward the perpetrator can be directed toward the multiple systems involved in a child abuse case, including police, court, social services, and treatment facilities. Immediately after a disclosure, parents are faced with the decision of whether to report the trauma. Although to some this may seem like an obvious decision, parents sometimes struggle with fears of retraumatizing their teen, reporting the crime only to have the perpetrator left uncharged or found not guilty, or being blamed by reporting agencies (Regehr, 1990). Andy described intense feelings of rage directed toward a police officer who suggested Andy's sexually assaulted daughter had been "unclear" about her intentions on a first date with her alleged perpetrator. Another mother–father dyad regretted their decision to follow through with charges after their daughter's perpetrator pleaded his case down from a felony to a misdemeanor, effectively denying their daughter the right to face her abuser.

When parents file charges with the police regarding sexual trauma, other child-protection departments and social service agencies become involved. Child Advocacy Centers, one such child-based social service organization, will often conduct forensic interviews with both the child and parents, followed by referrals for mental health treatment. Social Services Agencies (SSA) that receive and make decisions based on allegations of child abuse are also a frequent target of anger and frustration in the wake of a trauma. SSA can make any number of decisions in the interest of children at risk, with the most extreme being removal from the home. Their involvement can become a stressor for parents, particularly if the parent perceives the SSA workers as uncaring, meddlesome, or accusatory (DelPo & Koontz, 1991).

Although all of these systems are necessary parts of the legal process and designed to be helpful to the family from a judicial standpoint, many parents report that SSA's involvement is intrusive or even psychologically harmful (Manion et al., 1996). Indeed, the legal system, by its very design, is not always the most supportive of rights for victims of sexual trauma. As Judith Herman (2003) points out,

> The U.S. legal system is organized as an adversarial contest … Physical violence and intimidation are not allowed in court, whereas aggressive argument, selective presentation of the facts, and psychological attack are permitted, with the presumption that this ritualized, hostile encounter offers the best method of arriving at the truth. Constitutional limits on this form of conflict are designed to protect criminal defendants from the superior power of the state, but not to protect individual citizens from one another … The Constitution, therefore, offers strong guarantees for the rights of the accused, but no corresponding protection for the rights of crime victims. (p. 159)

Indeed, *many* of the parents and teens I have worked with report feeling attacked or retraumatized in some way during the course of court proceedings, although few ultimately regret their decision to report the trauma. One state attorney with whom I have worked on several cases told me he rarely puts a nonoffending parent on the stand, for fear of the way in which the defense might manipulate his/her testimony. Following her testimony, a parent remarked, "I was treated like a criminal [up there on the stand] … I realize [the defense attorney] was just doing his job, but I wonder how he sleeps at night, twisting around innocent people's words."

Despite all of the possible risks inherent in including SSA agencies, it is important to note that parents who do feel supported by SSA workers view this help as a valuable form of social support during the investigative process (McCourt & Peel, 1998). Other systems that can offer such assistance may include support groups, victim advocates, treatment providers, and/or school staff and personnel.

Parental Ambivalence

It may surprise, confuse, or anger you to learn that some parents struggle to consistently believe that their teen has been sexually abused and/or to respond congruently. Within the past six months, a mother, after weeks of therapy and interviews at the local child advocacy center following her teen son's allegations against a baseball coach, asked me, "Tell me the truth. Did this *really* happen?" Earlier in my training, this question would have angered me or made me feel protective of her son. Now, however, I can better understand her ambivalence. After all, admitting that her son's abuse really happened would force her to confront painful material that her ambivalence was enabling her to keep at bay.

Along these same lines, some research has suggested that ambivalence post disclosure is a normal phenomenon, resulting from the chaos that impacts life after trauma is revealed (Hooper & Humphreys, 1998), particularly when the costs of disclosure—financial, housing, relocation, social services involvement, and social support—are high (Bolen & Lamb, 2004). Hobfoll, Freedy, Green, and Solomon (1996) theorize that learning of a teen's trauma often (1) comes without warning, (2) attacks parents' beliefs that the world is safe, predictable, and just, (3) makes excessive demands, (4) inflicts painful trauma-related images and thoughts upon the parent, and (5) provides new terrain upon which parents have never needed resources to survive. In other words, the disclosure threatens resources and demands almost *constant* use of parents' coping skills, which in turn depletes adaptive coping and activates less effective skills. Once less effective coping skills are being used (e.g., missing work, isolating oneself, failing to show for case-related appointments), resources may become more difficult to obtain, leading to more stress and even less effective coping. In other words, parents may become ambivalent about their teen's disclosure as they (consciously or unconsciously) tally up the emotional costs and compare it against their coping abilities.

A parent may further struggle with ambivalence when the perpetrator is his/her partner, a primary provider of social support and, possibly, resources. Research has found that parents with an ambivalent attachment pattern seek out intense relationships; these parents experience great distress when their emotionally volatile relationships end. A teen's allegation of abuse against a parent's partner threatens the parent's relationship, one that he/she greatly fears losing (Bolen & Lamb, 2004). One mother told me, "I know I should hate him, and part of me does. But another part of me loves him and can't believe that he would do this to my daughter. How am I going to go on without him? He was my world. We loved each other so much."

Finally, some parents experience both the teen's trauma *and* his/her disclosure as traumatic (Landolt, Vollrath, Ribi, Gnehm, & Sennhauser, 2003), and subsequent ambivalence is reflective of avoidance features prominent in PTSD. I have had many parents tell me about intrusive thoughts and experiences related to the moment when they learned of the abuse. This, in some ways, was *their* trauma, and some avoid in an effort to cope. A father avoided his basement for months because, as he told me, "Everything down there reminds me of the night I learned that my little girl had been raped. I almost feel like, if I just don't go down there, maybe I dreamed the whole thing."

PARENTAL MENTAL HEALTH FACTORS FOLLOWING ADOLESCENT SEXUAL ABUSE

Nonoffending parents often report feeling alone in their experience (Deblinger, Hathaway, Lippmann, & Steer, 1993), and, not surprisingly, many report high rates of depression and overall distress, particularly when compared to parents whose children have not been sexually abused (Lipton, 1997; Mannarino, Cohen, Deblinger, & Steer, 2007; Santa-Sosa, Steer, Deblinger, & Runyon, 2013). Anxiety is also common, with many parents reporting a decreased sense of safety or a feeling of dread (Kilroy et al., 2014). Symptoms are often highest when the perpetrator is the parent's significant other (Deblinger et al., 1993; Mannarino et al., 2007). Studies estimate that between 25 and 50 percent of nonoffending parents display depressive symptoms (Mannarino et al., 2007; Santa-Sosa et al., 2013), and as many as 42 percent of parents meet the criteria for PTSD after their children's disclosures (Salloum, Stover, Swaidan, & Storch, 2015). These symptoms sometimes persist for years after the disclosure (Kelley, 1990).

Parents may be particularly susceptible to their teen's trauma when they themselves have experienced sexual abuse. Nonoffending parents with their own trauma histories are not uncommon; studies often find that mothers of sexually abused children were more likely to have been sexually abused than mothers of nonabused children (Oates, Tebbutt, Swanston, Lynch, & O'Toole, 1998). Such parents may be easily triggered by their teen's sexual trauma and likely to experience guilt for failing to protect their teens or worry even more about the negative impact sexual abuse will have on their teens (Kilroy et al., 2014; Oates et al., 1998). Parents' sexual abuse history can also impact parenting, particularly in the wake of their teen's trauma. Abused parents have more negative views of themselves as parents (Banyard, 1997), experience high levels of parenting stress (Ammerman et al., 2013; Cole, Woolger, Power, & Smith, 1992; Salloum et al., 2015), use less effective parenting strategies that involve overly punitive and/or permissive approaches (Ruscio, 2001), and provide less structure for their teens (Kim, Trickett, & Putnam, 2010).

Mental health and past trauma further complicate the already-complex reactions that nonoffending parents have after their teen's disclosure. When working with traumatized teens and their families, it is vital to understand the way in which parents' symptoms and experiences affect their emotional reactions. To determine what parents might need most—and when it might be time to make a referral for parents' individual therapy—Cyr, McDuff, and Hebert (2013) identified four profiles of nonoffending parents: resilient, avoidant coping, traumatized, and anger oriented (see table 7.1 for summary). These profiles highlight the heterogeneity of parents and suggest that trauma details and whether parents believe and protect their teens are only a couple of pieces of the puzzle. These profiles are a great starting point whenever you encounter a family recently rocked by a trauma disclosure.

Supporting Nonoffending Parents After Sexual Trauma

Parents are not only secondary victims of their children's traumas but also vitally important to their children's post-traumatic adjustment and recovery as their greatest potential "natural resource" (Heflin et al., 2000, p. 170). Parents report that they generally benefit from having a therapist available to listen objectively and without blame (McCourt & Peel, 1998). They may need support and assistance from you throughout specific post-traumatic stages, such as immediately after disclosure, throughout the reporting and investigation process, during their children's treatments, and, depending on the case, for the duration of any court proceedings. Essentially, your goal is to reduce parents' traumatization so that they can be emotionally, mentally, and physically prepared to address the needs of their teens (Corcoran, 2004).

1. Educate parents about trauma-related symptoms

Adolescents cope with trauma a little differently from both younger children and adults. In addition to psychophysiological changes experienced by many traumatized youth—increased heart rate, dysregulated hormones, cortisol levels, and startle reflexes[3]—teens often engage in avoidant symptoms—wishful thinking, detachment from others and memories of the trauma—and tension-reducing behaviors such as substance use, self-injury, and high-risk sexual encounters (Johnson & Kenkel, 1991). Depressive and anxious symptoms may also present themselves alongside trauma-specific behaviors; this is particularly true after sexual trauma (Kilpatrick et al., 2003). If parents can understand this, they can reconceptualize some of what they are seeing as trauma reactions rather than attempts at manipulation or attention-seeking. One parent, nearing his wits' end with his traumatized son, told me, "It's like he doesn't think we've been through enough this past year. Doesn't he get that every time he gets caught smoking pot, it just adds more stress to our

Table 7.1 Nonoffending Parent Profiles

Group	*Percentage of Sample*	*Belief of Child*	*Support of Child*	*Anger*	*Mental Health Symptoms*	*Life Stressors*	*Treatment Needs*
Resilient	32.7	Consistent	High general and trauma-specific emotional support	Lowest amount of anger toward perpetrator	Low	Low	Short-term educational approach
Avoidant Coping	32.7	10 percent did not believe child 16 percent did not protect from perpetrator 20 percent of children experienced physical violence during the abuse	Emotional support weak or absent		Moderate level of PTSD symptoms (e.g., avoidance)		Interventions designed to alleviate maternal symptoms, teach efficient coping strategies, and increase support of child
Traumatized	19.1		Adequate		May qualify for complex PTSD diagnosis	High	Interventions designed to help with current stressors as well as past trauma
Anger-Oriented	15.5	Consistent	Emotional support weak or absent	Highest amount of anger toward child			Interventions designed to modify parenting practices and foster a loving relationship with child

Source: Adapted from Cyr et al. (2013).

family? His [sexual assault] has caused enough of a strain on all of us." What this parent did not understand was that his son's marijuana use was an attempt to forget about the trauma and just "relax for a change."

Providing parents with information about the continuum upon which traumatized adolescents experience post-traumatic symptoms is often helpful. Many parents will already be familiar with the severe end—affective dysregulation, behavioral concerns, and self-esteem issues—and some of your teen clients will be exhibiting concerning behaviors.[4] However, despite the realities of suicide, depression, and high-risk behaviors after sexual trauma (Brown, Cohen, Johnson, & Smailes, 1999; Fergusson, Horwood, & Lynskey, 1996), negative assumptions are commonly made about sexually abused youth, sometimes by mental health professionals (Holm, Holguin, & Hansen, 2002, in Kouyoumdjian et al., 2009). Individuals often erroneously believe that sexual abuse unequivocally results in severe and chronic emotional, behavioral, and academic problems (see Kendall-Tackett, Williams, & Finkelhor, 1993, for a review), but the reality is that many traumatized teens do not develop PTSD. A recent meta-analysis found that only 16 percent of all traumatized youth develop PTSD; this percentage increases to 25 percent when only interpersonal traumas, such as sexual abuse, are considered (Alisic et al., 2014). Rates are even lower in samples of adolescents (without younger children): 6.3 percent in females and 3.7 percent in males (Kilpatrick et al., 2003). The higher rate of PTSD in females is due in part due to their greater exposure to sexual abuse, their stronger self-blame, or their more frequent experience of dissociation (Freyd, 1996; Janoff-Bulman, 1992; Tolin & Foa, 2006).

Interestingly, parents' expectations of the impact of sexual trauma on their teens are directly related to how their teens actually do in the months after their trauma disclosure (Kouyoumdjian et al., 2009); this may be especially true in cases where parents have their own sexual abuse history or PTSD (Ghesquiere et al., 2008). Depending on the strength and intensity of parents' negative expectancies, you may need to help parents develop awareness of their biases (Kouyoumdjian et al., 2009; Saathoff-Wells, Culp, & Yancey, 2005) and behaviors. As I have mentioned repeatedly throughout this book, do not be afraid to use the literature in these situations. Share findings that demonstrate that many traumatized youth show minimal (if any) post-traumatic symptoms, and more than half of symptomatic youth experience improvement or resolution of their symptoms twelve to eighteen months post-trauma (Kendall-Tackett et al., 1993). Ask parents about pretrauma functioning to help them differentiate between trauma reactions and possible preexisting mental health concerns or stressors.

2. Involve parents in trauma-focused treatment

The way in which you address sexual trauma in adolescents' therapy will depend on your theoretical orientation and treatment goals. Although there is no single "gold standard" treatment approach for adolescents affected by sexual trauma, trauma-focused psychotherapies are considered the minimal standard for treatment of youth with PTSD symptoms (American Academy of Child and Adolescent Psychiatry, 2010). Trauma-focused cognitive behavioral therapy (TF-CBT) has received the most empirical support and infuses *psychoeducation, relaxation skills, affective modulation skills, cognitive coping, exposures*, and *planning for future safety* with *parenting skills* (Cohen, Deblinger, Mannarino, & Steer, 2004). A stage-based approach to treating complex trauma[5] may also be appropriate, as it comprises many of the same skills as TF-CBT within a less structured, psychodynamic frame (Cohen, Mannarino, Kliethermes, & Murray, 2012). In the first stage, *safety and stabilization*, treatment goals are centered on symptom management, skill building, and the development of a strong therapeutic alliance. Teens may also start to recognize and discuss the role of trauma in high-risk and self-destructive behaviors. The second stage, *trauma processing*, involves processing traumatic memories through the development of a coherent trauma narrative, exploring distorted thinking patterns, and confronting avoided emotional experiences. In the third and final stage, teens *reconnect* with aspects of themselves, develop healthy interpersonal relationships, and identify goals for their future selves (Courtois & Ford, 2009; Herman, 1992).

Addressing the trauma head on is especially important when working with sexually traumatized adolescents who, as we just discussed, tend to utilize avoidance as a coping mechanism. Nevertheless, parents may have questions or concerns about a treatment that deals with sexual trauma so directly. It may be scary for them to think of their teen sharing the intimate details of his/her sexual trauma and using words like "rape" or "sexual abuse." When working with adolescent sexual trauma, I address these concerns directly, explain my rationale for a trauma-focused treatment, and encourage active parent participation from the very beginning.[6] The importance of careful pacing and timing to ensure that no teen is pushed too hard, too fast, and the prioritization of safety in the therapeutic relationship are *always* discussed, sometimes repeatedly throughout the course of treatment. Sometimes I explain the importance of using anatomically correct terms and trauma terminology (i.e., "rape" or "sexual abuse" versus "what happened") to decrease shame and begin desensitization to triggering words.

As the teen nears the second stage and prepares to tell his/her story, parents and I discuss the process openly, including possible responses before and after sessions and warning signs of destabilization. I proactively introduce the possibility that, as the trauma narrative is unfolding, parents or teens may not want to come back, and I normalize the feelings while also stressing the importance of continuing consistent treatment. Before teens share their narratives with parents—this is a component of the TF-CBT protocol (Cohen et al., 2004; Cohen, Mannarino, & Deblinger, 2006)—I share portions of the narrative with parents, without the teen present. In this session, parents can openly share their reactions, ask questions, and feel sadness and anger without fear of the way it will affect their teen.

Parents can be included in (or met separately for) safety planning as treatment enters its final stage. Galloway and Hogg (2008) stress the importance of establishing parents' commitment to their teen's protection. They caution,

> Our experience of working with non-abusing parents is that it is often difficult for parents initially to devise strategies for protection. This appears to be because it requires them to reflect on areas that they have previously not had to consider, or have taken for granted. (p. 234)

I have had similar experiences wherein parents tell me vaguely, "I'll never let anything like that happen again," but cannot give me any specific ideas as to how they will ensure safety. Crassati (2004) suggests that parental history of sexual trauma, history of poor parental relationships, patterns of abusive relationships, and mental health difficulties may interfere with parents' best intentions of protecting their teen (as cited in Galloway & Hogg, 2008).

3. Address the issue of blame

When you encounter a teen who has experienced sexual trauma, be prepared to address the issue of blame with parents. Research suggests that parental support factors into adolescents' recovery from trauma, even more so than the characteristics of the abuse, such as frequency or duration (Johnson & Kenkel, 1991). Unfortunately, adolescents are more at risk for having unsupportive parents than other traumatized youth, possibly because parents think their teen should have "known better" or because the parent views the teen as a willing participant. This dynamic plays out in court proceedings as well: younger children are often viewed as more credible witnesses (Rogers, Josey, & Davies, 2007; Tabak & Klettke, 2014), with teens regarded as adult rape victims who could have resisted and are more capable of lying (Klettke & Simonis, 2011). Michelle was sexually abused by her mother's live-in boyfriend for nearly a year. When her mother found out, her first reaction was to accuse her boyfriend of having an affair. To correspond with this accusation, she referred to Michelle, twelve at the time, as being a "mistress." Sadly, others have reported similar experiences with traumatized adolescents (Heriot, 1996).

Research has examined the role of victim resistance in blame attribution and found that, in general, victims who do not fight back or resist their perpetrator are blamed more often than those who resist (Davies, Rogers, & Bates, 2008). Countless times, parents have asked me why their teen did not fight back, scream, or call for help. This can be a *major* issue when teen boys report sexual trauma, especially if the boy is perceived as physically capable of fending off an attacker (Davies et al., 2008; Davies, Rogers, & Whitelegg, 2009). Although I am by no means a biologist, I have had to familiarize myself with the physiology behind stress responses to help parents understand why some victims fight back and other do not. Many people have a very basic working knowledge of the *fight or flight response* that individuals engage in during a threatening situation. However, fewer people know about a third possible response, known as the *freeze response.* In these cases, individuals shut down instead of fighting, often involuntarily. Elbert and Schauer's (2010) freeze-flight-fight-fright-flag-faint model illustrates that, in the face of danger, animals first experience a momentary decrease in heart rate and startle response (freeze), followed by an active attempt to either flee or fight. If fleeing is not possible, animals may experience tonic immobility where both of their nervous systems are activated in a last attempt to calm the body down. Finally, the body shuts down in a dissociative, numbed, detached state (flag) or may even faint in reaction to the stress. This explanation, while a little dense, can help parents understand the biological mechanisms behind trauma responses and dispels the belief that their teen simply chose not to fight, yell, or run.

Further compounding the issue of blame is the fact that the large majority of sexually traumatized teens do not disclose their trauma right away. In fact, less than a third of child sexual trauma victims disclose to someone within twenty-four hours (Schonbucher, Maier, Mohler-Kuo, Schnyder, & Landolt, 2012), and CPS is less consistently involved in adolescent cases than cases regarding younger children (Raissian, Dierkhising, Geiger, & Schelbe, 2014).[7] Many parents struggle to understand teens' decision to keep such an important secret, especially when the trauma occurred repeatedly. Parents may need help understanding reasons teens give for keeping sexual trauma a secret, which include fear of *burdening the parent*, fear of *parental sanctions* (in cases when the perpetrator was a peer, when drinking or drug use was involved, or when some consensual sexual activity had previously occurred), fear of *legal repercussions* for themselves and/or the perpetrator, fear of being *blamed* or not believed, and feelings of *shame*, *denial* (i.e., telling someone would make the trauma "real"), or *distrust* that disclosing would stop the abuse (Crisma, Bascelli, Paci, & Romito, 2004; Schonbucher et al., 2012; Smith & Cook, 2008). Other teens have described *ambivalence* about disclosing; one of my clients told me that she knew she would have felt better if she had told someone about the abuse, but she worried about her perpetrator being kicked out of the home. She did not want to be "responsible for someone being homeless."

Sadly, many teens report unsupportive responses following disclosure, and their parents may feel tremendous guilt when they realize they have responded unsupportively. I often explain the *just world view* as a way to normalize and help both parents and teens understand parents' negative responses. That is, it is difficult to accept that bad things happen to good, completely innocent people; this goes against a fundamental belief that the world is fair and just. Therefore, someone who experiences sexual trauma, for example, must have done something to deserve such a fate (Furnham, 2003; Lerner, 1980). Parents also engage in strategies that defend against the possibility that sexual trauma could happen again; this phenomenon is known as the *defensive attribution hypothesis* (Shaver, 1985). One parent admitted, "I know we shouldn't blame her, but holding her at least partially responsible [for drinking on the night of the sexual assault] means that maybe there is *something* we can do to prevent this from happening again to her or our other daughter."

ASSISTING PARENTS IN THE AFTERMATH OF SCHOOL VIOLENCE

I was a high school freshman in the spring of 1999 when the unprecedented tragedy of the Columbine High School shootings occurred, and I remember talking about it over and over again in our classes. Our sense of safety and of a just world had been violated, as I know it was for millions of teenagers throughout the country. Press fast forward, and I was a mother of a young child in 2012, when the Sandy Hook Elementary School shootings took place. Just as people can recall where they were when they heard about the 9/11 terrorist attacks, I vividly remember being at a work holiday party when I heard about the shootings, crying in my car as I listened to radio reports, and feeling that I desperately needed to be with my son right away and never wanted to let him out of my sight again.

I share these experiences because my memories and reactions at the time were vastly different. After the Sandy Hook shootings, which I experienced as a parent, I felt completely helpless and doubtful about adults' abilities to keep children safe. When I work with parents of teens whose lives have been affected by school violence, I hear similar sentiments and see adults who are attempting to both comfort their grieving teens and manage their own trauma reactions. Although these parents often have reactions similar to nonoffending parents of sexually abused youth, we have been discussing, I wanted to focus the final part of this trauma chapter on understanding and assisting parents after school violence occurs. The topic is timely; there has been a rapid escalation in the frequency and severity of school violence since 1997 (Shafii & Shafii, 2001), with the worst examples being rampage school shootings such as those at Columbine High School. As with any trauma, parental reactions in the aftermath of an incidence of school violence vary greatly, and the process of healing is not linear.

Negative Emotional Responses

Initially, parents are likely to experience feelings of confusion and disbelief. One parent told me, "It's like I couldn't comprehend what I was reading [from a text message]. A kid pulled out a gun in a classroom? It was like, huh?" Once parents register what is happening (or has already happened), they may report that their confusion turned to panic, or terror. In the days and weeks that follow, parents often report intense negative feelings that interfere with normal functioning. The limited studies of parents affected by school violence have found that feelings range from numbness to irritability, misery, anger, and guilt (Hawkins, McIntosh, Silver, & Holman, 2004; Mears, 2005; Schwarz & Kowalski, 1991). These parents, like parents in your office, struggled to accomplish their daily responsibilities, including caring for other, nontraumatized siblings and going to work, and they felt irritability toward their spouses, friends, and coworkers, particularly if they perceived any of these individuals as unsupportive.

Cognitive Responses

For many parents, school violence occupies a lot of space in their brains in the days and weeks after, and parents often struggle with ruminative thoughts (Mears, 2005; Schwarz & Kowalski, 1991). The frequency and intensity of the thoughts may even be worse than those of their directly exposed teens (Hawkins et al., 2004). This lines up with what I have seen in therapy as well; many parents complain of thinking about the incident when they do not want to, having difficulty stopping or controlling the thoughts, having an endless stream of "what ifs," and being unable to complete other tasks because of being distracted. Parents also complain that a lot of their energy goes toward managing these thoughts as well and that they are often unsuccessful. One parent told me that she randomly worried in the grocery store that someone might pull a weapon, as had happened in her son's school. Another parent thought about running into parents of the student who was responsible for the school violence; for hours after the thought, she would imagine and play out several different scenarios and responses.

Like parents of sexually traumatized teens, parents affected by school violence may also experience cognitions related to fairness, personal responsibility, foreshortened future, and attempts at meaning making (Hawkins et al., 2004; Lickel, Schmader, & Hamilton, 2003; Schwarz & Kowalski, 1991). Similarities can be drawn between these survivors and those who have experienced terrorist attacks; such experiences are nearly impossible to make sense of. Furthermore,

> [t]he most distressing aspect of the survivors' ordeal [can be] the shattering of their fundamental beliefs about themselves (invulnerability, immortality), the world (predictability, controllability, safety), and other people (trust, safety, isolation) that had previously shaped their lives. Many [are] angry that their fabric of belief in a just world [has] been rudely shredded. All [feel] isolated, in that others could not possibly understand what they had gone through. (Miller, 2003, pp. 263–264)

Parents' desires and efforts to make meaning of traumas such as school violence may be highly variable, with some parents actively seeking and finding meaning by understanding the motives of the offender, turning to spirituality, or asserting their family or community's strength in the face of trauma (Updegraff, Silver, & Holman, 2008). Other parents will not feel the need to search for meaning. The parents who tend to have the most difficulty are those who are searching for meaning but are unable to find any (Downey, Silver, & Wortman, 1990). Researchers suggest that these parents may get stuck, leaving them unable to gain mastery over the trauma and integrate it into a revised worldview that allows them to cope and heal. Similarly, forgiveness may or may not be something that parents are ready, willing, or able to discuss or consider.

Positive Emotional Responses

The trauma literature focuses heavily on post-traumatic negative emotions and reactions, and many media and nonprofessionals may be confused or surprised by positive reactions. Parents sometimes tell me that they feel judged if they demonstrate any degree of positive emotions after a trauma, or they may judge themselves. "I thought, 'what kind of mother can laugh [at a joke] after her child almost died?' and then I felt terrible," Courtney's mom told me after a peer pulled a weapon on Courtney in the cafeteria. She also told me that she found herself hugging her daughter more often and feeling an intense amount of affection, relief, and gratitude. Similarly, in Hawkins and colleagues' (2004) study of Columbine parents and students, affection was the most intense of all feelings reported in the weeks after the shootings.

Mears (2005) found that parents may also feel proud of their teens, pleased with the way the school handled a dangerous situation, or thankful for the people supporting them.

Guidelines for Working with Parents after School Violence

Like parents of sexually abused teens, parents who have survived an incident of violence at their child's school will need education, encouragement, and support. I would highly recommend that you include them in their teen's treatment every step of the way. Below are some additional guidelines that may be unique to those who have experienced community violence such as in the schools.

1. Educate parents on the variability of post-traumatic responses

As with nonoffending parents, education is key. Most parents will not know what to expect from their teens, and many will expect dramatic and negative reactions as is often portrayed in the media. Indeed, traumatized adolescents can experience adult-like post-traumatic symptoms and are at risk for self-injurious behaviors, aggression, and numbing (Murtonen, Suomalainen, Haravuori, & Marttunen, 2012), but negative reactions often occur within a broad spectrum. Furthermore, interviews of Columbine students revealed that they also experienced positive emotions such as gratitude, happiness, and love (Hawkins et al., 2004). Hawkins and colleagues note,

> Ironically, the traumatized individual's emotional response to the event may hinder social assistance … survivors who are not acting appropriately in the eyes of potential helpers (e.g., not sad enough, too happy, too irritable) may receive less support. Members of victim's social network may be confused by the desire for a hug one moment and an irritated replay at another. (p. 207)

It is important that parents are informed and aware of the continuum of responses their teens may display postviolence. When a community-wide incident occurs, parents often receive unsolicited advice and opinions from others, and it can be confusing or cause parents to second-guess what they are seeing from their teens. You may be one of the few supports in parents' lives who are adequately prepared to listen, understand, encourage, and educate parents as they endure the inevitable frustration and exhaustion that results from such inconsistent, unpredictable, and unexpected responses.

Finally, many trauma symptoms resemble typical behaviors and experiences for developing youth, and parents may struggle to differentiate between "normal" teen behavior and "trauma symptoms." I always encourage parents of traumatized teens to remember the skills they already possess. Prior to the school violence, what would have stood out to them as concerning? How would they have approached the symptoms with their teen then? Despite the fact that trauma challenges everything parents feel they know and trust, the same parenting skills that worked before can help parents after the event too.

2. Follow the family's lead with respect to funerals, memorials, community outreach, and so on

After a school violence incident, parents and teens may find it helpful to attend and/or participate in school- or community-based memorial or support services. Help parents and teens pay attention to their emotional and physical energy levels so that they can determine which events to attend or decline. Staying connected after a trauma is important, but so is self-care; both were highly emphasized by parents victimized in the Columbine shootings (Mears, 2005). Finally, you may need to assist parents and teens in deciding when it is time to resume a routine (Dyregrov, Gjestad, Bie Wikander, & Vigerust, 1999), as this is an important aspect of post-traumatic healing and adjustment.

3. Help parents recognize helpful and unhelpful involvement of others

Involvement with a social support has many benefits for parents and teens in the aftermath of a community trauma. Teens often look to their parents, family members, and friends as individuals who will listen, understand, and comfort them (Murtonen et al., 2012; Ringler & Hayden, 2000). Parents and their teens may need encouragement to spend time around friends, family, those directly affected by the incident, and those who were not (Hawkins et al., 2004). Physical affection helps ground individuals in the present moment (instead of getting lost in ruminative thoughts about the trauma) while also providing them with physical comfort and reassurance. School support after community trauma is often viewed positively by students (Dyregrov et al., 1999).

Parents must be equally aware of the unhelpful involvement of others so that they can set limits where necessary and process related feelings. As often as I hear about helpful responses from others, I hear about disappointment in friends and family who "haven't been there," irritability at those who are intrusive, and anger when people offer insensitive interpretations or judgments. After a scary bomb threat at her son's school, one mom recalled,

> I called [my neighbor] to tell her about it. I guess in retrospect, it wasn't *that* big of a deal because everyone was fine, but at the time, I was really scared, you know? She listened for about a week, and then one day she interrupted me and said, "Oh, God, everyone is fine! Stop being so dramatic." I was so hurt; she has *no* idea what this has been like for me and [my son].

Teens experience similar negativity from peers and other adults, and parents often turn to me for guidance on the best way to respond to their teens and/or address the situation with the person who was hurtful. Together, we are able to process the experience so that next steps can be decided upon.

4. Encourage parents to consider media requests and media exposure carefully

A variable that is somewhat unique to school violence is the intense, ongoing, and global media involvement. Although I have certainly worked on abuse cases that have made local news, and there are cases that make national news (e.g., the abuse allegations at Penn State University), the media frenzy that is caused by school violence is intense. Journalists often approach directly exposed victims quickly; studies have found that the majority is asked to consent to an interview (Haravuori, Suomalainen, Berg, Kiviruusu, & Marttunen, 2011; Thoresen, Jensen, & Dyb, 2014). This attention can be burdensome, annoying, and distressing, and exposure to news reports containing inaccuracies, exaggerating danger, and creating unnecessary fear can lead to increased post-traumatic distress (Haravuori et al., 2011; Maerker & Mehr, 2006; Neria, DiGrande, & Adams, 2011; Vasterman, Yzermans, & Dirkzwager, 2005). However, some victims' experience with media is positive and may even contribute positively to their healing (Englund, Forsburg, & Saveman, 2014). Thoresen et al. (2014) suggest,

> It may be that media participation is more difficult for individuals with a high symptom level, or that negative experiences with media participation may lead to an exacerbation of symptoms ... Individuals with a high symptom level may be less in control of their emotions and may have reduced available cognitive capacity to cope efficiently with interviews and be less able to set adequate limits for their disclosures to the public. (p. 644)

Parents may find themselves unsure about whether to agree to a media interview or to expose their family to media coverage of the events. Assist them in carefully evaluating their own mental health, considering their beliefs about media involvement, and determining what is most likely to promote well-being and recovery.

DYSFUNCTIONAL PARENTING STYLES AFTER SEXUAL TRAUMA[2]

The way in which parents respond to and support their teens after trauma largely impacts teens' mental health (Davies, 1995; Valentino, Berkowitz, & Stover, 2010). Research indicates that parental distress predicts children's post-traumatic stress responses (e.g., Deblinger, Stauffer, & Steer, 2001), perhaps even more than the potentially traumatic event itself (Scheeringa & Zeanah, 2001). Not surprisingly, many parents find parenting itself to be a challenging task following trauma (Alisic, Boeije, Jongmans, & Kleber, 2012), and they may vary in their abilities to adapt to their family's new reality. In some cases, dysfunctional parenting styles result and exacerbate teens' symptoms (Cohen, 2009). The model of *relational PTSD* (Scheeringa & Zeanah, 2001) describes three parenting patterns that can be impairing for a traumatized teen: withdrawn, overprotective, and frightening.

Withdrawn parents, also referred to as unresponsive or unavailable parents, are unable to attend to their teen's needs because of their own impairment (Valentino et al., 2010). These parents may have a personal trauma history that is triggered, or a preexisting mental health problem that limits their ability to accurately perceive and address their teen's needs. Teens' symptoms may become exacerbated as they attribute their parents' unavailability to being psychologically damaged and increase attention-seeking behaviors in an effort to elicit a response from their parents (Caffery & Erdman, 2000). *Overprotective* or constricting parents are cognitively preoccupied with the notion that their teen will be traumatized again. These parents may have difficulty remembering the importance of teen experiencing mastery and independence in the wake of a trauma (Valentino et al., 2010); they may also struggle to redevelop trusting and caring relationships with others. Scheeringa and Zeanah (2001) note that this type of parenting style may occur when a parent is present at the trauma but unable to protect the child. It may also occur when the parent believes his or her absence caused the traumatization. This could certainly apply in the case of school violence and is often the case with sexual abuse as well. Kimberly learned that her teen daughter's sexual abuse began around the time that Kimberly gave birth to her second child. She blamed herself for being "sexually unavailable" to her boyfriend and also for being "under the same roof sometimes" when the abuse occurred. Parents may also worry that their teen will blame the parent for failing to protect them (McCourt & Peel, 1998).

Finally, the *frightening*, reenacting, or endangering parental style mimics the intrusive symptoms many adults experience post-trauma. Parents may actually retraumatize their teens by consistently probing for more information related to the trauma. In the previously mentioned case of Jill, she thought she was promoting open communication by frequently asking her son about his trauma; however, he reported to his therapist that he felt fixated in his trauma whenever Jill introduced the subject. He found it difficult to discuss but continued to do so, as he believed it was helpful for Jill. Increased questioning by the parent can lead adolescents to attempt to set rigid personal and psychological boundaries in an effort at self-preservation (Scheeringa & Zeanah, 2001). This may lead to more secretive behavior, which puts them at risk for danger or even revictimization (Davies, 1995).

PARENT–TEEN ATTACHMENT AND TRAUMA

Trauma undoubtedly affects parents' and teens' relationships with family, friends, and one another. Parents and teens interviewed after the Columbine shooting reported feeling closer to their families (Hawkins et al., 2004), but interpersonal relationships can also be quite negatively impaired after trauma, particularly when feelings of trust and safety have been challenged. Regardless of how parents and teens may subjectively perceive their relationships, teens need their parents to provide a feeling of *belonging*—confidence, predictability, and a place within the family—and to exhibit *competence*—knowledge, helpfulness, accountability, and resourcefulness (Libo & Giffith, 1996). They need to feel believed and validated, so that they can communicate openly and work on coping without having to pretend that the trauma did not occur (Cook, Blaustein, Spinazzola, & van der Kolk, 2003). As we have discussed above, teens may not always receive support from those around them, including parents. By the time James, one of my former clients, entered treatment one year after being sexually abused at a school function, he had perfected his avoidance of traumatic material. It took nearly six months for him to acknowledge even one feeling related to the abuse. I learned that his parents had never spoken of the incident at home, and while they did not deny that the abuse happened, they frequently made comments such as "Do you really think this was even a big deal for him? He seems perfectly fine." Unintentionally, these parents had given James the message that he should not speak of the trauma and that it should not have any negative effect, and James had reinforced this viewpoint by not displaying any outward symptoms. The impact it had on their relationship became evident as he began talking about the trauma more and growing angrier with his parents for "sweeping it under the rug."

One of the challenges that James' parents faced was that, despite their minimization of the abuse, they had *very* strong feelings about their son's victimization, and neither parent was confident that they could "hold it together." Parents must be able to manage their emotional responses as well as tolerate their teens' emotions in order for the relationship to remain strong after trauma (Cook et al., 2003). As we have been discussing throughout this chapter, parents are experiencing post-traumatic reactions of their own, and may find it difficult to provide a secure, consistent, predictable base for their teens (Bugge, Darbyshire, Røkholt, Sulheim Haugstvedt, & Helseth, 2014). Many parents I work with struggle to strike a balance between acknowledging and processing their own feelings, while also being the parent their teens (and oftentimes other, nontraumatized children) need. Research suggests that as long as parents' distress does not override their teen's needs, they can remain a secure attachment figure (Deblinger & Heflin, 1996). Indeed, parenting effectively while managing intense post-traumatic feelings, thoughts, and symptoms can be physically, mentally, and emotionally exhausting.

Nonoffending parents and their traumatized children may also mirror one another's moods and needs (Bugge et al., 2014). In some cases, the similarities may help parents recognize, accept, and respond to their teens' symptoms and needs. In others, parents may be negatively affected when they see their teen having similar, difficult experiences. Be aware of the role teens take on when their parents are struggling. It is not uncommon or unhealthy for teens to recognize the commonalities and provide support for their parents, but you want to ensure that proper boundaries are being set and respected, particularly for a teen who has been sexually traumatized. In some cases, the emotional climate of the family is so interconnected that individual members have a difficult time moving far beyond the healing point of the rest of the members. Teens may begin avoiding or suppressing thoughts and feelings to protect parents or minimize their distress (Deblinger & Heflin, 1996). One client told me when her mom was having a bad day, she expected to have a bad day too. As treatment went on, she and I worked closely on ways to acknowledge and empathize with her mom's needs while also setting limits on the way in which it affected her day. I also worked with her mom on ways to continue processing her trauma without relying too heavily on her daughter; this included referring her for individual counseling.

COUNTERTRANSFERENCE ISSUES AND VICARIOUS TRAUMATIZATION

Therapists working with traumatized teens and their parents will inevitably experience countertransference reactions, sometimes of an intense nature. My most difficult cases have involved bearing witness to families' terrible experiences, enduring their negative feelings toward me when I am viewed as part of the flawed "system," supporting them during nasty trials and unsatisfying outcomes, and coping with my own feelings—both negative and positive—through it all. In order to be an effective trauma therapist, it is critical that you be able to manage countertransference issues.

When working with nonoffending parents, you will often experience distress that mirrors parents' distress; such distress can be both affective and physiological (e.g., nausea, physical exhaustion; Russo, 2015). Feelings of helplessness, fear, anger, sadness, and shock may be shared between you and parents. Watching parents as teens share their trauma narratives, for example, is usually an emotional experience for everyone involved, including me. You may become frustrated when parents test boundaries or even feel abusive when you enforce limits. It may be difficult to confront or challenge parents while they are in the midst of such a crisis. Anger, disappointment, confusion, or even disgust may flare up when parents are ambivalent, unsupportive, ineffective, or accusatory toward their teens. In these moments, it is important to assess whether you have assigned unrealistic expectations to the parents (McElroy & McElroy, 1991).

Personal identification with parents is also common; in recent years, much of my supervision and personal therapy has focused on being both a therapist and a parent. I would like to think that my job helps me be more in tune with my son's needs and more capable of meeting those needs. In many ways, I know this is true. However, I am also well aware of how overprotective I can be, and I know the child traumas I bear witness to play a role. As I have mentioned throughout this book, set and respect some limits for yourself. For example, several of my trauma colleagues have children, so we try to divide the cases so that no one has to take one with children too close to their own children's ages.

Vicarious Traumatization

Vicarious traumatization (VT) extends beyond countertransference and consists of a change in the way therapists experience themselves, others, and the world (McCann & Pearlman, 1990). VT results from therapists' repeated exposure to graphic and traumatic material, the reality of human cruelty, and clients' trauma reenactments during which they (or their parents) reenact elements of the initial trauma within therapy[8] (McCann & Pearlman, 1990; Pearlman & Saakvitne, 1995). Short- and long-term symptoms include intrusive imagery, hypervigilance, social withdrawal, cynicism, depressive symptoms, emotional numbness, decreased trust in others, and feeling easily overwhelmed. The culture of the workplace, coping style of the therapist, availability and utilization of supervision, awareness of VT, length and degree of exposure to traumatic material, extent of training, personal trauma history, and prioritization of self-care are some of the factors that contribute to VT (Saakvitne & Pearlman, 1996).

Self-Assessment and Management of VT

More than half of my caseload at any given time involves trauma, and I have come to recognize countertransference and VT symptoms in myself, particularly during especially difficult cases. This past spring, I attended a conference where Laura Pearlman, a most prominent name in the VT literature, presented to a room full of trauma therapists, some new and some seasoned. She had us all write down a few ways that VT affected us. Then she instructed us to walk around silently, with our papers displayed in front of us, so that we could read each other's lists. I got a lot of appreciative nods as therapists read my signs of VT; similarly, I identified with many of my colleagues' symptoms. It was fascinating to see how trauma work affected all of us, but I also found myself feeling very exposed. It was hard to concede that I was affected by trauma work in such profound ways.

Ongoing supervision, consultation with peers, and individual therapy can help therapists prevent and manage VT. Meichenbaum (2007) recommends considering the following questions and discussing them openly with someone you trust:[9]

- How am I doing?
- What do I need?
- What would I like to change?
- What is hardest about this work? What worries me most about my work?
- How have I changed since I began this work? (Consider positive and negative changes)
- What changes, if any, do I see in myself that I do not like?
- Am I experiencing any signs of VT? (See textbox 7.1)
- What is my sense of accomplishment in my work?
- What work barriers get in the way of my having more satisfaction?
- Have I talked to others about my concerns, feelings, and rewards of my job? If so, who did I talk to? What were their reactions? What did they say

Textbox 7.1 Signs of Vicarious Traumatization

Feelings

Overwhelmed, drained, overloaded, burnt out
Lingering anger and/or sadness about clients' traumas
Loss of pleasure
Loss of control
Depression
Distance, detachment, or alienation from colleagues
Guilty, ashamed, self-doubting
Hopeless, pessimistic

Cognitions

Preoccupation with thoughts of work outside of the office
Overidentification with clients
Cynicism

Questioning of competence and self-worth
Low job satisfaction
Altered beliefs about safety, trust, and relationships

Behavior

Distancing, numbing, and detachment from clients
Avoidance of traumatic material in session
Post-traumatic symptoms
Difficulty experiencing intimacy in personal relationships
Overextension of self
Difficulty maintaining professional boundaries with the client (Meichenbaum, 2007; Pearlman & Saakvitne, 1995; Rothschild, 2006)

or do that I found helpful (or unhelpful)? What were my reactions to their reactions?

- Is there anything about my work experience or other stressful events in my life that I have not told anyone? Why not?
- Is there anything about my experiences that I keep from myself? That I feel I cannot handle?

Additional suggestions for coping with VT include planning for self-care activities that promote physical and emotional well-being, engaging in rituals that assist you in transitioning from work to your personal life, normalizing your reactions, setting realistic expectations for yourself and your clients, challenging negativity, diversifying your caseload, and, when appropriate, sharing your reactions with clients gently and respectfully (Meichenbaum, 2007; Pearlman & Saakvitne, 1995; Saakvitne, Gamble, Pearlman, & Lev, 2000).

CONCLUSION

Nonoffending parents of traumatized teens are a special population that you will encounter more often than you would probably prefer. It is important to remember that these parents are experiencing a situation that no parent should *ever* need to endure, and their reactions at times may seem confusing, contradictory, or even dangerous. They may experience mental health symptoms or have their own trauma histories triggered. Normalizing parents' feelings about themselves, their teens, the perpetrator(s), and involved agencies will enable them to feel supported and safe within the working alliance. Keeping parents informed and involved in teens' trauma treatment is critical to its success. Remembering that there is no such thing as an "abnormal" reaction to trauma will assist you as you cope with countertransference feelings. Set limits for yourself so that you can withstand the trauma of being a trauma therapist and help parents and their teens work through their worst nightmares.

NOTES

1. For the purposes of this chapter, we will only discuss nonoffending parents of teen victims. However, there is a body of literature that discusses parents of teen sexual offenders as well. If you are interested in learning more about this, I would highly recommend Julie Bennett and Ron Frey's (2012) chapter in *Individual Trauma: Recovering from Deep Wounds and Exploring the Potential for Renewal.* The chapter is titled "The Deep Trauma of Secondary Victimisation: Parents of Sex Offenders," pages 115–138.
2. Copyright © 2013 by the Association for Play Therapy. Reproduced and adapted with permission. The official citation that should be used in referencing this material is Myrick, A. C., & Green, E. J. (2013). A play-based treatment paradigm for nonoffending caretakers: Evidence-informed secondary trauma treatment. *International Journal of Play Therapy*, *22*(4), 193–206. The use of this information does not imply endorsement by the publisher.
3. For a good review, see Kirsch, Wilhelm, and Goldbeck (2011).
4. See Cook et al. (2005) for a seminal discussion about the domains of functioning impaired by trauma. A colleague and I also reviewed these domains recently (Green & Myrick, 2014).
5. The term *complex trauma* refers to "both children's exposure to multiple traumatic events, usually of an invasive, interpersonal nature, and the wide-ranging, long-term impact of this exposure" (National Child Traumatic Stress Network, 2007, p. 34). Sexual abuse that occurs repeatedly would be considered complex trauma.
6. Research has shown that parental engagement in trauma treatment can have a positive effect not only on youth outcomes (Corcoron & Pillai, 2008) but also on parents' mental health post disclosure (Cohen et al., 2004).
7. It should be noted, however, that the inclusion of sexual abuse in a CPS report made a complaint 65 percent more likely to generate CPS involvement than a report involving an adolescent experiencing neglect or physical abuse without sexual abuse.
8. Reenactments are a challenging but important an aspect of trauma treatment to understand. I would highly recommend Michael Levy's (1998) article.
9. A complete list of questions, and the entire handout, are available at http://www.melissainstitute.org/handouts.html#Family07.

Chapter Eight

Knowing Your Limits

When to Make a Referral

"We're not the problem here." Throughout this book, I have aimed to present many scenarios you will encounter in your work with parents and teens. They all involve managing your role as a teen's therapist with legal and ethical responsibilities, parental expectations and barriers, and parents' needs as caregivers. There will be times, however, when you realize that your role as the teen's therapist is not quite enough to address the issues faced by your parents or the family as a whole. At that point, it is time to make a referral. Sometimes, you will refer parents for individual therapy or teens for more intensive treatment. Other times, you will recommend that parents and teens begin family therapy. In these cases, I highly recommend referring out so that your relationship with the parents and teens can remain the same. In this chapter, we will discuss family therapy involving teens, as well as an issue that typically prompts me to make a family therapy referral: psychological abuse (PA). We will also briefly talk about the process of referring cases, and the reactions this can stir up for you as the individual therapist.

FAMILY THERAPY FOR PARENTS AND ADOLESCENTS

Most parents that you meet will possess a belief about what makes up a "good family," and many will struggle to manage any deviations from this idealized image. In order to preserve their image as good parents, parents often blame adolescents for family issues (O'Reilly & Parker, 2014). They position the teen as the problem by describing extreme behaviors, employing diagnostic terms, and relying on third parties to validate their claims (O'Reilly, 2014, 2015). These behaviors are attempts to decrease parental accountability, which makes sense, but this can cause major problems for your client—their teen (O'Reilly, 2014). Family therapy challenges these types of beliefs and behaviors by carefully reframing parents' views of their teens as a systemic family difficulty and striving to maximize the strengths of the family so that it can operate more effectively as a whole (Johnston, 2005; O'Reilly, 2014).

Research support is strong for the use of family therapy with adolescents. Not only have studies demonstrated effectiveness for the treatment of various adolescent issues, but they also suggest that strengthening families' emotional resources can protect teens from future problems (Lampis, Agus, & Cacciarru, 2014). Treatment outcome studies have shown that as understanding, perspective taking, and communication improve among participating family members, parents and teens are better able to consider and tackle problems similarly and more effectively (Guo & Slesnick, 2013). The eating disorder and substance abuse fields have arguably contributed the most to the literature on adolescents in family therapy. The eating disorder literature has repeatedly found that high levels of family dysfunction—such as enmeshment, conflict avoidance, and rigidity—and low levels of cohesion and emotional support contribute to teens' eating disorders and are a necessary target of family therapy (Folse & Krawzak, 2013; Robinson, Strahan, Girz, Wilson, & Boachie, 2013). Likewise, the substance abuse literature supports various forms of family therapy to reduce conflict and improve communication (Baldwin, Christian, Berkeljon, Shadish, & Bean, 2012).

Before you make a referral for family therapy, it is important to remember that, despite its usefulness, family therapy is not easy. Families can be incredibly difficult to engage in therapy (Campbell, 2004), and little is known about the processes through which families reorganize their interactional patterns (Molinari, Everri, & Fruggeri, 2010). Furthermore, families are always alternating between stability and change, as new needs and demands present themselves, so therapeutic goals must be flexible (Molinari et al., 2010). Finally, many teens and parents present to therapy with polarized perceptions of their problems (Ferdinand, van der Ende, & Verhulst, 2004; Friedlander, Lee, Shaffer, & Cabrera, 2014), making goal setting a challenge for some families; this is particularly true in families experiencing high levels of conflict (Grills & Ollendick, 2003).

Although teens often need a forum to discuss complex issues with parents and other family members, they may be nervous to actually talk in family therapy (O'Reilly & Parker, 2013; Strickland-Clark, Campbell, & Dallos, 2000) or own the label of "the problem" (O'Reilly, 2015). While some parents can patiently listen while their teen answers questions or shares feelings, many of the families you refer for family therapy will struggle with this skill. Parents may be nervous to hear what teens will "air" in sessions, and, as a result, they talk more than their teens, interrupt, interject their own responses during exchanges between the therapist and teen, and/or speak negatively about their teens right in front of them (Molinari et al., 2010; O'Reilly, 2006, 2008; O'Reilly & Parker, 2014). These parents may also respond negatively if their teen interrupts anyone in the room or involves them less than other siblings (O'Reilly & Parker, 2013). I have heard many teens express concern over "what will happen" when they leave family therapy; there is often much anxiety about the car ride home after a session. Sometimes the anxiety is unfounded, but other times teens have had negative experiences after speaking up in the past (Strickland-Clark et al., 2000).

Once therapy actually begins, parents and teens may have vastly different views about the therapist, goals for treatment, or even the need for family therapy at all. Within-family alliance, or *shared sense of purpose* (Friedlander, Escudero, & Heatherington, 2006; Pinsof, 1995), is critical to family therapy's success, and the family therapist takes on the difficult task of getting all members "to 'sign on' without losing face" (Friedlander et al., 2006 in Friedlander et al., 2014, p. 42). Parents may struggle to accept a therapist's decision to meet with them without the children present or resent the therapist's suggestion that they are *detouring* marital difficulties onto the teen (Minuchin & Fishman, 1981)[1] or putting their teen in a position where they must mediate parents' conflicts (Peris et al., 2008). An effective family therapist is one who is able to meet the family where they are, accept their ambivalence about tackling difficult issues, and remain focused on the family's mutually agreed-upon goals (Friedlander et al., 2014).

A GAUGE FOR FAMILY THERAPY REFERRALS: THE FAMILY TIME-OUT

Some therapists are quick to make family therapy referrals, whereas others rarely do. I probably fall somewhere in the middle of these two extremes, which I have realized through countless conversations with colleagues. I think some of it depends on the field in which you work; as we discussed above, the eating disorder and substance abuse communities have long supported—and subsequently spent time and money researching—the use of family therapy with their adolescents. I also believe that it depends on your comfort level with doing conjoint family work within individual therapy.

In previous chapters, I have given you multiple examples of times when parents are invited into the work, and they are always included in the beginning and end of sessions, so oftentimes I try to do a little bit of parent–teen work to see how it is received. If it goes well and problems improve, great! This lets me know that the family is responsive and that continued parent–teen work or a referral to family therapy may be beneficial. When parents are completely opposed to the idea or unable to follow through with the plans we make in therapy, I can usually determine that they will be minimally cooperative with a family therapy referral (more on this below) and that treatment goals may be limited to what the teen and I can work on in individual sessions. Although the strength of my alliance with parents often gives me an idea of parents' receptivity and motivation, I have found that this is not always sufficient to determine which families are and which families are not good candidates for family therapy.

I love the idea of *family time-outs*, which is interesting because I do not typically recommend time-outs for parents of young clients. Time-outs, in essence, are activities "that interrupt a destructive pattern of behaviors so that constructive problem-solving can occur" (Veenstra & Scott, 1993, p. 72). There are multiple levels of time-outs:

1. Mental pause
2. Informal break
3. Formal truce
4. External intervention
5. Formal authority intervention
6. Prolonged separation

I used this intervention strategy with Shawna and her mother Stephanie, and I also kept their successes and struggles in mind as I assessed their appropriateness and readiness for family therapy. Prior to implementing a time-out plan, their arguments frequently escalated to the point of another family member intervening. Oftentimes, Shawna called her father, Stephanie's ex-husband, to come and get her when fights got out of hand.

The first level, the *mental pause*, involves taking a mental break to regain control of self and the situation. Shawna and Stephanie both identified body clues to anger and agreed to utilize deep breathing as a way to try and get their anger under control. We role-played different ways of reengaging after a mental pause, including restating the problem, clarifying each other's points, and trying to communicate their own messages as clearly as possible. "I feel ..." statements were also emphasized and practiced. We agreed that if the mental pause did not work, the next step would be an *informal break*, or a temporary, physical removal of oneself from the situation. Shawna acknowledged that she frequently felt like she needed to take a step out of the escalating argument to regain her composure and calm down—physically and emotionally. However, she complained that when she tried to do this, Stephanie viewed it as disrespectful and would follow Shawna around to continue the argument. Stephanie complained that Shawna would simply "walk out" in the middle of a fight without any explanation. After explaining the importance of physical space, I encouraged Stephanie to use these breaks as opportunities to disengage herself as well. She and Shawna agreed on a statement that temporarily paused the argument: "I think I need some space for a few minutes." The third level involves calling a *formal truce*. Here, Shawna and Stephanie decided that if one of them called a truce, the other would respect it for at least two days, enough time for everyone to "cool down" and readdress the issue at a later date. They also practiced limit-setting statements for situations where one of them was struggling to maintain the truce.

If teens and parents are able to respect established limits and use these skills, there are often great improvements. In cases where mental breaks, informal breaks, and formal truces are sufficient in the majority of situations, I feel comfortable continuing to work on the skills through individual therapy. Unfortunately, in cases where these skills are not sufficient, I begin to see some of the more dysfunctional family issues, and family therapy referrals become relevant. For Shawna and Stephanie, their arguments continued to escalate due to Stephanie's difficulties with the formal truce. For this reason, *external intervention* (level four) by Shawna's father remained a necessary aspect of Shawna's time-out needs. In other cases, *formal authority intervention* (e.g., law enforcement) or *prolonged separation* (e.g., staying with the noncustodial parent) may be warranted. Stephanie struggled to understand Shawna's decision to call her father and blamed Shawna for escalating the arguments further by involving him. The family was referred for family therapy to work on Shawna and Stephanie's frequent conflict and the father's role, and Shawna and I continued working on individual issues that contributed to their problems, including low self-esteem and anxiety. Over the course of our individual work, it became clear that many of Shawna's issues were related to the treatment she received at home, particularly since her mother and father had begun the divorce process. In fact, I soon learned that many of Stephanie's words and actions were psychologically abusive. Some of the things Shawna told me reminded me of another client I was currently working with and her family.

PSYCHOLOGICAL ABUSE: A PROMPT FOR FAMILY THERAPY

Whitney, age seventeen, entered treatment for self-reported depression, self-injurious behaviors, and low self-esteem. She came from an upper-class family where both parents worked outside of the home, and she had three younger siblings. From the outset of treatment, she described her parents as "assholes" who were "awful" to her. She told me that they vacillated between telling her to stay out of the house and criticizing her for never being home. They expected her to transport her siblings to practices and school, which she did, yet called her lazy and "a useless member of the family." She gave many examples of hurtful things that her siblings and parents said to her, including one instance when her brother told her to "just go cut [her]self" as her mother sat there watching. Whitney reported that her mother did nothing to stop or correct her brother's behavior. She also reported threatening and "scary" behavior that her father sometimes exhibited, including one instance when he broke her bedroom door off the hinges and then refused to repair it. "It was like he wanted me to feel scared all over again every time I walked into my room and saw that broken door," she told me.

About six months into our work together, I noticed the impact that a consistent, stable therapeutic relationship was having on Whitney. Her symptoms had improved, including a cessation of self-injury, and she began sharing stories of social and academic success in our sessions. However, her self-esteem and feelings of mastery remained somewhat low. Around the same time, I began noticing that her parents were becoming more and more withdrawn from therapy, rarely attending appointments or calling me to stay updated on her progress. They said all the right things—they were happy with her progress and relieved that she was no longer hurting herself—but Whitney reported that things were "worse than ever" at home. She and I talked at length about how difficult it was to maintain her treatment gains when her home life was so negative. It was becoming quickly apparent that Whitney's individual work was being threatened by her role in the family system.

Psychological abuse—also known as emotional abuse—is not a one-time event. Rather, it involves a repeated, sustained pattern of words and acts toward a child that causes or has a high probability of causing

> harm to the child's health or physical, mental, spiritual, moral, or social development. These acts must be reasonably within the control of the parent … Acts include restriction of movement, patterns of belittling, denigrating, scapegoating, threatening, scaring, discriminating, ridiculing, or other non-physical forms of hostile or rejecting treatment. (World Health Organization [WHO], 1999, p. 15)

Prevalence rates of PA are around 36 percent, with verbal abuse considered the most common form (Stoltenborgh, Bakermans-Kranenburg, Alink, & Van Ijzendoorn, 2012), and some have made the case that PA is at the core of all forms of abuse and neglect and the most damaging aspect of abuse (Boulton & Hindle, 2000; Navarre, 1987). Family stressors, including family conflict and parental mental health issues, are often associated with PA (Hibbard, Barlow, MacMillan, & Committee on Child Abuse and Neglect and American Academy of Child and Adolescent Psychiatry, 2012).

There are many ways that PA can manifest itself, but for the purposes of this chapter, we are going to stick with *scapegoating*. Scapegoats are the person at whom families direct their stress (Hollingsworth, Glass, & Heisler, 2007), and they are often described as "bad" or inadequate. Scapegoating is an efficient way to channel problems, and it relies on all family members (including the adolescent) to participate in the belief. Families who engage in scapegoating are often enmeshed, so any gains that result from therapy, such as the scapegoats' improved self-esteem, decreased symptomatology, or desire for autonomy, are seen as threats to the balance and homeostasis of the family (Hollingsworth et al., 2007). One of my clients, Jennifer, whom I discussed in chapter 5, noticed increased marital problems and arguing within the family once her own symptoms stabilized. She came to realize that her family was relying on her to stay mentally unwell to maintain stability as a whole system. As a result, it was difficult at times for her to remain committed to her own recovery. Repeatedly, she and I discussed her tendency to interact with family members in ways that solicited negative responses, which then triggered her self-injury and depression.

Scapegoats often have emotional reactions to their parents' hostile treatment of them, which parents use as further evidence that the teen is, in fact, the problem (James & MacKinnon, 2010). Furthermore, when a scapegoat refuses to continue playing such a role in the family, he/she may receive messages from their parents that they are no longer wanted, needed, or loved; they have become expendable (Sabbath, 1969). Both Whitney and Jennifer's cases illustrate this point; as their symptoms improved and they began to assert themselves in their family relationships, their parents seemed to "lose interest" in their treatment and their everyday lives.

Mental Health Effects on Teens

Not surprisingly, PA is associated with a wide range of teen issues, including interpersonal problems, academic achievement, internalizing disorders, and externalizing disorders (Ellis et al., 2014; Hibbard et al., 2012; Yahav & Sharlin, 2002). Expressed emotion (EE) likewise has been linked to internalizing problems, including depression and self-criticism, and externalizing behaviors, including self-harm and suicidality—particularly when parents are highly critical (Wedig & Nock, 2007). Some theorists have also suggested that parents' tendency to be critical makes them more likely to blame their teens for mental health issues and/or view them as intentionally causing difficulties for the family (Barrowclough & Hooley, 2003), possibly increasing the likelihood of scapegoating or other forms of PA.

Family Therapy for Psychological Abuse

It is difficult for family therapists to directly observe the pattern of ongoing psychologically abusive behavior, and James and MacKinnon (2010) refer to the behaviors observed in the room as merely the "tip of the iceberg." Because of this, therapists run the risk of over- or underestimating the extent to which PA is present. Unlike physical abuse, there are no visible signs of PA, so adolescents experiencing scapegoating and other forms of PA can benefit most from a family therapist who is closely attuned to and challenges the way parents and other family members are treating them. In these cases, the family therapist's role involves giving the teen a "fair shot" in therapy instead of simply accepting the negative view put forth by parents. Therapists assist teens in expressing their thoughts, feelings, and needs, while calling attention to psychologically abusive words and actions within the family (Bowling, Kearney, Lumadue, & St. Germain, 2002). Therapists also strive to work with parents to identify the ways in which their pasts affect their present struggles, to "own" individual problems rather than blaming the scapegoated teen, to recognize the appropriateness (or inappropriateness) of their parental expectations, and to reframe challenges within the family. All of these goals are addressed by the therapist, who delicately balances joining with parents in their concerns with refusing to participate in the belittlement of the teen (Boulton & Hindle, 2000; Copley, 1994).

Family therapy for PA may also involve identifying the roles family members play in the abuse. In one model, these interacting roles have been referred to as the *drama triangle* and include the Victim, Persecutor, and Rescuer (Karpman, 1968; L'Abate, 2009).[2] L'Abate (2009) explains,

> This pathogenic triangle is constituted by three intrinsically and simultaneously connected roles found in most, if not all, individuals involved in family dysfunctions. In such relationships all three roles are enacted by self and other parties at the same time, without an awareness of or control over their damaging consequences. Each participant in an intimate role plays the Victim, and can be perceived as a Persecutor or Rescuer at the same time, depending on who does or says what. For instance, one partner may perceive herself as the Victim, while being perceived as a Persecutor by the other partner who was seen originally as a Persecutor. (p. 2)

L'Abate goes on to say that these triangles are reactive and repetitive in families where abuse is present and that identifying the Victim and Persecutor is often easy. The Rescuer, on the other hand, may not be readily apparent, and any recognizable efforts may be "half-hearted, ineffective, discounted, or futile" (p. 8). In families where there is PA, roles may be in constant flux, even if the teen is the primary target of PA. For example, a teen who has become accustomed to PA by her father may respond to him aggressively at the dinner table. She has placed him permanently in the role of Persecutor and herself in the role of Victim; however, in this particular situation, he is likely to perceive her as the Persecutor and himself as the Victim. In an effort to protect himself, he may then respond by persecuting her in some way (e.g., name calling and inappropriate punishment), which places her back in the role of Victim. This dynamic continues in virtually all of their interactions.

Family therapy assists members in recognizing and understanding their roles. Over time, members' relinquishment of their roles in the triangle can enable them each to perform their roles as parents, children, siblings, and spouses more effectively. If, in the previous example, the daughter can give up her role as the Victim, she may feel less reactive during interactions with her father. As a direct result, he may "fire back" at her less often and no longer be the Persecutor. Similarly, if he can recognize the role that his persecution plays in their relationship, she may feel less like a Victim. If that happens, the need for persecution, victimization, and subsequent rescuing become less, PA is subsequently diminished or extinguished, and family functioning can improve (L'Abate, 2009).

Is it Psychological Abuse?

It can be difficult to differentiate poor parenting and relationship conflict from more severe PA. Some researchers have considered PA as the most severe level of nonphysical abuse, with verbal abuse and emotional abuse used to describe less chronic and severe behaviors (James & MacKinnon, 2010). In the literature, the term psychological abuse is assigned to any verbal or nonverbal behaviors that are cruel, over-controlling, or manipulative. These behaviors range from mild to severe and may include humiliation, terrorizing, cognitive disorientation, deprivation of basic needs or valued objects, denial of emotional responsiveness, extreme rejection, emotional blackmail, and/or exploitation/corruption (see table 8.1; Brassard & Donovan, 2006; Hart, Brassard, Binggeli, & Davidson, 2002; Moran, Bifulco, Ball, Jacobs, & Benaim, 2002). High levels of EE are also often indicative of PA. EE involves the emotional attitude of one family member (often a parent) toward another (often a child); specifically, measures of EE look at criticism, hostility, emotional over-involvement, and warmth (Hooley, 1985; Vaughn, 1989). Parents with high EE attitudes often present hostile, extreme, and negative descriptions about their teens, and are open about their high levels of frustration (Calam, Bolton, Barrowclough, & Roberts, 2002).

I use these terms and definitions to categorize what I see and hear. Generally speaking, I pay attention to statements and situations that mimic what I might see in an emotionally abusive intimate relationship. Constant put-downs,

Table 8.1 Nine Categories of Psychological Abuse

Category	*Key Feature*	*Severity Based On*	*Example*
Humiliation/ Degradation	Actions or comments that degrade or humiliate the child Potential to invoke shame	The amount of shame that would be invoked in most children (not self-reported shame) Public viewing would increase severity	Screaming at teen in front of peers
Terrorizing	Places teens in unpredictable/ chaotic situations Invokes intense fear or dread Calculated Excludes physical attacks	The amount of shame that would be invoked in most children (not self-reported shame)	Making disguised threatening phone calls to teen who is home alone (particularly if teen is afraid to stay home alone)
Cognitive Disorientation	Confuses or disorients the child in terms of (1) Belief in evidence of senses (e.g., hearing) (2) Memory (3) Sense of identity	Degree to which behavior mimics brainwashing	Repeatedly changing commands such that the teen feels as though they must just not be listening or, in extreme cases, are going crazy
Deprivation of Basic Needs/Isolating	Deprivation of needs such as light, sleep, food, or social interaction Intentionality will help distinguish from neglect	Level of deprivation	Refusing to allow teen to accompany family on vacation or at family meals

Deprivation of Valued Objects	Deprivation of a valued or treasured item (can be inanimate, alive, or abstract) May extend to significant others	Object is removed or destroyed in deliberate, cruel fashion, aimed at maximizing distress or disappointment	Throwing a teen's prized photo album in the fireplace (inanimate) Refusing to let teen see favorite aunt (alive) Telling a teen that they can try out for soccer and then, at the last minute, withdrawing the consent to participate (abstract)
Denying Emotional Responsiveness	Being detached or uninvolved Minimal interaction (only when necessary) Refusal to provide warmth, nurturance, or praise		
Extreme Rejection	Abandonment or indication that the parent wishes the teen was dead	Long periods of abandonment or explicit wishes of death	Leaving a teen on the side of the road at night after an argument in the car
Emotional Blackmail	Use of serious threats to ensure control and compliance	Degree of threat	Telling teen that she will be kicked out of the home if she tells her parent about the other parent's infidelity
Corruption/Exploitation	Forcing teen to take part in illicit activities Modeling or permitting antisocial behaviors	Risk of physical safety Sexual abuse	Having teen buy drugs for family member

Source: Adapted from Brassard and Donovan (2006), Hart et al. (2002), and Moran et al. (2002).

jokes at the teen's expense, hypercriticism, exclusion, conditional statements of love, withdrawal of verbal and/or physical affection, infliction of guilt and blame, invalidation of the teen's feelings, thoughts, and perspectives, and constant assertions of control are also signs that PA may be occurring within a family (James & MacKinnon, 2010). I notice whether or not teens withdraw or become passive when parents are in the room, and I also listen for teens who describe themselves as the "black sheep" in the family or who complain, more than the average teen, about unfair treatment in their home.

Mandated reporting of PA is more complicated than physical or sexual abuse reporting. Sadly, in cases where there is no clear evidence of impaired growth or development, many social service agencies will not accept a referral based solely on PA (Hibbard et al., 2012). This is one of my greatest frustrations as an adolescent therapist. When a teen comes into my office and describes being screamed at on the ride over, kicked out of the car, spat at, or otherwise treated horribly, I really struggle to manage my feelings. In one case, I pleaded with DSS to remove my teen client from an emotionally abusive home to no avail. Because DSS was already involved with the family due to an allegation of physical abuse, however, they were willing to add family therapy to the service agreement. It is always worth a call if you are concerned.

MAKING A REFERRAL TO FAMILY THERAPY

I could feel my anxiety mounting as I invited Kenny's mother into the room. Kenny had spent several sessions telling me about various forms of PA that he was enduring at home, but his recounting of a disagreement between him and his brother made me realize how badly the family needed therapy. Kenny was typically scapegoated in family interactions, but in this particular situation, Kenny's parents refused to intervene when Kenny's brother began punching and—by Kenny's report—hurting him. Kenny's parents responded later by telling him that he needed to "toughen up" and that he should not have provoked his brother. They ridiculed him for being weak, and I was concerned about both Kenny's safety and his parents' treatment of him. This was one of my first experiences with recommending family therapy, and, admittedly, I figured I could just mention it and have the family respond positively (they had been very open to therapy thus far). I was not prepared for Kenny's mother's response, which was to tell me I was wrong, that I was allowing Kenny to manipulate me, and I clearly did not know what their family needed. She stormed out, and I never saw Kenny or anyone in the family again.

What I did not realize then, but hope to impart to you now, is this: above all else, referring a family for therapy tells parents that you consider the family a part of, or a cause of, the teen's struggles (Haley, 1990, in Whiteside, 1993). Psychologically abusive parents may not be able to recognize their own behavior (Boulton & Hindle, 2000), and even parents who can acknowledge their role in the problem worry about being blamed. *No* parent wants to be perceived as "doing a bad job" or being "crap parents" (O'Reilly, 2015, p. 328). With your suggestion to attend family therapy, parents' fears of failure are confirmed. Whiteside (1993) discusses three types of family therapy referrals: maximum, intermediate, and minimal cooperation.

When parents are cooperative at a *maximum* level, they understand that the family as a whole needs help. Oftentimes, you have developed a strong working alliance with them, so an open, honest conversation can be a part of the referral process. In these cases, you express concerns, and parents agree with or add to them. Family therapy is easily discussed, and the majority of your time in the referral process involves helping parents find a good match for their family. I would highly recommend developing some connections with good family therapists; I have collaborated on cases with some wonderfully talented family therapists. Parents at the tier of maximum level of cooperation like to leave my office with a plan, and having a name (or names) is a great first step.

Parents at the *intermediate* level of cooperation are clearly interested in helping their teen, but you may be uncertain about their reaction to being named as part of the problem (Whiteside, 1993). These parents often realize that they need to seek help but might feel unready to do so for a number of reasons (remember our discussion in chapter 1). I approach this group gently, sometimes taking the emphasis off of the parents' hand in the problem and instead focusing on how beneficial it would be for the teen to have the parents' support. I am relatively straightforward, however. Parents may hear me say some hard truths, including, "I think we have made great progress in individual therapy, but I am not sure how much more progress we can make without a family component." I tell parents about the success I have seen when family therapy enters into the treatment equation; discussing past experiences also helps destigmatize the referral. Another reason for having a go-to list of family therapists is being able to share your personal experiences with family therapists in the area. Furthermore, hearing "This family therapist is wonderful; I really think s/he could help" often comforts parents. Like Whiteside (1993), I will also warn you that these parents may not seek family therapy the first time you recommend it, so be patient, and remember that if your referral is accurate, you will get another opportunity to suggest family work.

Kenny's mother represents the third, *minimally* cooperative group of parents. These parents react negatively to *any* insinuation that they play a role in their teen's problems (Whiteside, 1993). They may even redouble their efforts to blame the teen and present themselves as a "normal" family who has been burdened with a difficult teen (Boulton & Hindle, 2000). Such parents will be the ones who tell you, "Everyone in the family is fine; it is [teen] who is the problem. We'd be fine if it weren't for his/her issues." Minimally cooperative parents can also be sensitive to blame and preoccupied with personal issues. These families may be *multiproblem families*, or families that have problems on multiple levels of functioning, including teen, parent, child-rearing, family functioning, contextual, social network, and mental health care factors (see Bodden & Dekovic, 2016). Put bluntly, these are the parents who will make your heart rate go up just thinking about making a family therapy referral. Keeping a calm emotional climate is key when you broach the topic of family therapy with minimally cooperative parents; this can often be achieved by keeping the focus on everyone's shared interest: the teen. Beware of some of the issues we discussed in chapter 7; parental psychopathology can be a barrier to family therapy in the same way that it can interfere with teen's individual therapy. As a final note, be careful that you do not refer *all* of your minimally cooperative parents to family therapists you enjoying working with; just as you do not want your caseload to consist of all complex, difficult cases, your family therapist friends and colleagues do not either!

ATTACHMENT-BASED AND EMOTIONALLY FOCUSED FAMILY THERAPIES

Although there are many different theories and approaches to family therapy, I cannot say enough about the benefits of family therapies that target the attachment relationship. Throughout this book, we have talked about the role of attachment in adolescent therapy and the consideration that I feel it should be given when you are tackling issues throughout treatment. Two types of family therapy, Attachment-Based Family Therapy (ABFT) and Emotionally Focused Family Therapy (EFFT), are great options for parents and teens whose attachment relationship needs improvement.

ABFT aims to improve the quality of the parent–teen attachment through the repair of ruptures that have damaged trust between parents and adolescents. ABFT therapists assist adolescents in the expression of their hurts and needs and help parents respond in an empathic, supportive way. Over time, adolescents learn that their parents "care, are available, and can respond appropriately to their emotional needs" (Diamond, 2014, p. 15). Three core interventions are used in this type of family therapy: relational reframes, focusing on emotions and unmet attachment needs, and facilitation of corrective attachment experiences. Using *relational reframes*, therapists work to shift the focus of treatment away from teens' symptoms and more on the parent–teen relationship. Studies have found that ABFT helps parents view issues from a more interpersonal place (e.g., "He does not feel understood or supported by us" versus "He is always angry"), focus on these issues, and demonstrate improved understanding, empathy, and affirmation toward their adolescents (Diamond & Siqueland, 1998; Moran & Diamond, 2008; Moran, Diamond, & Diamond, 2005).

Next, ABFT therapists focus on *primary emotions and unmet attachment needs* so that they can understand times when the teen's attachment was ruptured, maybe through trauma or parental criticism. Once these ruptures are understood, therapists help adolescents express such feelings and experiences to parents so that *corrective attachment episodes* can occur. Therapists facilitate sessions in which adolescents can share their feelings and parents can respond to pain, disappointment, and needs supportively and nondefensively (Diamond, 2014). Parents may need a lot of help from therapists during this process. For example, psychologically abusive parents may belittle, blame, or withdraw when teens try to share their feelings; this blocks communication and does not give teens what they need: validation and acceptance of emotional experiences. Parents and teens may resist deepening their emotions for fear of intolerable vulnerability and/or rejection. Nevertheless, such a relational approach to family therapy can have a profound impact on the parent–teen attachment and related behaviors.

Similarly, EFFT strives to "facilitate the reestablishment of connection through encouraging new emotional and interactional experiences … by increasing emotional availability and responsiveness in an effort to improve attachment bonds" (Faber & Wittenborn, 2010, p. 97). EFFT assumes that rigid negative interaction patterns have limited family members' communication and security, leading to conflicts that are actually desperate attempts for attachment security or responses to a failed attempt at connection. In this type of family therapy, therapists help parents and adolescents de-escalate negative cycles of interaction, initiate more positive cycles of interaction, and incorporate such changes into daily life. These new emotional experiences and interactional patterns increase interpersonal connectedness within the family and individual well-being (Johnson, Maddeaux, & Blouin, 1998). When I am making a family therapy referral, I often look for a therapist who ascribes to either ABFT or EFFT. It is amazing to hear the impact that such relationship-focused work can have on my clients' symptoms, their sense of belonging and security, and their parents' investment and views of the therapeutic process.

COUNTERTRANSFERENCE ISSUES

We have talked throughout this book about the ways in which parents' behaviors and beliefs can push buttons for therapists and bring up strong reactions.

Observing and hearing about family-based interactions—communication issues, arguments, misunderstandings, and compromises—can initiate many reactions in us, especially as we consider our roles as partners, parents, and adults in our own families of origin (Heatherington, Friedlander, & Diamond, 2014). You may experience varying degrees of rescue fantasies in families where adolescents are horribly scapegoated and mistreated (Rosenberg, 2009). Dysfunctional families may injure your "good therapist" ego a bit; most of us want to believe that we are capable of helping the teens who come through our offices. It may be difficult to admit that the problems cannot be solved solely through individual work with you. Such a realization may also lead to feelings of helplessness and frustration (Mark, 1998). I have certainly worked with parents who make me want to scream at them, "How do you not understand what you are doing to your child?!" When these types of countertransference reactions come up, think about whether or not you are getting pulled into the family system. Consider the following examples:

- You are struggling to get a parent to recognize the role that his behaviors play in his son's aggressive behavior. You find yourself "giving up" and withdrawing from—or even avoiding—the parent during check-ins and check-outs. Your teen client has been describing grief over not having the father he wants.
- You feel frustrated that the only time you can get a teen's parents to come into therapy is when the teen is doing something unsafe. You notice yourself saying things like "If you want me to continue working with your daughter, you need to come in this week for an emergency session." Lately, you and your client have been discussing the fact that she only feels like her parents pay attention to her when she is in crisis.
- Despite the fact that they diligently bring their daughter to therapy each week, a couple does not make any effort to change their behaviors or parenting style. You notice yourself feeling angry and invisible. Their daughter complains that she feels ignored and misunderstood by her parents.

In each of these situations, countertransference reactions can give you a window into family dynamics. Depending on the severity and chronicity of patterns between parents and their teens, you may or may not decide it is time to refer for family therapy. Be prepared to experience such reactions when you make referrals and if/when family therapy begins. Splitting individual and family therapists (e.g., one is good, the other is bad), bad mouthing the family therapist, and idealizing your role (e.g., "Why can't we just see you? You have been so wonderful for our family") are all very real possibilities that will give you plenty of topics of conversation for peer consultation and supervision sessions.

CONCLUSION

Working with parents of teens can be a rewarding and exciting experience; however, there are times when you will realize that a family's needs outweigh what you can provide as the teen's individual therapist. Prior to making a referral, I often see what I am able to help families achieve in individual therapy; the family time-out is one assessment tool and intervention that I employ frequently. Understanding the complexities of family therapy will further assist you in determining if family therapy is warranted and if the family will be willing and/or able to do the work. Finally, like all of the topics we have discussed in this book, pay close attention to your countertransference reactions, as they will provide you with some important insights into the needs of the parents, teens, and family as a whole.

NOTES

1. Detouring involves parents focusing on the teen's problems rather than their issues with one another in the marriage.
2. This is simply one method of considering family dynamics. Virtually all family systems theories consider this issue in some way, and family therapists' style and theoretical background will largely determine how this addressed.

Chapter Nine

The Long Goodbye

Terminating with Parents and Their Teens

"Can't you just see us forever?" When the topic of termination comes up, many parents make a similar statement, sometimes with a laugh, but almost always with some seriousness behind it. After all we have talked about in this book, you can understand why. I find that many therapists also have a tendency to make light of termination and, interestingly, the topic does not get as much attention in the literature as you might think. Gil and Crenshaw (2016) suggest that one reason could be the shift toward briefer forms of therapy. In treatment episodes that only last a few sessions or months, it is reasonable that therapists may underestimate the termination phase of treatment; this may be true for therapists who work primarily in managed care settings and do not always have control over when clients finish their treatments. Nevertheless, research suggests that even therapeutic relationships—even brief ones—are vital to treatment success (Lilliengren, Falkenström, Sandell, Mothander, & Werbart, 2015; Mallinckrodt & Jeong, 2015; Shirk, Karver, & Brown, 2011; Shirk, Karver, Handelsman, Fields, & Bickman, 2006), and those of us who have worked with clients for a long time know what an intricate part of our clients' worlds we become. One client, as we celebrated our fifth holiday season together, remarked, "When we first started, I would have never thought I'd even still be around for five Christmases." She writes me a heartfelt Christmas card every year, and the gesture often acts as a catalyst for us to discuss her progress and her hopefulness for a bright future. Indeed, the termination process for this client, when she is ready, will be a lengthy and significant part of our work together.

Another possibility for the limited reading material on termination is that it is *uncomfortable*. It is a strange and sometimes painful feeling, saying goodbye to someone that you have seen weekly for an extended period of time. On the one hand, there can be so much joy because the client (and his/her parents) is doing well and do not need to come to counseling anymore.

On the other hand, I never get to see the successful directions their lives take. I often find myself wondering about some of my clients who have terminated and hoping they are doing well or worrying about them at certain times of year. It is so easy for me to minimize the role I have played in someone's life and, relatedly, minimize the effect they have had on mine.

In this chapter, I hope to shed some light on a powerful aspect of therapy: the goodbye. As we will discuss, some parents manage termination easily, while others fear it greatly. You will work with parents who insist therapy is over when you do not agree, and others who would, quite literally, see you forever if you let them. Termination can be a powerful time in treatment, and determining when it is time to terminate with teens and their families and how to conduct your final sessions is critically important. After all, these decisions will be your final ones as a provider for your clients. Keeping your own feelings and countertransference reactions in mind is also relevant, as they guide how and when you discuss termination.

This final chapter was a bittersweet one for me to write. I was reminded of many clients that I have said goodbye to and the feelings each termination evoked in me. Some left before any of us were ready, due to family relocations or placement changes; others terminated without warning, and I grieved the abrupt ends to those relationships. I went back and read e-mails and cards I have been sent by former, successfully terminated clients over the years and marveled at their journeys. I thought about my own personal experiences terminating with therapists and supervisors. Finally, I reflected on the process of writing this book, realizing that with the close of this chapter comes the end of one of the most challenging and rewarding experiences of my life so far.

INITIATION OF TERMINATION

Why Do We Have to Terminate, Anyway?

Termination is an important part of any therapeutic relationship. First, it extends the metaphor of the therapy room acting as a microcosm of clients' worlds. Throughout life, clients will say many hellos and goodbyes, and it is important that they value relationships and learn to experience and work through feelings of ambivalence, loss, and doubt. Oftentimes, this process is somewhat natural, with teens detaching themselves over time as symptoms remit and developmental milestones (e.g., identity development and independence) are reached. Treatment termination, then, marks the end of a particular chapter in the life of teens and their parents. I believe that a termination session, even in the case of a premature termination (PT), is necessary and should be requested whenever possible (more on that below) to provide closure. Second, termination emphasizes the finite nature of the therapeutic relationship, which is not designed to last forever and is defined in part by

> the presence and management of a frame … that explicitly differentiates it from other relationships, both personal and professional, defines its limits, marks its boundaries and so implicitly suggests its temporality. Unlike other relationships which, when all goes well, may last a lifetime, or which evolve and transform themselves in response to relatively predetermined milestones, [therapists and clients] engage in a relationship that is intended to be time limited … [h]owever indeterminate that time may be. (Bass, 2009, pp. 749–750)

Many clients and their parents begin treatment focused only on the *now:* presenting symptoms and the search for solutions. It may be difficult for them to think about anything other than the problems right in front of them, including the fact that at some point, it will be time to end treatment. Swift and Greenberg (2015) suggest that the promise of termination encourages clients to develop "clear and appropriate expectations," so that they can be "ready, and willing, to start thinking about the end of psychotherapy and what it is that they are trying to achieve while in treatment" (p. 93).

Along these lines, I do like to mention termination throughout treatment, both to begin desensitizing parents and teens to the idea and to remind them that treatment cannot continue forever. I often tell them that it is my job to "work myself out of a job" and that the goal is not to need to come in anymore. By talking about termination, we can openly discuss realistic expectations about the duration of treatment, assess progress and goals, and prepare for feelings that may arise as the termination date nears. This process is by no means linear—Bass (2009) refers to it as a "moving target"—and I often find myself revisiting the idea of termination *many* times with both teens and their parents.

Signs That It Is Time to Terminate

It is difficult to determine what merits "successful termination" when treating adolescents, and some propose that it is simply a pause in treatment before teens return as adult clients. I have certainly worked with clients who I anticipate will return to treatment at some point in their lives, while for others, I consider termination a true end to treatment. For these reasons, I like Delgado and Strawn's (2012) conceptualization of termination as

> the time when the adolescent and his or her parents end a therapeutic relationship with the therapist, which is marked by the adolescent's resumption of a course of healthy psychological development by the integration of the work achieved during the therapy and by improvement in the symptoms that originally brought the young patient to treatment … Termination is heralded by

> dysfunctional patterns no longer needing to be repeated, healthier relationships with new objects becoming apparent, and the relinquishing of pathological defenses. (p. 24)

When teens begin complaining that they have nothing left to talk about, telling you that they believe they are doing better, or wondering if sessions can become less frequent, they are likely beginning to consider termination. I would strongly encourage you to pay attention to these indirect signs; Delgado and Strawn (2012) suggest they may represent a teen's dilemma over feeling better but not quite wanting to end the therapeutic relationship or treatment. For many clients,

> the relationship with the [therapist] becomes meaningful and sustaining in its own right … [therapy] itself has become an enriching part of the [client]'s life, with ongoing benefits that go beyond any original expectations … making a decision to end the relationship a far more problematic challenge than could have been anticipated the day the [client] met the [therapist]. (Bass, 2009, p. 751)

Many teens come to care for their therapists and fear that broaching the conversation of termination will hurt their therapists' feelings. I have had many a termination conversation that began with "No offense, but …" or "You're great, but …" Missing appointments is another common sign that termination may be approaching, as some teens will do so to avoid the grief reactions that come with ending treatment.

Teens and I discuss termination when we can identify and agree upon the achievement of both tangible and intangible treatment goals. Oftentimes, early goals are comprised primarily as symptom relief and expand over time to include more overarching, identity-related, and interpersonally driven aims. Indeed, Shedler (2010) suggests,

> Successful treatment should not only relieve symptoms (i.e., get rid of something) but also foster the positive presence of psychological capacities and resources. Depending on the person and the circumstances, these might include the capacity to have more fulfilling relationships, make more effective use of one's talents and abilities, maintain a realistically based sense of self-esteem … and face life's challenges with greater freedom and flexibility. (p. 100)

When an adolescent client is able to demonstrate growth such as this, you have done your job, and it is time to talk about termination.

THE TERMINATION CONVERSATION AND ITS AFTERMATH

You might be thinking (or hoping) that your clients will just tell you when they are ready to finish treatment. Although I have had parents and their teens tell me that they are finished, more often, I have to initiate the conversation. Similarly, Grant (2000) found that therapists were usually the trigger for the termination conversation in family therapy, and he guessed that many families may have continued to meet indefinitely had the therapist not broached the subject.

Planned termination acts, in some ways, as a sort of sealant on the therapeutic work you have done and can be a positive growth experience if handled correctly (Nursten, 1997). Improvements can be solidified, and clients can leave feeling prepared to handle future problems (Maples & Walker, 2014). Indeed, many clients leave therapy feeling more positive than negative emotions (Quintana & Holahan, 1992). On the other hand, poorly executed endings can act as a "heavy, renewed cumulative trauma," particularly if clients and/or their parents feel as though you are no longer emotionally committed to your work together (Huntley, 2008, p. 62).

Timing and What to Say

As ready as you may see clients and their parents to terminate, remember that endings can be intimidating. For teens and parents, termination can go smoothly when a three-step process is followed (Grant, 2000). First, the therapist broaches the topic. I usually have been thinking about termination for a few sessions by the time I bring it up to clients, and I opt for a genuine and basic approach at the start of a session. I do this to leave plenty of time to discuss feelings and reactions without trying to squeeze it in at the end of the session and then sending the family away. I typically say something like,

> I've been thinking about your treatment and about how far you have come since you first started therapy. [I give a couple examples.] I've also noticed that we are having a little less to talk about, and sometimes our sessions feel a little casual. This isn't a bad thing! It means we are running out of things to talk about, and when that happens, it is usually time to start thinking about winding down therapy. How do you feel about that?

I like to pay attention to first responses to my message that I see them as ready to terminate; some clients and parents nod, as if they had been thinking the same thing, while others look panicked or shocked. If they are in the former group, clients and parents consider termination; I encourage them to decide if they think now is the right time and evaluate the productivity and necessity of recent sessions. If they agree with my assessment, they agree to terminate and negotiate what the end will look like. When we are all on the same page and moving forward with termination, we discuss the number of remaining sessions and options for a return to therapy in the future. If they do not think now is the right time or still think there is work to be done, then we have another conversation altogether. With teens, this conversation usually involves us deciding on a number of sessions to conduct before discussing termination again. We use the suggestion of termination as the impetus to explore their anxieties, views of self, and future goals. More often, in my experience, however, it is parents who are not ready, and we will discuss them later in this chapter.

But back to families who feel ready to terminate. Like so many other things in therapy, time constraints are somewhat arbitrary when it comes to deciding how much time to dedicate to termination. That being said, I almost *always* suggest two to four sessions after our initial discussion about ending treatment, a guideline recommended in interpersonal therapy as well (Weissman, Markowitz, & Klerman, 2000). Why two to four sessions? For one, I like to spend some time processing the termination plan in the next session. Some questions I might ask include the following:

- How were you feeling after you left here last session?
- Were you surprised when I brought up the idea of termination? (If I initiated the conversation) OR Were you surprised at my response when you brought up the idea of termination? (If they or their parents initiated the conversation)
- How are you feeling today about terminating?
- Do you feel like we have any unfinished business?

Over the next couple of sessions, we tend to do a "test run," spacing appointments out a little more so that teens (and their parents) can get some practice with managing situations and exploring solutions without me. In the remaining sessions, we address questions such as:

- What resources did you use? How do you think it went?
- How did it feel to work through that problem without my help?
- What does your handling of this situation tell you about your readiness to terminate?

Of course, flexibility is needed. I have extended termination dates to accommodate sudden break-ups, deaths in the family, and medication alterations. Certainly, dates can be changed, if need be, without losing sight of the goal of termination and autonomy (Delgado & Strawn, 2012).

The Role of Attachment

Attachment can be a useful framework for thinking about termination. Assuming the teen has developed a positive attachment with you, he internalizes, or incorporates, this relationship into his understanding of himself, the world, and relationships. The relationship guides his expectations, thoughts, feelings, and behaviors in close relationships (Hazan & Shaver, 1994). Bembry and Ericson (1999) suggest that in termination, adolescents work through the loss of the therapist but are able to think about relationships in new ways and tolerate subsequent losses. In other words, they are able to take what they have learned in therapy and experienced in the relationship, and they apply it to future situations. Clients sometimes tell me that they "hear my voice" when they are trying to make a decision or being too hard on themselves. After experiencing a positive therapeutic attachment, they seek out and build relationships that are founded upon mutual respect, equality, and kindness. In these ways, therapy facilitates a positive attachment experience and sets teens up for positive attachment experiences outside of therapy. It is time for termination when the strengths of the therapeutic alliance can be successfully transferred to other relationships.

Attachment style factors in when we think about responses to termination. As I just said, there can be a definite loss when termination occurs, a fact that surprises many parents and teens. After all, many clients come into treatment with the expectation that you will help them "fix" their problems and send them on their way. Few are adequately prepared for how important of a fixture you become in their families; Gil and Crenshaw (2016) call this becoming "faux extended family" (p. 192), and Bass (2009) beautifully articulates this concept when he says,

> [The] relationship with the [therapist] becomes meaningful and sustaining in its own right. [Therapy] itself has become an enriching part of the patient's life, with ongoing benefits that go beyond any original expectations of what [therapy] might bring, making a decision to end the relationship a far more problematic challenge than could have been anticipated the day the patient met the [therapist]. (p. 751)

This challenge will be encountered differently depending on attachment patterns. Securely attached parents and teens will often experience this feeling of loss but are able to work through the feelings and walk away with positive feelings about termination. On the other hand, ambivalent individuals may experience termination as rejection, abandonment, or traumatic loss. They may have a much harder time saying goodbye, especially if they have been in long-term treatment (Shulman, 1999). And what about parents and teens who never quite developed a close relationship with you, despite your best attempts to foster a healthy reliance on treatment and productive alliances? In termination, these individuals' avoidant attachment styles may manifest as expressing little to no feelings about termination, which can be frustrating for therapists (more on that below).

Anger may also present itself during the process of termination, and this, too, has been conceptualized as an attachment strategy. Although it is often considered a manifestation of insecure attachment—an attempt to make demands or withdraw from the therapist to express pain—some securely attached individuals will also express anger when threatened with separation from someone with whom they have grown attached (Dalenberg, 2004). I have noticed that I am often prepared for the anxiety and stress reactions, but less primed when clients or their parents meet my suggestion of termination with anger and/or accusation. After all, "So you are just done with us then?" is a pretty provocative way to respond to my reflection on therapy as successful. Considering this anger as an attempt to forestall abandonment rather than a personal attack allows me to address it with care in therapy, just as I do with anxiety and stress reactions.

WHEN THE PARENT ISN'T READY

When teens and their parents demonstrate self-awareness and insight, we can approach termination as a joint decision in which everyone is able to acknowledge the related feelings of loss and finality while also celebrating the success of treatment. Clients can leave treatment feeling calm and happy (Marx & Gelso, 1987). But what about parents who are not ready to say goodbye? These parents will panic, insisting that it is not the right time, and they will resist the notion that treatment is coming to an end. Recognizing what that panic can look like, understanding what might be contributing to it, and preparing parents to manage it will assist you in ending therapy the same way you have been conducting it all along—in a working alliance.

What You Can Expect to See

I review progress with parents and teens throughout treatment, and termination is always a part of that discussion. Specifically, we talk about treatment frequency (i.e., too frequent? Not frequent enough?) and when we should review again (e.g., family session in three months, ongoing parent sessions, revisit in a month and begin discussing plans for termination). Despite this part of treatment, some parents are truly surprised when their teen and I share with them our thoughts about termination. They may feel as though termination is happening *to* them, a passive experience rather than a collaborative decision to be made (Grant, 2000). They may express anger, feelings of abandonment, or fear. They may withdraw in the sessions that follow, physically or emotionally, or you may experience a passive aggressive comment or two (e.g., "I guess I can see your point; you aren't really doing much for us anymore"). Gil and Crenshaw (2016) share instances where parents encourage their children to ask to stay in treatment, find new problem areas to focus upon, and/or report regression in issues that have been considered resolved (p. 191).

Contributors to Termination Reluctance

It is not uncommon for parents to have a different perspective of teens' readiness to terminate treatment. Parents may believe there is more work to be done; they may suspect that their teen is not being honest with you (this includes only sharing successes between sessions), or they have other goals for treatment that the teen does not share. By this point, you will have a good understanding of your client's parents, and you have undoubtedly decided whether they are reliable reporters. Keep this in mind as you integrate parents' thoughts on termination into your own.

Also consider parents' emotions evoked in termination, which may be painful and/or difficult in nature. Many of parents' reactions will mirror those of teens and therapists during the termination process. Fear or sadness associated with saying goodbye is common. One of my clients' fathers is only now, five years later, able to tolerate the idea that treatment will end one day. This directly coincides with his daughter's fears, which have sabotaged her progress multiple times over the years. Parents may have unresolved feelings about their adolescents' progress in treatment, particularly if treatment has resulted in increasing autonomy, new parenting demands, or referrals for family therapy (Delgado & Strawn, 2012). Finally, some parents develop a dependency on their teen's therapist, and this overreliance leads to anxiety about managing future issues without the therapist there to walk them through it.

How to Manage Parents' Feelings

One of the first things I like to impress on parents is that their thoughts and feelings play a role in termination. Parents get to be a part of this—it is not a passive experience for them, and they are *not* being "kicked out" of therapy (Delgado & Strawn, 2012). To that end, parents can negotiate a termination that feels as safe and comfortable as possible.

Hirschberg (1969) suggests that parents will view termination more positively if they can manage several pieces of the process. First, parents must be able to recognize and support their teen's readiness to leave treatment. Understanding the reasons behind their teen's decision to terminate treatment is often helpful. Parents have admitted that they thought their teen was just "making a snap decision," but once they realized that termination was considered thoughtfully in treatment, they were more open to the idea. Second, parents must understand the range of emotions their teen may experience. I will often encourage teens to share their conflicting feelings about termination so that parents can be aware of ambivalence, possible self-sabotage, feelings of abandonment, anxiety, or sadness.

Third, I work to ensure that parents recognize and accept their teen's success in treatment; many times parents insist that their teen has not yet made enough progress. According to Hirschberg (1969),

> It is difficult for parents to realize that [treatment] does not have to do the job completely but that something can be left for the positive interplay between the child, the parents, the environment, and its resources … [P]arents must be helped to direct their attention not only to the problem areas of the patient but to his problem-free areas also. It is important for parents to realize that [treatment] is a means toward helping the child and not a cure for the child or his problems. (pp. 364–365)

In this same vein, parents may also need approval and assistance in accepting their parenting accomplishments. Fourth, parents must be able to discuss their own feelings about termination. This includes being able to tolerate feelings of loss without experiencing the end of therapy as abandonment (Delgado & Strawn) and awareness of angry feelings. Hirschberg (1969) discusses parents' tendency to have the "illogical but deeply felt thought, 'If you really liked my child and if you really liked me, you would not be willing to let us go. It makes me angry that you do not insist on holding onto us. I thought we meant more to you than this …'" (p. 368).

Fifth, I try to be genuine with parents in sharing my own feelings about termination with their adolescent. It is comforting for parents to know that I am experiencing a feeling of loss as well as they are, and sometimes I have found that it normalizes their experience. I often say something like "This is both the best and hardest part of my job! I am so proud of my families when they have done the work and are ready to move on, but I am sad to say goodbye and no longer be a part of their lives." Related to this, and as a final step in the termination process, I emphasize the fact that the teen and parents will be "substituting their own relationship as well as other meaningful relationships for the ones that previously existed between teen and parents and [therapist]" (Hirschberg, 1969, p. 369). I *always* encourage families to let me know how they are doing and share good news. I find that this helps me process my loss (more on that below) but also highlights the faith that I have in the teen's ability to use the knowledge and skills gained in treatment, the parent–teen relationship, and parents' capacity to problem-solve and make good decisions. Just a few weeks ago, I received an e-mail from a mother whose teen had just completed her first winter track season, something she would never have been able to do (and her mother would have never been able to support) prior to intensive trauma treatment.

COMING BACK: TUNE-UPS

Terminations can seem a bit less scary to parents and adolescents when there is an understanding that the family can return to treatment if future problems arise. I completely agree with Eliana Gil (Gil & Crenshaw, 2016) when she says that having ongoing contact with clients throughout different stages in their lives and development can be incredibly rewarding. Sometimes, I reconnect with the parents when they bring another one of their children to treatment, and my former clients will accompany their siblings just to say "hi." Other times, my original client returns for a session or two. I call these sessions *tune-ups* and I frame them as positive, healthy check-ups. A former client, Ava, whose sister I now see on a regular basis, likes to come in for tune-ups. If she is having a tough time, her mom will ask her if she wants to schedule an appointment with me, and Ava will say, "I'm not ready to go yet." I give her parents so much credit for respecting her self-assessment! Once she is ready, Ava will tell her mom, "It's time to give Amie a call," and we will schedule an appointment. It seems that she is both comforted and challenged by my presence. She seems to like coming in on *her* terms, and I believe that our work is more productive when she can recognize her needs and seek me out to help her with them.

Another advantage to the *open-door terminations*, as they are often called in the literature, is that therapists can be flexible with clinical goals and approaches. I think this is probably its greatest "selling point" when it comes to working with teenagers. Many times, adolescents are referred to treatment for specific problems, and although I can see how deeper issues may be related, teens are not ready to do the work. The option to come back into treatment, if needed, emphasizes that there is more work to be done while respecting the client's limits. Should the family return, you already have some contextual knowledge that you can draw upon in the "next round." Furthermore, Gil and Crenshaw (2016) suggest the teen may be more likely to initiate a return to therapy than the first time, and that those who return

> often engage in more determined and meaningful work than in the initial period. One reason for this is that developmentally they may be better equipped emotionally and cognitively to engage in and to benefit from the therapy. Another is that they are returning to a familiar setting and person—usually positive associations have been made. (p. 36)

Finally, I am careful to frame a return to treatment as a positive step, *not* a failure. Many clients fear that they will fail when they leave treatment, and parents experience anxiety, disappointment, and even shame when they find themselves once again in need of a child therapist. Therefore, I explain tune-ups simply as a parent and/or teen's recognition that things are not working and emphasize that self-awareness, interdependence, and help-seeking are all great strengths that keep a person from returning to "square one." I always take time with parents and teens to discuss "warning signs" that it might be time to return to treatment. Together, we identify four or five signs, such as

- thoughts about suicide or incidents of self-harm;
- feeling sad or anxious more days than not for a couple of weeks;
- coping skills that have been working are no longer working; and
- new problems that feel bigger than parents and teens can handle.

There can be drawbacks to an open-door approach as well, including a minimization of termination-related feelings, or a perception on the part of teens or parents that the therapist is not confident about their future success. Clients may be sending you an important message that they are not quite ready to terminate when they demonstrate overwhelming relief at the option to return (Gil & Crenshaw, 2016). However, in my opinion, all of these issues can be addressed as you prepare for termination; feelings about the end can still be elicited, discussions about my confidence in their future success can be had, and clients' anxieties about life without the "safety net" of therapy can be processed. To me, the advantages of open-door terminations far outweigh the disadvantages.

PREMATURE TERMINATION: WHEN THE TEEN AND THERAPIST ARE NOT READY

We have all had it happen: things seem to be going well, treatment is progressing, and then, all of a sudden, the family stops attending sessions or refuses to participate in treatment. Sometimes we have an inkling as to why it has happened; other times, we are blindsided. There are many reasons why treatment ends before it is time, including managed care restrictions, unexpected job loss or family relocations, and the therapist leaving his/her position (Delgado & Strawn, 2012; Gil & Crenshaw, 2016). For the purposes of this section, however, we are going to focus on PT by the family—specifically, by the parents. PT can be defined as

> the idea that the client has not completed a full course of treatment … has unilaterally decided to stop attending sessions without the therapist's agreement and/or without discussing the decision with the therapist, and … a significant amount of relief from the client's original problems has not been met. (Swift, Greenberg, Whipple, & Kominiak, 2012, p. 379)

PT is relatively common in child and adolescent therapy and has been attributed to a variety of youth, parent, and therapy/therapist factors (de Haan,

Boon, de Jong, Hoeve, & Vermeiren, 2013). As we discussed in chapter 1, parents play an important role in getting teens into treatment, so it would stand to reason that they are a salient factor in whether teens *stay* in treatment.

Before we get into reasons why parents prematurely terminate, let me stress that parents have *every* right to terminate treatment. When they think their teen has made sufficient improvement, parents are often able to articulate that they are happy with the progress and ready to terminate. They permit you to close out therapy in a positive, paced way that gives you and their teen time to accommodate. In these cases, you can present the idea of tune-ups should the teen or family wish to return later to do additional work. Parents may also choose to end treatment due to financial, transportation, and availability issues (Garcia & Weisz, 2002). I recently had a client whose parents were going through a messy, expensive divorce. As I do not take insurance, they informed me that they would be seeking a therapist within their network. When treatment must end, I try to work with parents to have at least one more session to terminate with their teen, and when possible, I assist them in finding a new provider.

Parents who terminate unexpectedly—without any input from the therapist and before any improvements have been made—are different. For these parents, expectations often play a big role. In the same way that some parents want their teen to continue treatment indefinitely because they are not yet "fixed," they may want to terminate because their teen has not been "fixed" (Grant, 2000). Many times, this expectation that therapy can fix their child corresponds with their consideration of their teen as "the problem." These parents may have struggled to accept the role of the parent–teen relationship, parent variables, and family dynamics in the teen's difficulties. Or, more simply, they may have expected rapid improvement sooner than was realistic; studies have found that many clients expect to recover much more quickly than treatment outcome research suggests (see Swift & Greenberg, 2015, for a review).

Parents who are struggling to form a working alliance with their teen's therapist are also at risk for PT. Their perceptions of treatment are important when it comes to whether or not it will continue; that is, when parents do not think you are doing the right thing, care about them or their teen, or are meeting their needs, they may quit therapy (Burns, 2004; Burns, Cortell, & Wagner, 2008; Desrosiers, Saint-Jean, & Breton, 2015; Joyce, Piper, Ogrodniczuk, & Klein, 2007). Parental psychological characteristics, including depressive symptoms, paranoia, and personality issues like we discussed in chapter 6, are also risk factors for teens' treatment (Desrosiers et al., 2015; King, Hovey, Brand, & Wilson, 1997; Venable & Thompson, 1998). When parents are struggling with personality disorders, they may be hostile, struggle to see the purpose of treatment or to manage feelings evoked by the therapy, fail to empathize with their teen, and/or see you as an ally rather than a competitor (Desrosiers et al., 2015; Venable & Thompson, 1998). Furthermore, they may be unwilling or unable to change their relationship to better meet their teen's needs. Boundary issues, including overprotectiveness and an overestimation of teen's autonomy, can also impact whether or not teen's treatment continues (Desrosiers et al., 2015).

Suggestions to Reduce Premature Termination[1]

1. Provide parents and teens with information about duration and patterns of change

Parents often expect symptoms to remit much more quickly than they actually do, and unrealistically high expectations for treatment duration and recovery have been linked time and time again with treatment dropout (Swift & Greenberg, 2015; Swift et al., 2012). Parents who think treatment should be progressing more quickly may feel disappointed, which can prevent them from seeing the potential benefits of treatment or small changes that have occurred. In the majority of my cases, I tell parents that I plan for at least three months so that we all have time to build a relationship, the teen has time to learn and practice some new skills, and I have time to understand the problem from as many different angles as possible. Then, as we near the end of those three months, we discuss my impressions, progress, challenges, and next steps. I have found that giving practical estimates of treatment gives parents some realistic ideas about treatment duration and reduces the likelihood that they give up too soon.

Swift and colleagues (2012) also recommend sharing potential courses of change with clients. This includes the possibility that some clients feel better after only a few sessions but that it typically takes longer for overall functioning to improve. They suggest that this may prevent parents and teens from terminating prematurely before addressing issues completely, only to return frustrated when gains are not maintained or new issues replace the old. Another possibility is that, on the course to recovery, some clients feel worse before they feel better. If clients are not prepared for this, they may think treatment is not working. Indeed, even after sharing this risk, I *still* have to remind parents that treatment is working even when it seems that things are getting worse. A former therapist of mine once told me, "Sometimes you will leave here feeling better, and sometimes you will leave here feeling worse. It is important to remember that it is *all* part of the journey. If you trust the process, we will get you where you want to go." I have shared a similar sentiment with parents and teens many times, especially after a trauma when I am preparing them for the difficult work ahead, or in cases where a teen begins expressing himself for the first time after being silently compliant for years.

2. Provide realistic role expectations

Help parents and teens know what to expect from therapy with you. This might include explanations of how sessions will be structured, who will do most of the talking, and what approach you will use and why. Ask parents and teens what their experiences have been in the past; if this is their first time in treatment, ask them what they were expecting when they came to your office, or what others have told them about therapy. Parents may be surprised to learn that they will not be in the room for the majority of the session, for example, or, at the opposite end of the spectrum, may not realize that you expect them to be present for check-ins and check-outs. Parents and teens may worry that they are "doing it wrong" when it comes to out of office contact, disclosures, or asking for guidance. Similarly, they may think *you* are doing it wrong if you do not engage in advice giving or will not accept calls at 3 a.m. Remember the boundaries I mentioned in the first chapters of the book, and make them clear early on so that families know what to expect. While some parents and teens will come into therapy with relatively accurate expectations of the process, others will need much more guidance and clarification (Swift et al., 2012).

3. Incorporate client and parent preferences

Clients and their parents will always have preferences, particularly if they have past experience with therapy. Just by choosing you and not another therapist from an online search or referral list, they have already demonstrated a preference. I like to find out why clients choose me as their therapist to ensure that I will be able to accommodate their preferences. For example, one parent told me that I "didn't seem too stuffy" and they liked that I "acted like a real person during our intake session" but "seemed to know [my] stuff." What I heard in those statements was that they wanted someone genuine and approachable, yet someone who was also knowledgeable and able to help.

I try my best to accommodate parent and client preferences, but there are times when I am unable to do so. The issues I encounter the most often are boundary-related, such as frequent and lengthy out of session contact, parental preferences to "stay out of" treatment, or addressing goals that are in direct opposition to the treatment plan. One parent in particular comes to mind as I write this. She was educated and had been successful in individual therapy, and she was convinced that her daughter, Andie, had an eating disorder. She admitted that her own struggles with an eating disorder were probably factoring in as well, but insisted I was failing by not addressing the problem as an eating disorder. I had a different perception of Andie's relationship with food, and I believed that working on her negative self-talk and depressive symptoms would enable her to develop healthy self-care rituals. Her mother and I had a couple of pretty heated conversations over this issue. I respected her viewpoints and right to change providers if she wanted to take a different approach. I also expressed my own concerns about overestimating the food component and underestimating the depressive component.

Ultimately, I left it up to Andie and her mother to decide their preferences about treatment approach and provider. We compromised on the approach: We would try addressing the depression as primary and pay close attention to the eating behaviors. If the eating behaviors worsened or new symptoms that pointed to an eating disorder diagnosis emerged, we would change course. Andie's mother seemed happy to be collaborating on the treatment plan, and they stayed in treatment. Over time, Andie's depressive symptoms and food difficulties improved, and her mother's anxieties about an eating disorder dissipated. More than once, Andie's mother reflected that, had I taken a hard-nosed approach to the treatment plan, they would have left treatment, but that our arrangement had made her feel heard and respected.

4. Strengthen early hope

In order to commit to and stay in treatment, parents must have a general hope that therapy can help their teen (and family) get better. One way that I try to instill hope is to express my own confidence and hopefulness that treatment will work. Expressing confidence in the client and parents' abilities to enact change is also important (Constantino, Glass, Arnkoff, & Ametrano, 2011). I usually point out how difficult it is to make and attend the first appointment, giving them credit for taking the first step toward healing.

My work with trauma clients has convinced me of the value of careful pacing in treatment. Much has been written about the phases of treatment, the first of which involves *remoralization*, or increases in subjective well-being that enable clients to reduce symptoms and learn long-term coping strategies (Howard, Lueger, Maling, & Martinovich, 1993; Lambert & Ogles, 2004). For many of my clients, spending time developing alliances enables both clients and parents to feel understood, accepted, and trusting, which in turn, often helps them feel hopeful about the work ahead. This hope and their relationships with me protect them from being overwhelmed and alone and help them stay in treatment.

5. Foster the working and therapeutic alliances
After dedicating an entire chapter to this topic, I do not have too much more to add here. Remember everything we talked about in chapter 2, and prioritize the working and therapeutic alliances, as they are the foundation of all of the work you will do with your teen clients.

6. Assess and discuss treatment progress
It makes sense that parents want to know how treatment is going. As we have discussed in previous chapters, parents like to have a sense of what is going on in sessions. Regular check-ins and check-outs help keep parents in the loop and assist them in understanding and recognizing the multidimensional aspects of problems as they are revealed in treatment (Grant, 2000). During these times, research suggests that it may also be helpful to compare actual progress to parents' expectations of progress and what is expected for progress to continue (Howard, Moras, Brill, Martinovich, & Lutz, 1996). Something as simple as "How are you feeling about the progress we've made so far? Were you hoping we'd be further along?" or "I think something that might help us make more progress would be more follow-through on the homework. What ideas do you have for increasing how often the homework is getting done?" can go a long way toward keeping everyone involved in the process and decreasing the likelihood of dropout.

COUNTERTRANSFERENCE

As I have mentioned repeatedly throughout this book, I strive to be genuine with my clients. Oftentimes in the termination process, this takes the form of self-disclosure about my feelings. I find that it helps parents and teens normalize their own affective experiences, feel comfortable to express ambivalence or anxiety, and assertively express what they need to be successful in the process. Of course, in order to be genuine, I have to first understand what it is that I am feeling and then make a clinical decision about whether to share it. In this section, we are going to focus on negative reactions, but I wanted to point out that I have *many* positive emotions regarding my clients' treatment endings as well. I feel genuine hopefulness, excitement, and relief. I also experience pride; after all, who doesn't love a good success story? In some ways, I rely on those stories during times when it seems that all of my clients are having a tough time, or when a family unexpectedly terminates. As we have been discussing throughout this book, adolescent treatment can be a long, complicated marathon, and termination is the finish line. What a rewarding experience to agree together that your work is done.

Negative Emotional Reactions

Kramer (1982) found that the most commonly endorsed therapist reaction to termination was sadness, suggesting that therapists have their own experiences of loss when termination nears (in Maples & Walker, 2014). In addition to the loss of a meaningful, rewarding relationship, therapists may experience anxiety about their clients' future success, concern for their client who is experiencing termination anxiety. It is important to recognize that you can feel sadness about ending but still follow through with it. Like some clients and parents, you may also have a hard time admitting that it is time for termination and setting a final session date. Temporary setbacks or crises may have you second-guessing your decision, even if your client is able to manage such situations effectively.

You may also find yourself having reactions to parents' and teens' nonreactions. I remember a client with whom I had worked for over a year; as readiness for termination became more evident, I began bracing myself for the discussion. I was sure that my suggestion would be met with resistance; this was an anxious mom who admitted that she struggled with change, and a daughter who regularly told me that she waited all week for her sessions. When I broached the topic of termination, however, they nodded, said they had been talking about the same subject on the ride over to the appointment, and asked how we should move forward. I was stunned and, admittedly, a little hurt. Weren't they sad to end treatment? Hadn't this relationship mattered to them at all? Was I silly to be sad? Remember that not all clients will be sad, and that this is okay and actually quite normal, although some clients will display "pre-protest" wherein they show little to no emotion, only to experience a full grief reaction as termination gets closer (Swanson & Schaefer, 1993). Maples and Walker (2014) consider that

> [t]he descriptive literature has typically devoted an overwhelming majority of discussion of termination reactions to negative reactions with little or no discussion of possible positive reactions … In contrast to the historical emphasis on loss in the termination process, extant research suggests that many clients experience the termination phase favorably. (p. 106)

I cannot emphasize enough how invaluable good colleagues and supervisors are during the termination process. Two years ago, two of my grandparents passed away within one month of each other. Around that time, I had a couple of clients nearing termination, and I was acutely aware of my desire to avoid the end, coupled with the thought, "I just can't handle *another* goodbye." As we have discussed, termination is largely a subjective decision. I wanted to make sure that I was not keeping anyone in treatment to avoid additional losses or dismissing ambivalent feelings about termination that might be signaling that it was not yet time. I was able to process these feelings and use my supervisors and colleagues as sounding boards as I teased apart how much my recent losses were playing into my decisions. In the end, I approached the termination conversation with one client and waited with the other; in time, I had meaningful, largely positive endings with both.

Issues that you have identified throughout treatment, such as parental barriers to treatment, may once again rear their ugly heads. Narcissistic parents, for example, may stir up feelings of resentment or a desire to highlight your achievements, as they seek to show you that their parenting abilities "outdo" yours. Remember that the ability of parents and teens to see themselves as capable of success without therapy *is* a positive thing, even if the parents' style is frustrating or makes you feel like your role has been minimized.

Responses after Premature Termination

Unfortunately, premature termination can intensify countertransference reactions, especially when you do not get an opportunity for closure due to sudden, unexpected endings. I always encourage parents to bring their teens in for one more session so that we can (sort of) terminate, but they (or their teens) are not always willing or able. In one case, a mother and I experienced an abrupt rupture in our alliance.[2] She began cancelling appointments at the last minute, complaining to her son's social worker about it, and largely disengaging from our sessions. As time went on, we had a couple of heated discussions where she was verbally abusive toward me and unhappy when I set some limits on her behavior. This mother refused to pay "one more penny" for her son and I to terminate and would not consider even a brief phone call or short (nonbillable) session. I felt so much anxiety, anger, and sadness for her son; after all, we were right in the middle of some difficult work when she "pulled the plug." In situations such as these, Gil and Crenshaw (2016) highly recommend seeking your own closure process, through supervision, expressive art activities, journaling/writing a letter, or engaging in some extra self-care so that you have the time and energy to process your loss experience. I spent some time processing this experience with my supervisor and was eventually able to make peace with the fact that although I might have done something, unknowingly, to offend or hurt the mother, it was not my responsibility to read minds, and that I could not *make* her continue treatment if she was unwilling. I had to accept that I had done my best, recognize that premature termination is always a risk, address my ambivalent feelings regarding the client and his mom, and hope that he had a positive enough experience in treatment that he might return to therapy one day as an adult.

SPECIAL CONSIDERATION: TERMINATION WITH PARENTS AND TEENS AFFECTED BY TRAUMA

Without a doubt, trauma complicates the termination process. Depending on the nature of trauma, you may be one of the first people whom your adolescent clients could trust; thus, termination's success is critically important, as it may act as their first healthy "good-bye" (Kliethermes & Wamser, 2012). For others, you may be one of the few people who believed them when they disclosed. To parents, you may represent safety, security, hope, and understanding. Remember, you entered their lives at a time when everything had changed and many losses had been sustained (remember chapter 7), and the thought of termination often arouses similar feelings and conflicts. Indeed, it is my trauma clients and parents who come to view me as "faux extended family" (Gil & Crenshaw, 2016, p. 192), which makes a goodbye all the more challenging. Be prepared for heightened countertransference reactions including feelings of responsibility, guilt, and sadness. Make referrals for parents to individual therapy if they still are experiencing significant distress, utilizing the rapport you have spent many sessions building and highlighting the necessity of parental mental health to maintain teens' treatment gains (Pearlman, Schwalbe, & Cloitre, 2010).

Finally, beware of the risk for premature termination among traumatized teens and their parents. In addition to all of the reasons we have already talked about that lead parents and teens to prematurely terminate, trauma research has found that avoidance symptoms, single incident traumas, traumas that did not involve threat to life or physical injury, and peer-perpetrated violence are associated with greater premature termination (Chasson, Mychailyszyn, Vincent, & Harris, 2013; Chasson, Vincent, & Harris, 2008).

CONCLUSION

Termination is a necessary part of treatment, and yet it can pose some interesting challenges for therapists, parents, and teens, whether treatment has lasted months or years. Although some clients do initiate the termination conversation, you will often find yourself in a position where you are required to get parents and teens thinking about ending treatment. Some parents and teens will share your opinion and readily negotiate the end of treatment with you, while others will not be ready. When it comes to termination, you can expect a myriad of feelings ranging from pride to anxiety for everyone involved. Sometimes, you will come to work only to find out that your client has unexpectedly and prematurely terminated treatment, and you will experience feelings about that as well. Focusing on the working and therapeutic alliances, being open to clients' preferences and goals, and instilling hope throughout treatment can help keep parents and teens engaged in treatment. While termination can be difficult, it can be one of the most rewarding moments in treatment with both teens and their parents.

NOTES

1. From Swift et al. (2012).
2. I still, to this day, do not know exactly what caused the rift, although I suspect it had to do with some difficult material her son and I were uncovering, symptoms that had improved but not remitted despite significant work in treatment, and some of the mom's personality issues.

Bibliography

Adam, K. S., Sheldon-Keller, A. E., & West, M. (1996). Attachment organization and history of suicidal behavior in clinical adolescents. *Journal of Consulting and Clinical Psychology*, *64*, 264–272.

Adshead, G. (2003). Dangerous and severe parenting disorder? Personality disorder, parenting and new legal proposals. *Child Abuse Review*, *12*, 227–237.

Afifi, T. D. (2003). "Feeling caught" in stepfamilies: Managing boundary turbulence through appropriate communication privacy rules. *Journal of Social & Personal Relationships*, *20*(6), 729–755.

Afifi, T. D., & McManus, T. (2010). Divorce disclosures and adolescents' physical and mental health and parental relationship quality. *Journal of Divorce & Remarriage*, *51*(2), 83–107. doi:10.1080/10502550903455141

Afifi, T. D., & Schrodt, P. (2003). Uncertainty and the avoidance of the state of one's family in stepfamilies, postdivorce single-parent families, and first-marriage families. *Human Communication Research*, *29*(4), 516–532.

Afifi, T. D., Afifi, W. A., & Coho, A. (2009). Adolescents' physiological reactions to their parents' negative disclosures about the other parent in divorced and nondivorced families. *Journal of Divorce & Remarriage*, *50*(8), 517–540.

Afifi, T. D., Hutchinson, S., & Krouse, S. (2006). Toward a theoretical model of communal coping in postdivorce families and other naturally occurring groups. *Communication Theory (10503293)*, *16*(3), 378–409. doi:10.1111/j.1468-2885.2006.00275.x

Afifi, T. D., McManus, T., Hutchinson, S., & Baker, B. (2007). Inappropriate parental divorce disclosures, the factors that prompt them, and their impact on parents' and adolescents' well-being. *Communication Monographs*, *74*(1), 78–102.

Aidane, E., Wendland, J., Rabain, D., & Marie, P. (2009). An atypical therapeutic approach: Therapeutic co-constructions of the early relationship between a borderline mother and her infant. *Psychiatrie de l'Enfant*, *52*, 131–166.

Ainsworth, M. D. S., & Wittig, B. A. (1969). Attachment and exploratory behavior of one-year-olds in a strange situation. In B. M. Foss (Ed.), *Determinants of infant behavior* (pp. 111–136). London, England: Methuen.

Alexander, P. C. (2003). Parent-child role reversal: Development of a measure and test of an attachment theory model. *Journal of Systemic Therapies*, *22*, 31–43.

Alisic, E., Boeije, H. R., Jongmans, M. J., & Kleber, R. J. (2012). Supporting children after single-incident trauma: Parents' views. *Clinical Pediatrics*, *51*(3), 274–282. doi:10.1177/0009922811423309

Alisic, E., Zalta, A. K., van Wesel, F., Larsen, S. E., Hafstad, G. S., Hassanpour, K., & Smid, G. E. (2014). Rates of post-traumatic stress disorder in trauma-exposed children and adolescents: Meta-analysis. *The British Journal of Psychiatry*, *204*, 335–340.

Almeida, D. M., Wethington, E., & Chandler, A. L. (1999). Daily transmission of tensions betwen marital dyads and parent-child dyads. *Journal of Marriage & Family*, *61*, 49–61.

Alvarez, K. M., Donohue, B., Kenny, M. C., Cavanagh, N., & Romero, V. (2005). The process and consequences of reporting child maltreatment: A brief overview for professionals in the mental health field. *Aggression and Violent Behavior*, *10*(3), 311–331.

Alvarez, K. M., Kenny, M. C., Donohue, B., & Carpin, K. M. (2004). Why are professionals failing to initiate mandated reports of child maltreatment, and are there any empirically based training programs to assist professionals in the reporting process? *Aggression and Violent Behavior*, *9*(5), 563–578.

American Academy of Child and Adolescent Psychiatry. (2010). Practice parameter for the assessment and treatment of children and adolescents with posttraumatic stress disorder. *Journal of the American Academy Child & Adolescent Psychiatry*, *49*(4), 4145–4430.

American Counseling Association. (2014). *ACA Code of Ethics*. Alexandria, VA: Author.

American Psychiatric Association. (2013a). *Diagnostic and Statistical Manual of Mental Disorders, Fifth Edition*. Washington, DC: American Psychiatric Publishing.

American Psychiatric Association. (2013b). Personality disorders. Retrieved from http://www.dsm5.org/Documents/Personality Disorders Fact Sheet.pdf

American Psychological Association. (2002). American Psychological Association ethical principles of psychologists and code of conduct. Retrieved from http://www.apa.org/ethics/code2002.html

Amianto, F., Daga, G. A., Bertorello, A., & Fassino, S. (2013). Exploring personality clusters among parents of ED subjects. Relationship with parents' psychopathology, attachment, and family dynamics. *Comprehensive Psychiatry*, *54*(7), 797–811. doi:10.1016/j.comppsych.2013.03.005

Ammerman, R. T., Shenk, C. E., Teeters, A. R., Noll, J. G., Putnam, F. W., & Van Ginkel, J. B. (2013). Multiple mediation of trauma and parenting stress in mothers in home visiting. *Infant Mental Health Journal*, *34*, 234–241.

Andrews, J. A., Hops, H., Ary, D. V., Tildesley, E., & Harris, J. (1993). Parental influence on early adolescent substance use: Specific and nonspecific effects. *Journal of Early Adolescence*, *13*(3), 285–310. doi:10.1177/0272431693013003004

Anthony, K. H. (1997). Bitter homes and gardens: The meanings of home to families of divorce. *Journal of Architectural and Planning Research*, *14*(1), 1–19.

Asano, M., Esaki K., Wakamatsu A., Kitajima T., Narita T., Naitoh H., Ozaki N., & Iwata N. (2013). Maternal overprotection score of the Parental Bonding Instrument predicts the outcome of cognitive behavior therapy by trainees for depression. *Psychiatry & Clinical Neurosciences*, *67*(5), 340–344. doi:10.1111/pcn.12054

Ashley, O. S., & Foshee, V. A. (2005). Adolescent help-seeking for dating violence: Prevalence, sociodemographic correlates, and sources of help. *Journal of Adolescent Health*, *36*(1), 25–31. doi:10.1016/j.jadohealth.2003.12.014

Assor, A., & Tal, K. (2012). When parents' affection depends on child's achievement: Parental conditional positive regard, self-aggrandizement, shame and coping in adolescents. *Journal of Adolescence*, *35*, 249–260. doi:10.1016/j.adolescence.2011.10.004

Assor, A., Roth, G., & Deci, E. L. (2004). The emotional costs of perceived parents' conditional regard: A self-determination theory analysis. *Journal of Personality*, *72*, 47–89.

Assor, A., Roth, G., Israeli, M., Freed, A., & Deci, E. L. (2007). Parental conditional positive regard: Another harmful type of parental control. Paper presented at the Society for Research in Child Development, Boston, MA.

Assor, A., Vansteenkiste, M., & Kabuth, B. (2009). Identified and introjection approach and introjection avoidance motivations in school and in sport: The limited benefits of self-worth strivings. *Journal of Educational Psychology*, *101*, 482–497.

Aunola, K., Stattin, H., & Nurmi, J.-E. (2000). Parenting styles and adolescents' achievement strategies. *Journal of the Study of Alcohol and Drugs*, *71*, 539–543.

Baetens, I., Claes, L., Martin, G., Onghena, P., Grietens, H., Van Leeuwen, K., … Griffith, J. W. (2014). Is nonsuicidal self-injury associated with parenting and family factors? *Journal of Early Adolescence*, *34*(3), 387–405. doi:10.1177/0272431613494006

Baetens, I., Claes, L., Muehlenkamp, J., Grietens, H., & Onghena, P. (2011). Non-suicidal and suicidal self-injurious behavior among Flemish adolescents: A web-survey. *Archives of Suicide Research*, *15*(1), 56–67. doi:10.1080/13811118.2011.540467

Bahr, S. J., & Hoffman, J. (2010). Parenting style, religiosity, peers, and adolescent heavy drinking. *Journal of the Study of Alcohol and Drugs*, *71*, 539–543.

Baiocco, R., Fontanesi, L., Santamaria, F., Ioverno, S., Marasco, B., Baumgartner, E., … Laghi, F. (2014). Negative parental responses to coming out and family functioning in a sample of lesbian and gay young adults. *Journal of Child and Family Studies*, *24*, 1490–1500. doi:10.1007/s10826-014-9954-z

Baker, A. J. L., & Ben Ami, N. (2011). To turn a child against a parent is to turn a child against himself. *Journal of Divorce and Remarriage*, *52*, 472–489.

Baker, A. J. L., & Brassard, M. R. (2013). Adolescents caught in parental loyalty conflicts. *Journal of Divorce & Remarriage*, *54*(5), 393–413. doi:10.1080/10502556.2013.800398

Baldwin, S. A., Christian, S., Berkeljon, A., Shadish, W. R., & Bean, R. (2012). The effects of family therapies for adolescent delinquency and substance abuse: A meta-analysis. *Journal of Marital and Family Therapy*, *38*(1), 281–304. doi:10.1111/j.1752-0606.2011.00248.x

Ballash, N., Leyfer, O., Buckley, A., & Woodruff-Borden, J. (2006). Parental control in the etiology of anxiety. *Clinical Child & Family Psychology Review*, *9*(2), 113–133. doi:10.1007/s10567-006-0007-z

Banyard, V. L. (1997). The impact of childhood sexual abuse and family functioning on four dimensions of women's later parenting. *Child Abuse and Neglect*, *21*(11), 1095–1107.

Barber, B. K. (2002). *Intrusive parenting: How psychological control affects children and adolescents*. Washington, DC: American Psychological Association.

Barber, B. K., & Harmon, E. L. (2002). Violating the self: Parental psychological control of children and adolescents. In B. K. Barber (Ed.), *Psychological control of children and adolescents* (pp. 15–52). Washington, DC: American Psychological Association.

Barfield-Cottledge, T. (2015). The triangulation effects of family structure and attachment on adolescent substance use. *Crime & Delinquency*, *61*(2), 297–320. doi:10.1177/0011128711420110

Barnes, D. H., Pazur, D., & Lester, D. (2014). Parents' views of their child's death by suicide. *Illness, Crisis, & Loss*, *22*(3), 181–193. doi:10.2190/IL.22.3.b

Barrowclough, C., & Hooley, J. M. (2003). Attributions and expressed emotion: A review. *Clinical Psychology Review*, *23*, 849–880.

Barth, F. D. (2014). Social media and adolescent development: Hazards, pitfalls and opportunities for growth. *Clinical Social Work Journal*, *43*(2), 201–208.

Bartimole, C. R. (2009). Teens who attempt suicide: Profile of survivors. (70), ProQuest Information & Learning, US. Retrieved from http://search.ebscohost.com/login.aspx?direct=true&db=psyh&AN=2009-99211-058&site=ehost-live&scope=site

Bass, A. (2009). It ain't over 'til it's over: Infinite conversations, imperfect endings, and the elusive nature of termination. *Psychoanalytic Dialogues*, *19*, 744–759.

Baumeister, R. F. (1990). Suicide as an escape from self. *Psychological Review*, *97*, 90–113.

Baumeister, R. F., & Leary, M. R. (1995). The need to belong: Desire for interpersonal attachments as a fundamental human motivation. *Psychological Bulletin*, *117*, 497–529.

Baumrind, D. (1968). Authoritarian vs. authoritative parental control. *Adolescence*, *3*(11), 255–272.

Baumrind, D. (1971). Current patterns of parental authority. *Developmental Psychology, 148 Monograph*, *4*(1) Part 2, 1–103.

Baumrind, D. (1991). The influence of parenting style on adolescent competence and substance use. *Journal of Early Adolescence*, *11*(1), 56–95.

Baumrind, D. (2003). Effects of authoritative parental control on child behavior. National Institute of Mental Health, U.S. Public Health Service, 888–892.

Beaver, K. M., da Silva Costa, C., Poersch, A. P., Freddi, M. C., Stelmach, M. C., Connolly, E. J., & Schwartz, J. A. (2014). Psychopathic personality traits and their influence on parenting quality: Results from a nationally representative sample of Americans. *Psychiatric Quarterly*, *85*(4), 497–511. doi:10.1007/s11126-014-9308-4

Beck, A. T., Rush, A. J., Shaw, B. F., & Emery, G. (1979). *Cognitive theory of depression*. New York, NY: Guilford Press.

Bedi, R. P., Davis, M. D., & Williams, M. W. (2005). Critical incidents in the formation of the therapeutic alliance from the client's perspective. *Psychotherapy: Theory, Research, Practice, Training*, *42*(3), 311–323. doi:10.1037/0033-3204.42.3.311

Begle, A. M., Hanson, R. F., Danielson, C. K., McCart, M. R., Ruggiero, K. J., Amstadter, A. B., ... Kilpatrick, D. G. (2011). Longitudinal pathways of victimization, substance use, and delinquency: Findings from the National Survey of Adolescents. *Addictive Behaviors*, *36*(7), 682–689. doi:10.1016/j.addbeh.2010.12.026

Behrman, R. (1994). Children and divorce: Overview and analysis. *The Future of Children*, *4*(1), 4–14.

Berger, L. E., Jodi, K. M., McElhaney, K. B., & Kuperminc, G. P. (2005). When adolescents disagree with others about their symptoms: Differences in attachment organization as an explanation of discrepancies between adolescent, parent, and peer reports of behavior problems. *Development and Psychopathology*, *17*, 509–528.

Betan, E., Heim, A. K., Zittel Conklin, C., & Westen, D. (2005). Countertransference phenomena and personality pathology in clinical practice: An empirical investigation. *The American Journal of Psychiatry*, *162*, 890–898.

Bhola, P., & Kapur, M. (2013). The development and role of the therapeutic alliance in supportive psychotherapy with adolescents. *Psychological Studies*, *58*(3), 207–215.

Bifulco, A., Schimmenti, A., Moran, P., Jacobs, C., Bunn, A., & Rusu, A. C. (2014). Problem parental care and teenage deliberate self-harm in young community adults. *Bulletin of the Menninger Clinic*, *78*(2), 94–114.

Black, B. M., Weisz, A. N., Preble, K. M., & Sharma, B. (2015). Parents' awareness of and anticipated responses to their teens' reports of dating violence. *Journal of Family Social Work*, *18*(1), 3–20. doi:10.1080/10522158.2014.968941

Bleakley, A., Jordan, A. B., & Hennessy, M. (2013). The relationship between parents' and children's television viewing. *Pediatrics*, *132*(2), e364–e371. doi:10.1542/peds.2012-3415

Block, A. M., & Greeno, C. G. (2011). Examining outpatient treatment dropout in adolescents: A literature review. *Child & Adolescent Social Work Journal*, *28*(5), 393–420.

Bobova, L., Finn, P. R., Rickert, M. E., & Lucas, J. (2009). Disinhibitory psychopathology and delay discounting in alcohol dependence: Personality and cognitive correlates. *Experimental and Clinical Psychopharmacology*, *17*, 51–61.

Bodden, D. H. M., & Dekovic, M. (2016). Multiproblem families referred for youth mental health: What's in a name? *Family Process*, *55*(1), 31–47.

Bogacki, D. F., & Weiss, K. J. (2007). Termination of parental rights: Focus on defendants. *Journal of Psychiatry and Law*, *35*, 25–45.

Bolen, R. M., & Lamb, J. L. (2004). Ambivalence of nonoffending guardians after child sexual abuse disclosure. *Journal of Interpersonal Violence*, *19*(2), 185–211. doi:10.1177/0886260503260324

Bordin, E. (1979). The generalizability of the psychoanalytic concept of the working alliance. *Psychotherapy: Theory, Research, and Practice*, *16*, 252–260.

Bornstein, R. F. (2012). From dysfunction to adaption: An interactionist model of dependency. *Annual Review of Clinical Psychology*, *8*, 291–316.

Bos, H., & Sandfort, T. (2010). Children's gender identity in lesbian and heterosexual two-parent families. *Sex Roles*, *62*(1/2), 114–126. doi:10.1007/s11199-009-9704-7

Boulton, S., & Hindle, D. (2000). Emotional abuse: The work of a multidisciplinary consultation group in a child psychiatric service. *Clinical Child Psychology & Psychiatry*, *5*(3), 439–452.

Bowlby, J. (1982). *Attachment and loss: Vol. 1. Attachment* (2nd ed.). New York, NY: Basic Books.

Bowling, S. W., Kearney, L. K., Lumadue, C. A., & St. Germain, N. R. (2002). Considering justice: An exploratory study of family therapy with adolescents. *Journal of Marital and Family Therapy*, *28*(2), 213–223. doi:10.1111/j.1752-0606.2002.tb00358.x

Bramsen, R. H., Lasgaard, M., Koss, M. P., Elklit, A., & Banner, J. (2012). Adolescent sexual victimization: A prospective study on risk factors for first time sexual assault. *European Child & Adolescent Psychiatry*, *21*(9), 521–526. doi:10.1007/s00787-012-0290-9

Brassard, M. R., & Donovan, K. L. (2006). Defining psychological maltreatment. In M. M. Feerick, J. F. Knutson, P. K. Trickett, & S. M. Flanzer (Eds.), *Child abuse and neglect: Definitions, classifications, and a framework for research* (pp. 3–27). Baltimore, MD: Paul H. Brookes.

Brennan, K. A., & Shaver, P. R. (1998). Attachment styles and personality disorders: Their connections to each other and to parental divorce, parental death, and perceptions of parental caregiving. *Journal of Personality*, *66*(5), 835–878. doi:10.1111/1467-6494.00034

Brent, D. A., Moritz, G., Liotus, L., Schweers, J., Balach, L., Roth, C., & Perper, J. A. (1998). Familial risk factors for adolescent suicide: A case-control study. In R. J. Kosky, H. S. Eshkevari, R. D. Goldney, & R. Hassan (Eds.), *Suicide prevention: The global context* (pp. 41–50). New York, NY: Plenum Press.

Brestan, E., & Payne, H. (2004). Behavioral parent training interventions for conduct disordered children. In B. E. Saunders, L. Berliner, & R. F. Hanson (Eds.), *Child physical and sexual abuse: Guidelines for treatment* (pp. 61–65). Charleston, SC: National Crime Victims Research and Treatment Center.

Briere, J., & Gil, E. (1998). Self-mutilation in clinical and general population samples: Prevalence, correlates, and functions. *American Journal of Orthopsychiatry*, *68*, 609–620.

Briggs, S. (2003). *Working with adolescents: A contemporary psycho-dynamic perspective*. New York, NY: Palgrave Macmillan.

Broad, K. L. (2011). Coming out for parents, families and friends of lesbians and gays: From support group grieving to love advocacy. *Sexualities*, *14*(4), 399–415. doi:10.1177/1363460711406792

Bromfield, R. (2005). *Teens in therapy: Making it their own*. New York, NY: Norton.

Brook, J. S., Brook, D. W., de la Rosa, M., Duque, L. F., Rodriguez, E., Montoya, I. D., & Whiteman, M. (1998). Pathways to marijuana use among adolescents: Cultural/

ecological, family, peer, and personality influences. *Journal of the American Academy of Child & Adolescent Psychology*, *37*, 759–766.

Brown, J., Cohen, P., Johnson, J. G., & Smailes, E. M. (1999). Childhood abuse and neglect: Specificity of effects on adolescent and young adult depression and suicidality. *Journal of American Academy of Child and Adolescent Psychiatry*, *38*(12), 1490–1496.

Brown, S. L. (2004). Family structure and child well-being: The significance of parental cohabitation. *Journal of Marriage and Family*, *66*(2), 351–367. doi:10.1111/j.1741-3737.2004.00025.x

Budd, E. (2012). The impact of a parent's personality disorder. *Family Advocate*, *34*(4), 34–39.

Bugge, K. E., Darbyshire, P., Rokholt, E. G., Sulheim Haugstvedt, K. T., & Helseth, S. (2014). Young children's grief: Parents' understanding and coping. *Death Studies*, *38*, 36–43.

Buist, K. L., Dekovic, M., Meeus, W., & van Aken, M. A. G. (2004). The reciprocal relationship between early adolescent attachment and internalizing and externalizing problem behavior. *Journal of Adolescence*, *27*, 251–266.

Bureau, J. F., Martin, J., Freynet, N., Poirier, A. A., Lafontaine, M. F., & Cloutier, P. (2010). Perceived dimensions of parenting and non-suicidal self-injury in young adults. *Journal of Youth and Adolescence*, *39*, 484–494.

Burns, C. D. (2004). Factors influencing treatment compliance among adolescents after suicide attempts and the relationship to later suicidal ideation. (64), ProQuest Information & Learning, US. Retrieved from http://search.ebscohost.com/login.aspx?direct=true&db=psyh&AN=2004-99010-218&site=ehost-live&scope=site

Burns, C. D., Cortell, R., & Wagner, B. M. (2008). Treatment compliance in adolescents after attempted suicide: A 2-year follow-up study. *Journal of the American Academy of Child & Adolescent Psychiatry*, *47*(8), 948–957. doi:10.1097/CHI.0b013e3181799e84

Burke, M. (2012). How families interact on Facebook. Retrieved from http://www.facebook.com/notes/facebook-data-science/how-families-interact-on-facebook/10151208188528859?utm_source=Labnotes+Newsletter&utm_campaign=b12bf56f38-Labnotes&utm_medium=email

Burton, C. W., Halpern-Felsher, B., Rehm, R. S., Rankin, S., & Humphreys, J. C. (2013). "It was pretty scary": The theme of fear in young adult women's descriptions of a history of adolescent dating abuse. *Issues in Mental Health Nursing*, *34*(11), 803–813. doi:10.3109/01612840.2013.827286

Byng-Hall, J. (2002). Relieving parentified children's burdens in families with insecure attachment patterns. *Family Process*, *41*(3), 375–388.

Byng-Hall, J. (2008). The significance of children fulfilling parental roles: Implications for family therapy. *Journal of Family Therapy*, *30*(2), 147–162. doi:10.1111/j.1467-6427.2008.00423.x

Byrne, S., Morgan, S., Fitzpatrick, C., Boylan, C., Crowley, S., Gahan, H., … Guerin, S. (2008). Deliberate self-harm in children and adolescents: A qualitative study exploring the needs of parents and carers. *Clinical Child Psychology and Psychiatry*, *13*(4), 493–504.

Caffery, T., & Erdman, P. (2000). Conceptualizing parent-adolescent conflict: Applications from systems and attachment theories. *The Family Journal*, *8*(1), 14–21. doi:10.1177/1066480700081004

Calafat, A., García, F., Juan, M., Becoña, E., & Fernández-Hermida, J. R. (2014). Which parenting style is more protective against adolescent substance use? Evidence within the European context. *Drug and Alcohol Dependence*, *138*, 185–192. doi:10.1016/j.drugalcdep.2014.02.705

Calam, R., Bolton, C., Barrowclough, C., & Roberts, J. (2002). Maternal expressed emotion and clinician ratings of emotional maltreatment potential. *Child Abuse & Neglect*, *26*(10), 1101–1106. doi:10.1016/S0145-2134(02)00373-3

Callahan, M. R., Tolman, R. M., & Saunders, D. G. (2003). Adolescent dating violence victimization and psychological well-being. *Journal of Adolescent Research*, *18*(6), 664–681.

Campbell, A. (2004). How was it for you? Families' experiences of receiving behavioral family therapy. *Journal of Psychiatric & Mental Health Nursing*, *11*, 261–267.

Carlton, P. A., & Deane, F. P. (2000). Impact of attitudes and suicidal ideation on adolescents' intentions to seek professional psychological help. *Journal of Adolescence*, *23*, 35–45.

Carnelley, K. B., Hepper, E. G., Hicks, C., & Turner, W. (2011). Perceived parental reactions to coming out, attachment, and romantic relationship views. *Attachment & Human Development*, *13*(3), 217–236. doi:10.1080/14616734.2011.563828

Cash, S. J., Thelwall, M., Peck, S. N., Ferrell, J. Z., & Bridge, J. A. (2013). Adolescent suicide statements on MySpace. *Cyberpsychology, Behavior, and Social Networking*, *16*(3), 166–174. doi:10.1089/cyber.2012.0098

Caughlin, J. P., Afifi, W. A., Carpenter-Theune, K. E., & Miller, L. E. (2005). Reasons for, and consequences of, revealing personal secrets in close relationships: A longitudinal study. *Personal Relationships*, *12*(1), 43–59. doi:10.1111/j.1350-4126.2005.00101.x

Centers for Disease Control and Prevention (CDC). (2007). Youth Risk Behavioral Surveillance—United States. MMWR2008; *57*(SS#4).

Centers for Disease Control and Prevention (CDC). (2011). Leading causes of death. Retrieved from http://www.cdc.gov/injury/wisqars

Centers for Disease Control and Prevention (CDC). (2012). Youth risk behavior surveillance—United States, 2011. *MMWR*, *61*(SS-4), 1–168.

Chapple, C. L. (2003). Examining intergenerational violence: Violent role modeling or weak parental controls? *Violence & Victims*, *18*(2), 143–162.

Chasson, G. S., Mychailyszyn, M. P., Vincent, J. P., & Harris, G. E. (2013). Evaluation of trauma characteristics as predictors of attrition from cognitive-behavioral therapy for child victims of violence. *Psychological Reports*, *113*(3), 734–753.

Chasson, G. S., Vincent, J. P., & Harris, G. E. (2008). The use of symptom severity measured just before termination to predict child treatment dropout. *Journal of Clinical Psychology*, *64*(7), 1–14.

Chen, F. P., Gearing, R. E., DeVylder, J. E., & Oh, H. Y. (2016). Pathway model of parental help seeking for adolescents experiencing first-episode psychosis. *Early Intervention in Psychiatry*, *10*(2), 122–128.

Child, J. T., Petronio, S., Agyeman-Budu, E. A., & Westermann, D. A. (2011). Blogg scrubbing: Exploring triggers that change privacy rules. *Computers in Human Behavior*, *27*, 2017–2027.

Childress, B. L. (1992). Thinking about parents and rescuing children. *Residential Treatment for Children & Youth*, *9*(4), 29–42. doi:10.1300/J007v09n04_03

Christofides, E., Muise, A., & Desmarais, S. (2009). Information disclosure and control on Facebook: Are they two sides of the same coin or two different processes? *Cyber Psychology and Behavior*, *12*, 341–345. doi:10.1089/cpb.2008.0226

Church, E. (1994). The role of autonomy in adolescent psychotherapy. *Psychotherapy*, *31*, 101–108.

Cleveland, H. H., Herrera, V. M., & Stuewig, J. (2003). Abusive males and abused females in adolescent relationships: Risk factor similarity and dissimilarity and the role of relationship seriousness. *Journal of Family Violence*, *18*(6), 325–339. doi:10.1023/A:1026297515314

Clinton, B. K., Silverman, B. C., & Brendel, D. H. (2010). Patient-targeted googling: The ethics of searching online for patient information. *Harvard Review of Psychiatry*, *18*(2), 103–112. doi:10.3109/10673221003683861

Cobham, V. E., Dadds, M., & Spence, S. H. (1998). The role of parental anxiety in the treatment of childhood anxiety. *Journal of Consulting & Clinical Psychology*, *66*, 893–905.

Coburn, K. L. (2006). Organizing a ground crew for today's helicopter parents. *About Campus*, *11*(3), 9–16.

Cohen, E. (2009). Parent in the throes of traumatic events: Risks and protection. In D. Brom, R. Pat-Horenczyk, & J. D. Ford (Eds.), *Treating traumatized children* (pp. 72–84). New York, NY: Routledge.

Cohen, J. A., Deblinger, E., Mannarino, A. P., & Steer, R. A. (2004). A multisite, randomized controlled trial for children with sexual abuse-related PTSD symptoms. *Journal of the American Academy of Child & Adolescent Psychiatry*, *43*(4), 393–402. doi:10.1097/00004583-200404000-00005

Cohen, J. A., Mannarino, A. P., & Deblinger, E. (2006). *Treating trauma and traumatic grief in children and adolescents*. New York, NY: Guilford Press.

Cohen, J. A., Mannarino, A. P., Kliethermes, M., & Murray, L. A. (2012). Trauma-focused CBT for youth with complex trauma. *Child Abuse and Neglect*, *36*(6), 528–541. doi:10.1016/j.chiabu.2012.03.007

Cohen, O. (1998). Parental narcissism and the disengagement of the non-custodial father after divorce. *Clinical Social Work Journal*, *26*(2), 195–215.

Cole, C. L., & Cole, A. L. (1999). Boundary ambiguities that bind former spouses together after the children leave home in post-divorce families. *Family Relations*, *48*(3), 271.

Cole, P. M., Woolger, C., Power, T. G., & Smith, K. D. (1992). Parenting difficulties among adult survivors of father-daughter incest. *Child Abuse & Neglect*, *16*(2), 239–249. doi:10.1016/0145-2134(92)90031-L

Colli, A., Tanzilli, A., Dimaggio, G., & Lingiardi, V. (2014). Patient personality and therapist response: An empirical investigation. *The American Journal of Psychiatry*, *171*, 102–108.

Conley, C. L. (2011). Learning about a child's gay or lesbian sexual orientation: Parental concerns about societal rejection, loss of loved ones, and child well being. *Journal of Homosexuality*, *58*, 1022–1040.

Conner, K. R., & Goldston, D. B. (2007). Rates of suicide among males increase steadily from age 11 to 21: Developmental framework and outline for prevention. *Aggression and Violent Behavior*, *12*(2), 193–207. doi:10.1016/j.avb.2006.07.002

Connor, J., & Rueter, M. (2009). Predicting adolescent suicidality: Comparing multiple informants and assessment techniques. *Journal of Adolescence*, *32*(3), 619–631. doi:10.1016/j.adolescence.2008.06.005

Constantino, M. J., Glass, C. R., Arnkoff, D. B., & Ametrano, R. M. (2011). Expectations. In J. C. Norcross (Ed.), *Psychotherapy relationships that work* (2nd ed., pp. 354–376). New York, NY: Oxford University Press.

Cook, A., Blaustein, M., Spinazzola, J., & van der Kolk, B. (Eds.). (2003). Complex trauma in children and adolescents: White paper. National Child Traumatic Stress Network. Retrieved July 2005 from http://www.NCTSN.org/

Cook, A., Spinazzola, J., Ford, J. D., Lanktree, C., Blaustein, M., Cloitre, M., … van der Kolk, B. A. (2005). Complex trauma in children and adolescents. *Psychiatric Annals*, *35*(5), 390–398.

Copley, B. (1994). Introducing families to family work. In S. Box & B. Copley (Eds.), *Crisis at adolescence: Object relations therapy with the family* (pp. 51–65). Lantham, MD: Jason Aronson.

Corcoran, J. (2004). Treatment outcome research with the non-offending parents of sexually abused children: A critical review. *Journal of Child Sexual Abuse: Research, Treatment, & Program Innovations for Victims, Survivors, & Offenders*, *13*(2), 59–84. doi:10.1300/J070v13n02_04

Corrigan, P. W. (2004). How stigma interferes with mental health care. *American Psychologist*, 59, 614–625.

Costello, E. J., He, J. P., Sampson, N. A., Kessler, R. C., & Merikangas, K. R. (2014). Services for adolescents with psychiatric disorders: 12-month data from the National Comorbidity Survey-Adolescent. *Psychiatric Services*, *65*(3), 359–366. doi:10.1176/appi.ps.201100518

Courtois, C. A., & Ford, J. D. (Eds.). (2009). *Treating complex traumatic stress disorders: An evidence-based guide*. New York: Guilford Press.

Cox, B. J., Fleet, C., & Stein, M. B. (2004). Self-criticism and social phobia in the US national comorbidity study. *Journal of Affective Disorders*, *82*(2), 227–234.

Coyne, L. W., & Wilson, K. G. (2004). The role of cognitive fusion in impaired parenting: An RFT analysis. *International Journal of Psychology and Psychological Therapy*, *4*(3), 469–486.

Coyne, S. M., Padilla-Walker, L. M., Day, R. D., Harper, J., & Stockdale, L. (2014). A friend request from dear old dad: Associations between parent–child social networking and adolescent outcomes. *Cyberpsychology, Behavior, and Social Networking*, *17*(1), 8–13. doi:10.1089/cyber.2012.0623

Cramer, D. W., & Roach, A. J. (1988). Coming out to mom and dad: A study of gay males and their relationships with their parents. *Journal of Homosexuality*, *15*, 79–91.

Crawford, A. M., & Manassis, K. (2001). Familial predictors of treatment outcome in childhood anxiety disorders. *Journal of the American Academy of Child & Adolescent Psychiatry*, *40*, 1182–1189.

Crenshaw, D. A., & Kenney-Noziska, S. (2014). Therapeutic presence in play therapy. *International Journal of Play Therapy*, *23*(1), 31–43.

Crenshaw, W. B., Lichtenberg, J. W., & Bartell, P. A. (1993). Mental health providers and child sexual abuse: A multivariate analysis of the decision to report. *Journal of Child Sexual Abuse: Research, Treatment, & Program Innovations for Victims, Survivors, & Offenders*, *2*(4), 19–42.

Crisma, M., Bascelli, E., Paci, D., & Romito, P. (2004). Adolescents who experience sexual abuse: Dears, needs, and impediments to disclosure. *Child Abuse and Neglect*, *28*, 1035–1048.

Crosby Budinger, M., Drazdowski, T., & Ginsburg, G. (2013). Anxiety-promoting parenting behaviors: A comparison of anxious parents with and without social anxiety disorder. *Child Psychiatry & Human Development*, *44*(3), 412–418. doi:10.1007/s10578-012-0335-9

Cuijpers, P., Weitz, E., Karyotaki, E., Garber, J., & Andersson, G. (2015). The effects of psychological treatment of maternal depression on children and parental functioning: A meta-analysis. *European Child & Adolescent Psychiatry*, *24*(2), 237–245.

Cundy, L. (2015). Attachment, self-experience, and communication technology: Love in the age of the Internet. In L. Cundy (Ed.), *Love in the age of the Internet: Attachment in the digital era* (pp. 1–29). London, UK: Karnac Books.

Cyr, M., McDuff, P., & Hebert, M. (2013). Support and profiles of nonoffending mothers of sexually abused children. *Journal Child and Sex Abuse*, *22*(2), 209–230.

Cyr, M., McDuff, P., & Wright, J. (2006). Prevalence and predictors of dating violence among adolescent female victims of child sexual abuse. *Journal of Interpersonal Violence*, *21*(8), 1000–1017. doi:10.1177/0886260506290201

Dalenberg, C. J. (2004). Maintaining the safe and effective therapeutic relationship in the context of distrust and anger: Countertransference and complex trauma. *Psychotherapy: Theory, Research, Practice, Training*, *41*(4), 438–447. doi:10.1037/0033-3204.41.4.438

Dank, M., Lachman, P., Zweig, J. M., & Yahner, J. (2014). Dating violence experiences of lesbian, gay, bisexual, and transgender youth. *Journal of Youth and Adolescence*, *43*(5), 846–857. doi:10.1007/s10964-013-9975-8

Darling, N., & Dowdy, B. (2010). Trust, but verify: Knowledge, disclosure, and mothers' beliefs about adolescents' trustworthiness. In K. J. Rotenberg (Ed.), *Interpersonal trust during childhood and adolescence* (pp. 203–222). New York, NY: Cambridge University Press.

Darling, N., & Steinberg, L. (1993). Parenting style as context: An integrative model. *Psychological Bulletin*, *113*, 487–496.

Darling, N., Cumsille, P., Caldwell, L. L., & Dowdy, B. (2006). Predictors of adolescents' disclosure to parents and perceived parental knowledge: Between- and within-person differences. *Journal of Youth and Adolescence*, *35*(4), 667–678.

D'Augelli, A. R., Grossman, A. H., & Starks, M. T. (2008). Families of gay, lesbian, and bisexual youth: What do parents and siblings know and how do they react? *Journal of GLBT Family Studies*, *4*(1), 95–115. doi:10.1080/15504280802084506

Davies, M. G. (1995). Parental distress and ability to cope following disclosure of extra-familial sexual abuse. *Child Abuse and Neglect*, *19*, 399–408.

Davies, M. G., Rogers, P., & Bates, B.-A. (2008). Blame towards male rape victims as a function of victim sexuality and degree of resistance. *Journal of Homosexuality*, *55*, 533–544.

Davies, M. G., Rogers, P., & Whitelegg, L. (2009). Effects of victim gender, victim sexual orientation, victim response and respondent gender on judgements of blame in a hypothetical adolescent rape. *Legal & Criminological Psychology*, *14*(2), 331–338. doi:10.1348/978185408X386030

De Bellis, M. D., Broussard, E. R., Herring, D. J., Wexler, S., Moritz, G., & Benitez, J. G. (2001). Psychiatric co-morbidity in caregivers and children involved in maltreatment: A pilot research study with policy implications. *Child Abuse & Neglect*, *25*, 923–944.

de Haan, A. M., Boon, A. E., de Jong, J. T. V. M., Hoeve, M., & Vermeiren, R. R. J. M. (2013). A meta-analytic review on treatment dropout in child and adolescent outpatient mental health care. *Clinical Psychology Review*, *33*(5), 698–711. doi:10.1016/j.cpr.2013.04.005

de Leeuw, R. N. H., Scholte, R. H. J., Vermulst, A. A., & Engels, R. C. M. E. (2013). The associations of anticipated parental reactions with smoking initiation and progression in adolescents. *The American Journal on Addictions*, *22*(6), 527–534. doi:10.1111/j.1521-0391.2013.12020.x

Deane, F. P., Skogstad, P., & Williams, M. W. (1999). Impact of attitudes, ethnicity, and quality of prior therapy on New Zealand prisoners' intentions to seek professional psychological help. *International Journal for the Advancement of Counseling*, *21*, 55–67.

Deblinger, E., Hathaway, C. R., Lippmann, J., & Steer, R. (1993). Psychosocial characteristics and correlates of symptom distress in nonoffending mothers of sexually abused children. *Journal of Interpersonal Violence*, *8*(2), 155–168. doi:10.1177/088626093008002001

Deblinger, E., & Heflin, A. H. (1996). *Treating sexually abused children and their nonoffending parents: A cognitive behavioral approach.* Thousand Oaks, CA: Sage.

Deblinger, E., Stauffer, L. B., & Steer, R. A. (2001). Comparative efficacies of supportive and cognitive behavioral group therapies for young children who have been sexually abused and their nonoffending mothers. *Child Maltreatment*, *6*(4), 332.

DeChello, P. (2008). *Understanding self-injury*. Middlefield, CT: D & S Associates.

Dehue, F., Bolman, C., Vollink, T., & Pouwelse, M. (2012). Cyberbullying and traditional bullying in relation to adolescents' perception of parenting. *Journal of Cybertherapy and Rehabilitation*, *5*(1), 25–34.

DeJong, S. M. (2014). Professionalism and adolescent psychiatry in the digital age. *Adolescent Psychiatry*, *4*(2), 64–72.

Deković, M. (1999). Risk and protective factors in the development of problem behavior during adolescence. *Journal of Youth and Adolescence*, *28*, 667–685.

Delgado, S. V., & Strawn, J. R. (2012). Termination of psychodynamic psychotherapy with adolescents: A review and contemporary perspective. *Bulletin of the Menninger Clinic*, *76*(1), 21–52.

DelPo, E. G., & Koontz, M. A. (1991). Group therapy with mothers of incest victims, Part II: Therapeutic strategies, recurrent themes, interventions, and outcomes. *Archives of Psychiatric Nursing*, *5*(2), 70–75.

Dempsey, A. F., Singer, D. D., Clark, S. J., & Davis, M. M. (2009). Adolescent preventative health care: What do parents want? *Journal of Pediatrics*, *155*, 689–694.

Dempster, R., Wildman, B., & Keating, A. (2013). The role of stigma in parental help-seeking for child behavior problems. *Journal of Clinical Child and Adolescent Psychology*, *42*(1), 56–67.

Desrosiers, L., Saint-Jean, M., & Breton, J. J. (2015). Treatment planning: A key milestone to prevent treatment dropout in adolescents with borderline personality disorder. *Psychology and Psychotherapy: Theory, Research and Practice*, *88*(2), 178–196. doi:10.1111/papt.12033

Diamond, G., & Siqueland, L. (1998). Emotions, attachment and the relational reframe: The first session. *Journal of Systemic Therapies*, *17*(2), 36–50. Retrieved from http://search.ebscohost.com/login.aspx?direct=true&db=psyh&AN=1998-10088-003&site=ehost-live&scope=site

Diamond, G. M. (2014). Attachment-based family therapy interventions. *Psychotherapy*, *51*, 15–19.

Diamond, G. M., Liddle, H. A., Hogue, A., & Dakof, G. A. (1999). Alliance-building interventions with adolescents in family therapy: A process study. *Psychotherapy*, *36*, 355–368.

DiCaccavo, A. (2002). Investigating individuals' motivations to become counselling psychologists: The influence of early caretaking roles within the family. *Psychology and Psychotherapy: Theory, Research and Practice*, *75*, 463–472.

DiCaccavo, A. (2006). Working with parentification: Implications for clients and counselling psychologists. *Psychology and Psychotherapy: Theory, Research and Practice*, *79*, 469–478.

DiFilippo, J. M., & Overholser, J. C. (2000). Suicidal ideation in adolescent psychiatric inpatients as associated with depression and attachment relationships. *Journal of Clinical Child Psychology*, *29*, 155–166.

DiGiuseppe, R., Linscott, J., & Jilton, R. (1996). Developing the therapeutic alliance in child-adolescent psychotherapy. *Applied and Preventive Psychology*, *5*(2), 85–100.

DiLillo, D., & Gale, E. B. (2011). To Google or not to Google: Graduate students' use of the Internet to access personal information about clients. *Training and Education in Professional Psychology*, *5*(3), 160–166. doi:10.1037/a0024441

Dishion, T. J., & McMahon, R. J. (1998). Parental monitoring and the prevention of child and adolescent problem behavior: A conceptual and empirical formulation. *Clinical Child and Family Psychology Review*, *1*, 61–75.

Disney, K. L. (2013). Dependent personality disorder: A critical review. *Clinical Psychology Review*, *33*, 1184–1196.

dosReis, S., Mychailyszyn, M. P., Myers, M., & Riley, A. W. (2007). Coming to terms with ADHD: How urban African-American families come to seek care for their children. *Psychiatric Services*, *58*(5), 636–641.

Doty, J., & Dworkin, J. (2014). Parents' of adolescents use of social networking sites. *Computers in Human Behavior*, *33*, 349–355. doi:10.1016/j.chb.2013.07.012

Dowell, K. A., & Ogles, B. M. (2010). The effects of parent participation on child psychotherapy outcome: A meta-analytic review. *Journal of Clinical Child and Adolescent Psychology*, *39*(2), 151–162.

Downey, G., Silver, R. C., & Wortman, C. B. (1990). Reconsidering the attribution-adjustment relation following a major negative event: Coping with the loss of a child. *Journal of Personality and Social Psychology*, *59*, 925–940.

Drake, J. A., Price, J. H., Maziarz, L., & Ward, B. (2012). Prevalence and correlates of sexting behavior in adolescents. *American Journal of Sexuality Education*, *7*, 1–15.

Dubus, N. (2014). Texting: The third client in the room. *Clinical Social Work Journal*, *43*(2), 209–214.

Duchesne, S., & Larose, S. (2007). Adolescent attachment to mother and father and academic motivation and performance in early adolescence. *Journal of Applied Social Psychology*, *37*, 1501–1521.

Duncan, B. L., & Moynihan, D. W. (1994). Applying outcome research intentional utilization of the client's frame of reference. *Psychotherapy: Theory, Research, Practice, Training*, *31*, 294–301.

Duncan, D. T., & Hatzenbuehler, M. L. (2014). Lesbian, gay, bisexual, and transgender hate crimes and suicidality among a population-based sample of sexual-minority adolescents in Boston. *American Journal of Public Health*, *104*(2), 272–278.

Duncan, R. E., Vandeleur, M., Derks, A., & Sawyer, S. (2011). Confidentiality with adolescents in the medical setting: What do parents think? *Journal of Adolescent Health*, *49*, 428–430.

Dwairy, M., Achoui, M., Abouserie, R., & Farah, A. (2006). Adolescent-family connectedness among Arabs: A second cross-regional research study. *Journal of Cross-Cultural Psychology*, *37*, 248–261.

Dyregrov, A., Gjestad, R., Bie Wikander, A., & Vigerust, S. (1999). Reactions following the sudden death of a classmate. *Scandinavian Journal of Psychology*, *40*, 167–176.

Earley, L., & Cushway, D. J. (2002). The parentified child. *Clinical Child Psychology & Psychiatry*, *7*(2), 163.

East, P. L., Chien, N. C., Adams, J. A., Hokoda, A., & Maier, A. (2010). Links between sisters' sexual and dating victimization: The roles of neighborhood crime and parental controls. *Journal of Family Psychology*, *24*(6), 698–708. doi:10.1037/a0021751

Eaton, D. K., Davis, K. S., Barrios, L., Brener, N. D., & Noonan, R. K. (2007). Associations of dating violence victimization with lifetime participation, co-occurrence, and early initiation of risk behaviors among U.S. high school students. *Journal of Interpersonal Violence*, *22*(5), 585–602. doi:10.1177/0886260506298831

Ehrenberg, M. F., Hunter, M. A., & Elterman, M. F. (1996). Shared parenting agreements after marital separation: The roles of empathy and narcissism. *Journal of Consulting and Clinical Psychology*, *64*(4), 808–818. doi:10.1037/0022-006X.64.4.808

Elbert, T., & Schauer, M. (2010). Dissociation following traumatic stress. *Zeitschrift für Psychologie / Journal of Psychology, 218*(2), 109–127. doi:10.1027/0044-3409/a000018

Elizur, Y., & Mintzer, A. (2001). A framework for the formation of gay male identity: Processes associated with adult attachment style and support from family and friends. *Archives of Sexual Behavior, 30*, 143–167.

Elliot, A. J., & Thrash, T. (2004). The intergenerational transmission of fear of failure. *Personality and Social Psychology Bulletin, 30*, 957–971.

Elliott, A. N., & Carnes, C. N. (2001). Reactions of nonoffending parents to the sexual abuse of their child: A review of the literature. *Child Maltreatment, 6*(4), 314–331. doi:10.1177/1077559501006004005

Ellis, A. J., Portnoff, L. C., Axelson, D. A., Kowatch, R. A., Walshaw, P., & Miklowitz, D. J. (2014). Parental expressed emotion and suicidal ideation in adolescents with bipolar disorder. *Psychiatry Research, 216*, 213–216.

Ellison, R., Rhodes, P., Madden, S., Miskovic, J., Wallis, A., Baillie, A., ... Touyz, S. (2012). Do the components of manualized family-based treatment for anorexia nervosa predict weight gain? *International Journal of Eating Disorders, 45*, 609–614.

Englund, L., Forsberg, R., & Saveman, B.-I. (2014). Survivors' experiences of media coverage after traumatic injury events. *International Emergency Nursing, 22*, 25–30.

Epstein, M., Hill, K. G., Bailey, J. A., & Hawkins, J. D. (2013). The effect of general and drug-specific family environments on comorbid and drug-specific problem behavior: A longitudinal examination. *Developmental Psychology, 49*(6), 1151–1164. doi:10.1037/a002930910.1037/a0029309.supp (Supplemental).

Erkolahti, R., & Nyström, M. (2009). The prevalence of transitional object use in adolescence: Is there a connection between the existence of a transitional object and depressive symptoms? *European Child & Adolescent Psychiatry, 18*(7), 400–406. doi:10.1007/s00787-009-0747-7

Esbjørn, B. H., Sømhovd, M. J., Nielsen, S. K., Normann, N., Leth, I., & Reinholdt-Dunne, M. L. (2014). Parental changes after involvement in their anxious child's cognitive behavior therapy. *Journal of Anxiety Disorders, 28*, 664–670. doi:10.1016/j.janxdis.2014.07.008

Evans, S. (2014). The challenge and potential of the digital age: Young people and the internet. *Transactional Analysis Journal, 44*(2), 153–166.

Evenson, R. J., & Simon, R. W. (2005). Clarifying the relationship between parenthood and depression. *Journal of Health and Social Behavior, 46*, 341–358.

Eyrich-Garg, K. M. (2008). Strategies for engaging adolescent girls at an emergency shelter in a therapeutic relationship: Recommendations from the girls themselves. *Journal of Social Work Practice, 22*(3), 375–388.

Faber, A. J., & Wittenborn, A. K. (2010). The role of attachment in children's adjustment to divorce and remarriage. *Journal of Family Psychotherapy, 21*(2), 89–104. doi:10.1080/08975353.2010.483625

Fairburn, C. G., Cooper, Z., Doll, H. A., & Welch, S. L. (1999). Risk facts for anorexia nervosa: Three integrated case-control comparisons. *Archives of General Psychiatry, 56*, 468–476.

Federal Policy Brief. (2012). LGBTQ youth national policy statement. National Alliance to End Homelessness. Retrieved from http://www.endhomelessness.org/library/entry/lgbtq-youth-national-policy-statement

Feeney, J. A. (2005). Hurt feelings in couple relationships: Exploring the role of attachment and perceptions of personal injury. *Personal Relationships*, *12*(2), 253–271.

Feinberg, M., & Hetherington, E. M. (2001). Differential parenting as a within-family variable. *Journal of Family Psychology*, *15*(1), 22–37. doi:10.1037/0893-3200.15.1.22

Feng, J.-Y., Chen, Y.-W., Fetzer, S., Feng, M.-C., & Lin, C.-L. (2012). Ethical and legal challenges of mandated child abuse reporters. *Children and Youth Services Review*, *34*, 276–280.

Ferdinand, R. F., van der Ende, J., & Verhulst, F. C. (2004). Parent-adolescent disagreement regarding psychopathology in adolescents from the general population as a risk factor for adverse outcome. *Journal of Abnormal Psychology*, *113*, 198–206.

Fergusson, D. M., Horwood, J., & Lynskey, M. T. (1996). Childhood sexual abuse and psychiatric disorder in young adulthood; II: Psychiatric outcomes of childhood sexual abuse. *Journal of American Academy of Child and Adolescent Psychiatry*, *35*(10), 1365–1374.

Finkelhor, D., Ormrod, R., Turner, H., & Hamby, S. (2005). The victimization of children and youth: A comprehensive, national survey. *Child Maltreatment*, *10*, 5–25.

Finkenauer, C., Engels, R. C. M. E., & Meeus, W. (2002). Keeping secrets from parents: Advantages and disadvantages of secrecy in adolescence. *Journal of Youth and Adolescence*, *31*(2), 123–136.

Finkenauer, C., Engels, R. C. M., & Kubacka, K. E. (2008). Relational implications of secrecy and concealment in parent-adolescent relationships. In M. Kerr, H. Stattin, & R. C. M. Engels (Eds.), *What can parents do? New insights into the role of parents in adolescent problem behavior* (pp. 43–64). New York, NY: John Wiley & Sons.

Finkenauer, C., Frijns, T., Engels, R. C. M., & Kerkhof, P. (2005). Perceiving concealment in relationships between parents and adolescents: Links with parental behavior. *Personal Relationships*, *12*, 387–406.

Finzi, R., Ram, A., Har-Even, D., Shnit, D., & Weizman, A. (2001). Attachment styles and aggression in physically abused and neglected children. *Journal of Youth and Adolescence*, *30*(6), 769–786. doi:10.1023/A:1012237813771

Fisher, M. A. (2013). *The ethics of conditional confidentiality: A practice model for mental health professionals*. New York, NY: Oxford University Press.

Flaherty, E. G., Sege, R., Price, L. L., Christoffel, K. K., Norton, D. P., & O'Connor, K. G. (2006). Pediatrician characteristics associated with child abuse identification and reporting: Results from a national survey of pediatricians. *Child Maltreatment*, *11*(4), 361–369.

Fleet, D., & Mintz, R. (2013). Counsellors' perceptions of client progression when working with clients who intentionally self-harm and the impact such work has on the therapist. *Counselling & Psychotherapy Research*, *13*(1), 44–52. doi:10.1080/14733145.2012.698421

Fliege, H., Grimm, J.-R., Grimm, A., & Klapp, B. F. (2009). Risk factors and correlates of deliberate self-harm behavior: A systematic review. *Journal of Psychosomatic Research, 66*, 477–493.

Folse, V. N., & Krawzak, K. M. (2013). Family experience with eating disorders scale: A systematic way to engage the family in treatment. *Perspectives in Psychiatric Care, 49*(4), 269–277.

Fontaine, D., & Nolin, P. (2012). Personality disorders in a sample of parents accused of physical abuse or neglect. *Journal of Family Violence, 27*(1), 23–31. doi:10.1007/s10896-011-9403-3

Ford, C. A., Millstein, S., Halpern-Felsher, B. L., & Irwin, C. E. (1997). Influence of physician confidentiality assurances on adolescents' willingness to disclose information and seek future health care: A randomised controlled trial. *Journal of American Medical Association, 278*, 1029–1034.

Ford, C. A., Thomsen, S. L., & Compton, B. (2001). Adolescents' interpretations of conditional confidentiality assurances. *Journal of Adolescent Health, 29*(3), 156–159.

Fortunato, L., Young, A. M., Boyd, C. J., & Fons, C. E. (2010). Hook-up sexual experiences and problem behaviors among adolescents. *Journal of Child & Adolescent Substance Abuse, 19*(3), 261–278. doi:10.1080/1067828X.2010.488965

Foshee, V. A., Bauman, K. E., Greene, W. F., Koch, G. G., Linder, G. F., & MacDougall, J. E. (2000). The Safe Dates Program: 1-year follow-up results. *American Journal of Public Health, 90*(10), 1619–1622.

Foshee, V. A., Benefield, T. S., Ennett, S. T., Bauman, K. E., & Suchindran, C. (2004). Longitudinal predictors of serious physical and sexual dating violence victimization during adolescence. *Preventive Medicine, 39*, 1007–1016.

Foshee, V. A., Reyes, H. L. M., Ennett, S. T., Cance, J. C., Bauman, K. E., & Bowling, J. M. (2012). Assessing the effects of families for safe dates, a family-based dating abuse prevention program. *Journal of Adolescent Health, 51*(4), 349–356.

Freedman, M. R., Rosenberg, S. J., Gettman-Feizien, D., & Van Scoyk, S. (1993). Evaluator countertransference in child custody evaluations. *American Journal of Forensic Psychology, 11*(3), 61–73.

Freeman, A., Breitmeyer, A., & Flint, M. (2013). The challenges in diagnosing narcissistic personality disorder: Difficult to define, but "we know it when we see it." *The Behavior Therapist, 36*(7), 179–184.

Frew, A. (2014). Predictive characteristics of styles of parenting and attachment in mothers. (75), ProQuest Information & Learning, US. Retrieved from http://search.ebscohost.com/login.aspx?direct=true&db=psyh&AN=2014-99160-263&site=ehost-live&scope=site

Freyd, J. J. (1996). *Betrayal trauma: The logical of forgetting childhood abuse*. Cambridge, MA: Harvard University Press.

Freyd, J. J. (2008). Betrayal trauma. In G. Reyes, J. D. Elhai, & J. D. Ford (Eds.), *Encyclopedia of psychological trauma* (p. 76). New York, NY: John Wiley & Sons.

Friedlander, M. L., Escudero, V., & Heatherington, L. (2006). *Therapeutic alliances with couples and families: An empirically-informed guide to practice*. Washington, DC: American Psychological Association.

Friedlander, M. L., Lee, H.-H., Shaffer, K. S., & Cabrera, P. (2014). Negotiating therapeutic alliances with a family at impasse. *Psychotherapy, 51*(1), 41–52. doi:10.1037/a0032524

Frijns, T., Finkenauer, C., & Keijsers, L. (2013). Shared secrets versus secrets kept private are linked to better adolescent adjustment. *Journal of Adolescence, 36*(1), 55–64. doi:10.1016/j.adolescence.2012.09.005

Frijns, T., Finkenauer, C., Vermulst, A. A., & Engels, R. C. M. E. (2005). Keeping secrets from parents: Longitudinal associations of secrecy in adolescence. *Journal of Youth and Adolescence, 34*(2), 137–148.

Frijns, T., Keijsers, L., Branje, S., & Meeus, W. (2010). What parents don't know and how it may affect their children: Qualifying the disclosure–adjustment link. *Journal of Adolescence, 33*(2), 261–270.

Furey, W. M., & Basili, L. A. (1988). Predicting consumer satisfaction in parent training for noncompliant children. *Behavior Therapy, 19*, 555–564.

Furnham, A. (2003). Belief in a just world: Research progress over the past decade. *Personality and Individual Differences, 34*(5), 795–817.

Gabel, S., & Bemporad, J. (1994). Variations in countertransference reactions in psychotherapy with children. *American Journal of Psychotherapy, 48*(1), 111–119.

Gabriel, T. (2010, August 22). Students, welcome to college: Parents, go home. *The New York Times.*

Gaines, R. (2003). Therapist self-disclosure with children, adolescents, and their parents. *Journal of Clinical Psychology, 59*(5), 569–580.

Gallopin, C., & Leigh, L. (2009). Teen perceptions of dating violence, help-seeking, and the role of schools. *Prevention Researcher*, 16(1), 17–20.

Galloway, S., & Hogg, N. (2008). Non-abusing parents and their role in risk management. In J. Houston & S. Galloway (Eds.), *Sexual offending and mental health: Multidisciplinary management in the community* (pp. 229–247). Philadelphia, PA: Jessica Kingsley.

Garcia, J. A., & Weisz, J. R. (2002). When youth mental health care stops: Therapeutic relationship problems and other reasons for ending youth outpatient treatment. *Journal of Consulting and Clinical Psychology, 70*, 439–443.

García, F., & Gracia, E. (2009). Is always authoritative the optimum parenting style? Evidence from Spanish families. *Adolescence, 44*(173), 101–131.

Gartrell, N. K., Bos, H., & Goldberg, N. G. (2011). Adolescents of the US National Longitudinal Lesbian Family Study: Sexual orientation, sexual behavior, and sexual risk exposure. *Archives of Sexual Behavior, 40*, 1199–1209.

Gaskin, D. J., Kouzis, A., & Richard, P. (2008). Children's and adolscents' use of mental health care is a family matter. *Medical Care Research and Review, 65*, 748–762.

Gatta, M., Spoto, A., Svanellini, L., Lai, J., Toldo, I., Testa, C. P., & Battistella, P. A. (2012). Alliance with patient and collaboration with parents throughout the psychotherapeutic process with children and adolescents: A pilot study. *Journal of Psychopathology / Giornale di Psicopatologia, 18*(1), 28–34.

Gay Lesbian and Straight Education Network [GLSEN]. (2010). 2009 National School Climate Survey. Retrieved from http://www.glsen.org/cgi-bin/iowa/all/news/record/2624.html

Géhin, A., Kabuth, B., Pichené, C., & Vidailhet, C. (2009). Ten year follow-up study of 65 suicidal adolescents. *Journal of the Canadian Academy of Child and Adolescent Psychiatry / Journal de l'Académie canadienne de psychiatrie de l'enfant et de l'adolescent, 18*(2), 117–125.

Geller, S. M., & Greenberg, L. S. (2002). Therapeutic presence: Therapists' experience of presence in the psychotherapeutic encounter. *Person-Centered and Experiential Psychotherapies, 1*, 71–86. doi:10.1080/14779757.2002.9688279

Geller, S. M., & Greenberg, L. S. (2010). *Therapeutic presence: An essential way of being*. Washington, DC: American Psychological Association.

Geller, S. M., Greenberg, L. S., & Watson, J. C. (2010). Therapist and client perceptions of therapeutic presence: The development of a measure. *Psychotherapy Research, 20*, 599–610. doi:10.1080/ 10503307.2010.495957

Gerdes, A. C., Lawton, K. E., Haack, L. M., & Schneider, B. W. (2014). Latino parental help seeking for childhood ADHD. *Administration and Policy in Mental Health and Mental Health Services Research, 41*(4), 503–513.

Ghesquiere, A., Fan, M.-Y., Berliner, L., Rivara, F. P., Jurkovic, G. J., Russo, J., … Zatzick, D. F. (2008). Adolescents' and parents' agreement on posttraumatic stress disorder symptoms and functioning after adolescent injury. *Journal of Traumatic Stress, 21*(5), 487–491.

Gibbs, D. (2011). Assessing suicidal cognitions in adolescents: Establishing the reliability and validity of the Suicide Cognitions Scale. (71), ProQuest Information & Learning, US. Retrieved from http://search.ebscohost.com/login.aspx?direct=true&db=psyh&AN=2011-99080-377&site=ehost-live&scope=site

Gil, E., & Crenshaw, D. A. (2016). *Termination challenges in child psychotherapy*. New York, NY: Guilford Press.

Giordano, P. C., Soto, D. A., Manning, W. D., & Longmore, M. A. (2010). The characteristics of romantic relationships associated with teen dating violence. *Social Science Research, 39*(6), 863–874. doi:10.1016/j.ssresearch.2010.03.009

Glazebrook, K., Townsend, E., & Sayal, K. (2015). The role of attachment style in predicting repetition of adolescent self-harm: A longitudinal study. *Suicide and Life-Threatening Behavior, 45*(6), 664–678. doi:10.1111/sltb.12159

Glenn, C. R. (2013). The functions of nonsuicidal self-injury in an adolescent clinical sample: Frequency, structure, and psychological correlates. (74), ProQuest Information & Learning, US. Retrieved from http://search.ebscohost.com/login.aspx?direct=true&db=psyh&AN=2013-99160-584&site=ehost-live&scope=site

Godress, J., Ozgul, S., Owen, C., & Foley-Evans, L. (2005). Grief experiences of parents whose children suffer from mental illness. *Australian and New Zealand Journal of Psychiatry, 39*, 88–94.

Goldberg, A. E. (2010). *Lesbian and gay parents and their children: Research on the family life cycle*. Washington, DC: American Psychological Association.

Golish, T. D. (2003). Stepfamily communication strengths. *Human Communication Research, 29*(1), 41.

Golombok, S. (2000). *Parenting: What really counts?* Philadelphia, PA: Taylor and Francis.

Goodrich, K. M. (2009). Mom and dad come out: The process of identifying as a heterosexual parent with a lesbian, gay, or bisexual child. *Journal of LGBT Issues in Counseling*, *3*(1), 37–61.

Gottlieb, L. (2011). How to land your kid in therapy. *The Atlantic*. Retrieved from http://www.theatlantic.com/magazine/archive/2011/07/how-to-land-your-kid-in-therapy/308555/

Grant, H. B., Jr. (2000). Termination: How families experience the end of family therapy. (60), ProQuest Information & Learning, US. Retrieved from http://search.ebscohost.com/login.aspx?direct=true&db=psyh&AN=2000-95009-185&site=ehost-live&scope=site

Gratz, K. L. (2006). Risk factors for deliberate self-harm among female college students: The role and interaction of childhood maltreatment, emotional inexpressivity, and affect intensity/reactivity. *American Journal of Orthopsychiatry*, *79*, 238–250.

Gratz, K. L., Conrad, S. D., & Roemer, L. (2002). Risk factors for deliberate self-harm among college students. *American Journal of Orthopsychiatry*, *72*, 128–140.

Green, E. J., & Myrick, A. C. (2014). Treating complex trauma in adolescents: A phase-based, integrative approach for play therapists. *International Journal of Play Therapy*, *23*(3), 131–145. doi:10.1037/a0036679

Green, J. (2006). Annotation: The therapeutic alliance—A significant but neglected variable in child mental health treatment studies. *Journal of Child Psychology and Psychiatry*, *47*, 425–435.

Green, N. (2001). Outwardly mobile: Young people and mobile technologies. In J. Katz (Ed.), *Machines that become us: The social context of personal communication technology* (pp. 201–218). New Brunswick, NJ: Transaction.

Green, R. (2000). Lesbians, gay men, and their parents: A critique of LaSala and the prevailing clinical "wisdom." *Family Process*, *39*, 257–266.

Greene, R. W. (2001). *The explosive child: A new approach for understanding and parenting easily frustrated, chronically inflexible children*. New York, NY: HarperCollins.

Grills, A. E., & Ollendick, T. H. (2003). Multiple informant agreement and the anxiety disorders interview schedule for parents and children. *Journal of the American Academy of Child & Adolescent Psychiatry*, *42*, 30–40.

Grolnick, W. S. (2003). *The psychology of parental control: How well-meant parenting backfires*. Mahwah, NJ: Erlbaum.

Grosz, C. A., Kempe, R. S., & Kelly, M. (2000). Extrafamilial sexual abuse: Treatment for child victims and their families. *Child Abuse & Neglect*, *24*(1), 9–23.

Gunnoe, M. L., Hetherington, E. M., & Reiss, D. (2006). Differential impact of fathers' authoritarian parenting on early adolescent adjustment in conservative protestant versus other families. *Journal of Family Psychology*, *20*(4), 589–596. doi:10.1037/0893-3200.20.4.589

Gunsberg, L. (2013). Betrayal of the family: The parental affair as family incest. In L. Gunsberg & P. Hymowitz (Eds.), *A handbook of divorce and custody: Forensic, developmental, and clinical perspectives* (pp. 91–108). Hoboken, NJ: Taylor and Francis.

Guo, X., & Slesnick, N. (2013). Family versus individual therapy: Impact on discrepancies between parents' and adolescents' perceptions over time. *Journal of Marital & Family Therapy*, *39*(2), 182–194.

Guseh, J. S., Brendel, R. W., & Brendel, D. H. (2009). Medical professionalism in the age of online social networking. *Journal of Medical Ethics, 35*, 584–586.

Gutner, C. A., Rizvi, S. L., Monson, C. M., & Resick, P. A. (2006). Changes in coping strategies, relationship to the perpetrator, and posttraumatic distress in female crime victims. *Journal of Traumatic Stress, 19*(6), 813–823. doi:10.1002/jts.20158

Hair, E. C., Moore, K. A., Garrett, S. B., Ling, T., & Cleveland, K. (2008). The continued importance of quality parent–adolescent relationships during late adolescence. *Journal of Research on Adolescence, 18*(1), 187–200.

Hallab, L., & Covic, T. (2010). Deliberate self-harm: The interplay between attachment and stress. *Behaviour Change, 27*(2), 93–103. doi:10.1375/bech.27.2.93

Halpern, C. T., Oslak, S. G., Young, M. L., Martin, S. L., & Kupper, L. L. (2001). Partner violence among adolescents in opposite-sex romantic relationships: Findings from the National Longitudinal Study of Adolescent Health. *American Journal of Public Health, 91*, 1679–1685.

Halpern, C. T., Spriggs, A. L., Martin, S. L., & Kupper, L. L. (2009). Patterns of intimate partner violence victimization from adolescence to young adulthood in a nationally representative sample. *Journal of Adolescent Health, 45*(5), 508–516. doi:10.1016/j.jadohealth.2009.03.011

Hamburger, M. E., Leeb, R. T., & Swahn, M. H. (2008). Childhood maltreatment and early alcohol use among high-risk adolescents. *Journal of Studies on Alcohol and Drugs, 69*(2), 291–295.

Hannah, M. (2010). Cyberbullying education for parents: A guide for clinicians. *Journal of Social Sciences, 6*, 532–536.

Hanville, C., & Snyder, A. (2012). *Internet marketing for therapists made easy*. Cathy Hanville.

Haravuori, H., Suomalainen, L., Berg, N., Kiviruusu, O., & Marttunen, M. (2011). Effects of media exposure on adolescents traumatized in a school shooting. *Journal of Traumatic Stress, 24*, 70–77.

Hargie, O., & Dickson, D. (2004). *Skilled interpersonal communication: Research, theory, and practice* (4th ed.). London, England: Routledge.

Harper, G., & Irvin, E. (1985). Alliance formation with parents: Limit-setting and the effect of mandated reporting. *American Journal of Orthopsychiatry, 55*(4), 550–560.

Harries, M. (2002). Mandatory Reporting of Child Abuse: Evidence and Options. http://www.uwa.edu.au/__data/assets/pdf_file/0009/1102131/MRFinalReport.pdf

Harrison, D., & Albanese, P. (2012). The "parentification" phenomenon as applied to adolescents living through parental military deployments. *Canadian Journal of Family and Youth, 4*(1), 1–27.

Hart, S. N., Brassard, M. R., Binggeli, N. J., & Davidson, H. A. (2002). Psychological maltreatment. In J. E. B. Myers, L. A. Berliner, J. N. Briere, C. T. Hendrix, T. A. Reid, & C. A. Jenny (Eds.), *The APSAC handbook on child maltreatment*. Thousand Oaks, CA: Sage.

Haskett, M. E., Scott, S. S., Willoughby, M., Ahern, L., & Nears, K. (2006). The Parent Opinion Questionnaire and child vignettes for use with abusive parents: Assessment of psychometric properties. *Journal of Family Violence, 21*, 137–151.

Haut, M. W., & Muehleman, T. (1986). Informed consent: The effects of clarity and specificity on disclosure in a clinical interview. *Psychotherapy: Theory, Research, Practice, Training, 23*(1), 93–101.

Hawk, S. T., Hale, W. W., III, Raaijmakers, Q. A. W., & Meeus, W. (2008). Adolescents' perceptions of privacy invasion in reaction to parental solicitation and control. *Journal of Early Adolescence, 28*(4), 583–608.

Hawkins, N. A., McIntosh, D. N., Silver, R. C., & Holman, E. A. (2004). Early responses to school violence: A qualitative analysis of students' and parents' immediate reactions to the shootings at Columbine High School. *Journal of Emotional Abuse, 4*, 197–223.

Hawley, K. M., & Garland, A. F. (2008). Working alliance in adolescent outpatient therapy: Youth, parent and therapist reports and associations with therapy outcomes. *Child & Youth Care Forum, 37*(2), 59–74.

Hawley, K. M., & Weisz, J. R. (2005). Youth versus parent working alliance in usual clinical care: Distinctive associations with retention, satisfaction, and treatment outcome. *Journal of Clinical Child & Adolescent Psychology, 34*(1), 117–128. doi:10.1207/s15374424jccp3401_11

Hazan, C. & Shaver, P. R. (1994). Attachment as an organizational framework for research on close relationships. *Psychological Inquiry, 5*, 1–22.

Heatherington, L., Friedlander, M. L., & Diamond, G. M. (2014). Lessons offered, lessons learned: Reflections on how doing family therapy can affect therapists. *Journal of Clinical Psychology: In Session, 70*(8), 760–767.

Heflin, A. H., Deblinger, E., & Fisher, C. D. (2000). Child sexual abuse. In F. M. Dattilio & A. Freeman (Eds.), *Cognitive-behavioral strategies in crisis intervention* (pp. 166–195). New York, NY: Guilford Press.

Helitzer, D. L., Sussman, A. L., Urquieta de Hernandez, B., & Kong, A. S. (2011). The "ins" and "outs" of provider-parent communication: Perspectives from adolescent primary care providers on challenges to forging alliances to reduce adolescent risk. *Journal of Adolescent Health, 48*(4), 404–409.

Henderson, S. H., Hetherington, E. M., Mekos, D., & Reiss, D. (1996). Stress, parenting, and adolescent psychopathology in nondivorced and stepfamilies: A within-family perspective. In E. M. Hetherington & E. A. Blechman (Eds.), *Stress, coping, and resiliency in children and families* (pp. 39–66). Mahwah, NJ: Lawrence Erlbaum Associates.

Herek, G. M. (2014). Not equal yet: Building upon foundations of relationship equality: Evaluating the methodology of social science research on sexual orientation and parenting: A tale of three studies. *UC Davis Law Review*, 48, 583.

Heriot, J. (1996). Maternal protectiveness following the disclosure of intrafamilial child sexual abuse. *Journal of Interpersonal Violence, 11*(2), 181–194. doi:10.1177/088626096011002003

Herman, J. L. (1992). *Trauma and recovery*. New York, NY: Basic Books.

Herman, J. L. (2003). The mental health of crime victims: Impact of legal interventions. *Journal of Traumatic Stress, 16*(2), 159–166.

Herrenkohl, T. I., McMorris, B. J., Catalano, R. F., Abbott, R. D., Hemphill, S. A., & Toumbourou, J. W. (2007). Risk factors for violence and relational aggression in adolescence. *Journal of Interpersonal Violence, 22*(4), 386–405. doi:10.1177/0886260506296986

Hessler, D. M., & Katz, L. F. (2010). Brief report: Associations between emotional competence and adolescent risky behavior. *Journal of Adolescence*, *33*, 241–246.

Hetherington, E. M., Henderson, S. H., Reiss, D., Anderson, E. R., Bridges, M., Chan, R. W., ... Taylor, L. V. (1999). Adolescent siblings in stepfamilies: Family function and adolescent adjustment. *Monographs of the Society for Child Development*, *64*(4, Serial No. 222).

Hewitt, P. L., Caelian, C. F., Chen, C., & Flett, G. L. (2014). Perfectionism, stress, daily hassles, hopelessness, and suicide potential in depressed psychiatric adolescents. *Journal of Psychopathology and Behavioral Assessment*, *36*(4), 663–674. doi:10.1007/s10862-014-9427-0

Hibbard, R., Barlow, J., MacMillan, H., & Committee on Child Abuse and Neglect and American Academy of Child and Adolescent Psychiatry. (2012). Psychological maltreatment. *Pediatrics*, *130*, 372–278.

Highet, G. (2005). Alcohol and cannabis: Young people talking about how parents respond to their use of these two drugs. *Drugs: Education, Prevention & Policy*, *12*(2), 113–124. doi:10.1080/09687630412331315125

Himmelstein, K. E. W., & Bruckner, H. (2011). Criminal-justice and school sanctions against nonheterosexual youth: A national longitudinal study. *Pediatrics*, *127*(1), 49–57.

Hines, M., Brook, C., & Conway, G. S. (2004). Androgren and psychosexual development: Core gender identity, sexual orientation, and recalled childhood gender role behavior in women and men with congenital adrenal hyperplasia (CAH). *Journal of Sex Research*, *41*, 75–81.

Hinshaw, S. P. (2005). The stigmatization of mental illness in children and parents: Developmental issues, family concerns, and research needs. *Journal of Child Psychology and Psychiatry*, *46*, 714–734.

Hirschberg, J. C. (1969). Termination of residential treatment of children with emphasis on the process with the parents. *Bulletin of the Menninger Clinic*, *33*(6), 364–369. Retrieved from http://search.ebscohost.com/login.aspx?direct=true&db=psyh&AN=1970-10680-001&site=ehost-live&scope=site

Hobfoll, S. E., Freedy, J. R., Green, B. L., & Solomon, S. D. (1996). Coping in reaction to extreme stress: The roles of resource loss and resource availability. In M. Zeidner & N. S. Endler (Eds.), *Handbook of coping: Theory, research, applications* (pp. 322–349). New York, NY: John Wiley & Sons.

Hock, E., Eberly, M., Bartle-Haring, S., Ellwanger, P., & Widaman, K. F. (2001). Separation anxiety in parents of adolescents: Theoretical significance and scale development, *Child Development*, *71*(1), 284–298.

Hogue, A., Dauber, S., Stambaugh, L. F., Cecero, J. J., & Liddle, H. A. (2006). Early therapeutic alliance and treatment outcome in individual and family therapy for adolescent behavior problems. *Journal of Consulting and Clinical Psychology*, *74*, 121–129.

Holi, M. M., Pelkonen, M., Karlsson, L., Tuisku, V., Kiviruusu, O., Ruuttu, T., & Marttunen, M. (2008). Detecting suicidality among adolescent outpatients: Evaluation of trained clinicians' suicidality assessment against a structured diagnostic assessment made by trained raters. *BMC Psychiatry*, 8, 97.

Hollander, M. (2008). *Helping teens who cut: Understanding and ending self-injury.* New York, NY: Guilford Press.

Hollingsworth, J., Glass, J., & Heisler, K. W. (2007). Empathy deficits in siblings of severely scapegoated children: A conceptual model. *Journal of Emotional Abuse*, *7*(4), 69–88. doi:10.1300/J135v7n04_04

Holtzen, D. W., Kenny, M. E., & Mahalik, J. R. (1995). Contributions of parental attachment to gay or lesbian disclosure to parents and dysfunctional cognitive processes. *Journal of Counseling Psychology*, *42*(3), 350–355. doi:10.1037/0022-0167.42.3.350

Hooley, J. M. (1985). Expressed emotion: A review of the critical literature. *Clinical Psychology Review*, *5*, 119–139.

Hooley, J. M. (2007). Expressed emotion and relapse in psychopathology. *Annual Review of Clinical Psychology*, *3*, 349–372.

Hooper, C., & Humphreys, C. (1998). Women whose children have been sexually abused: Reflections of a debate. *British Journal of Social Work*, *28*, 565–580.

Hooper, L. (2007). Expanding the discussion regarding parentification and its varied outcomes: Implications for mental health research and practice. *Journal of Mental Health Counseling*, *29*(4), 322–337.

Horesh, N., Nachshoni, T., Wolmer, L., & Toren, P. (2009). A comparison of life events in suicidal and nonsuicidal adolescents and young adults with major depression and borderline personality disorder. *Comprehensive Psychiatry*, *50*(6), 496–502. doi:10.1016/j.comppsych.2009.01.006

Horne, S. (1998). *The role of parental narcissism and depression in predicting adolescent empathy, marcissism, self-esteem, pleasing others, and peer conflict*. Doctoral dissertation (PhD), University of Georgia.

Horowitz, A. V. (1978). Family, kin, and friend networks in psychiatric help-seeking. *Social Science & Medicine*, *12*, 297–304.

Horvath, A. O., & Bedi, R. P. (2002). The alliance. In J. C. Norcross (Ed.), *Psychotherapy relationships that work* (pp. 36–69). London, England: Oxford University Press.

Horwath, J., & Morrison, T. (2010). Assessing parental motivation to change. In J. Horwath (Ed.), *The child's world: The comprehensive guide to assessing children in need* (2nd ed., pp. 98–113). London, England: Jan Kingsley.

Houck, C. D., Barker, D., Rizzo, C., Hancock, E., Norton, A., & Brown, L. K. (2014). Sexting and sexual behavior in at-risk adolescents. *Pediatrics*, 133, e276–e282.

Hougaard, E. (1994). The therapeutic alliance: A conceptual analysis. *Scandinavian Journal of Psychology*, *35*, 67–85.

Howard, K., Lueger, R., Maling, M., & Martinovich, Z. (1993). A phase model of psychotherapy outcome: Causal mediation of change. *Journal of Consulting & Cinical Psychology*, *61*(4), 678–685.

Howard, K., Moras, K., Brill, P. L., Martinovich, Z., & Lutz, W. (1996). Evaluation of psychotherapy: Efficacy, effectiveness, and patient progress. *American Psychologist*, *51*, 1059–1064.

Howard, D. E., Wang, M. Q., & Yan, F. (2007). Prevalence and psychosocial correlates of forced sexual intercourse among U.S. high school adolescents. *Adolescence*, *42*(168), 629–643.

Howard, M. S., & Medway, F. J. (2004). Adolescents' attachments and coping with stress. *Psychology in the Schools*, *41*, 391–402. http://www.theatlantic.com/magazine/archive/2011/07/how-to-land-your-kid-in-therapy/308555/

Hudson, J. L., & Rapee, R. M. (2004). From anxious temperament to disorder: An etiological moel. In R. G. Heinberg, C. L. Turk, & D. S. Mennin (Eds.), *Generalized anxiety disorder: Advances in research and practice* (pp. 51–74). New York, NY: Guilford Press.

Hudson, J. L., Newall, C., Rapee, R. M., Lyneham, H. J., Schniering, C. C., Wuthrich, V. M., … Gar, N. S. (2014). The impact of brief parental anxiety management on child anxiety treatment outcomes: A controlled trial. *Journal of Clinical Child and Adolescent Psychology, 43*(3), 370–380.

Hunter, M., & Gerber, P. (1990). Use of the terms "victim" and "survivor" in the grief stages commonly seen during recovery from sexual abuse. In M. Hunter (Ed.), *The sexually abused male, Volume 2: Application of treatment strategies* (pp. 79–89). Lexington, MA: Lexington Books.

Huntley, M. (2008). Relationship-based social work: How do endings impact on the client? *Practice: Social Work in Action, 14*(2), 59–66.

Iannos, M., & Antcliff, G. (2013). The application of motivational interviewing techniques for engaging "resistant" families. Retrieved from https://aifs.gov.au/cfca/publications/application-motivational-interviewing-techniques

Im-Bolter, N., Zadeh, Z. Y., & Ling, D. (2013). Early parenting beliefs and academic achievement: The mediating role of language. *Early Child Development and Care, 183*, 1811–1826.

Jackson, S. (2002). Abuse in dating relationships: Young people's accounts of disclosure, non-disclosure, help-seeking and prevention education. *New Zealand Journal of Psychology, 31*(2), 79–86.

Jacobson, C. M., & Gould, M. F. (2007). The epidemiology and phenomenology of non-suicidal self-injurious behavior among adolescents: A critical review of the literature. *Archives of Suicide Research, 11*, 129–147.

Jacobson, K. C., & Crockett, L. J. (2000). Parental monitoring and adolescent adjustment: An ecological approach. *Journal of Research on Adolescence, 10*, 65–97.

James, D., & Hawton, K. (1985). Overdoses: Explanations and attitudes of self-poisoners and significant others. *British Journal of Psychiatry, 146*, 481–485.

James, K., & MacKinnon, L. (2010). The tip of the iceberg: A framework for identifying non-physical abuse in couple and family relationships. *Journal of Feminist Family Therapy: An International Forum, 22*(2), 112–129. doi:10.1080/08952831003787867

Janoff-Bulman, R. (1992). *Shattered assumptions: Towards a new psychology of trauma*. New York, NY: The Free Press.

Jent, J. F., Eaton, C. K., Merrick, M. T., Englebert, N. E., Dandes, S. K., Chapman, A. V., & Hershorin, E. R. (2011). The decision to access patient information from a social media site: What would you do? *Journal of Adolescent Health, 49*(4), 414–420. doi:10.1016/j.jadohealth.2011.02.004

Jobes, D. A. (2006). *Managing suicidal risk: A collaborative approach*. New York, NY: Guilford Press.

Johnson, B. J., & Kenkel, M. (1991). Stress, coping, and adjustment in female adolescent incest victims. *Child Abuse and Neglect, 15*, 292–305.

Johnson, D. W. (1990). *Reaching out* (4th ed.). Englewood Cliffs, NJ: Prentice-Hall.

Johnson, J., Cohen, P., Kasen, S., & Brook, J. (2008). Psychiatric disorders in adolescence and early adulthood and risk for child-rearing difficulties during middle adulthood. *Journal of Family Issues*, *29*(2), 210–233.

Johnson, S. M., Maddeaux, C., & Blouin, J. (1998). Emotionally focused family therapy for bulimia: Changing attachment patterns. *Psychotherapy: Theory, Research, Practice, Training*, *35*(2), 238–247. doi:10.1037/h0087728

Johnston, J. R. (2005). Clinical work with parents in entrenched custody disputes. In L. Gunsberg & P. Hymowitz (Eds.), *A handbook of divorce and custody: Forensic, developmental, and clinical perspectives* (pp. 343–363). New York, NY: The Analytic Press/Taylor & Francis.

Johnston, L. D., O'Malley, P. M., Bachman, J. G., & Schulenberg, J. E. (2011). *Monitoring the future national survey results on drug use, 1975–2010*. (Volume I: Secondary school students, 2010). Bethesda, MD: National Institute on Drug Abuse.

Joiner, T., Pettit, J. W., Walker, R. L., Voelz, Z. R., Cruz, J., Rudd, M. D., & Lester, D. (2002). Perceived burdensomeness and suicidality: Two studies on the suicide notes of those attempting and those completing suicide. *Journal of Social and Clinical Psychology*, *21*, 531–545.

Jordan, A. B., Hershey, J., McDevitt, J., & Heitzler, C. (2006). Reducing children's television-viewing time: A qualitative study of parents and their children. *Pediatrics*, *18*, e1301–e1310.

Jouriles, E. N., Mueller, V., Rosenfield, D., McDonald, R., & Dodson, M. C. (2012). Teens' experiences of harsh parenting and exposure to severe intimate partner violence: Adding insult to injury in predicting teen dating violence. *Psychological Violence*, *2*(2), 125–138. doi:10.1037/a0027264

Joyce, A. S., Piper, W. E., Ogrodniczuk, J. S., & Klein, R. H. (2007). Patient characteristics and variations in termination processes and outcomes. *Termination in psychotherapy: A psychodynamic model of processes and outcomes* (pp. 109–131). Washington, DC: American Psychological Association.

Jurkovic, G. J., Morell, R., & Thirkield, A. (1999). Assessing childhood parentification: Guidleines for researchers and practitioners. In N. Chase (Ed.), *Burdened children: Theory, research, and treatment parentification* (pp. 92–113). London, England: Sage.

Kaess, M., Parzer, P., Mattern, M., Plener, P. L., Bifulco, A., Resch, F., & Brunner, R. (2013). Adverse childhood experiences and their impact on frequency, severity, and the individual function of nonsuicidal self-injury in youth. *Psychiatry Research*, *206*(2–3), 265–272.

Kahn, A. S., Fricker, K., Hoffman, J., Lambert, T., Tripp, M., & Childress, K. (2000). Hooking up: Dangerous new dating methods? Paper presented at the Annual Meeting of American Psychological Association, Washington, DC.

Kaiser Family Foundation. (2010). *Generation M2: Media in the lives of 8- to 18-year olds*. Menlo Park, CA: Author.

Kandel, D. B., & Yamaguchi, K. (2002). Stages of drug involvement in the U.S. population. In D. B. Kandel (Ed.), *Stages and pathways of drug involvement: Examining the Gateway Hypothesis* (pp. 65–89). New York, NY: Cambridge University Press.

Kandel, D. B., Hu, M.-C., & Griesler, P. C. (2013). Epidemiology of substance use disorders. In D. S. Charney, J. D. Buxbaum, P. Sklar, & E. J. Nestler (Eds.), *Neurobiology of mental illness* (4th ed., pp. 772–787). New York, NY: Oxford University Press.

Kanter, M., Afifi, T., & Robbins, S. (2012). The impact of parents "friending" their young adult child on Facebook on perceptions of parental privacy invasions and parent–child relationship quality. *Journal of Communication*, *62*(5), 900–917. doi:10.1111/j.1460-2466.2012.01669.x

Karavasilis, L., Doyle, A., & Markiewicz, D. (2003). Associations between parenting style and attachment to mother in middle childhood and adolescence. *International Journal of Behavioral Development*, *27*, 153–164.

Karpman, S. B. (1968). Fairy tales and script drama analysis. *Transactional Analysis*, *24*, 214–215.

Katz, J., & Aakhus, M. (2002). *Perpetual contact: Mobile communication, private talk, public performance*. Cambridge, UK: Cambridge University Press.

Kazdin, A. E., Holland, L., & Crowley, M. (1997). Family experiences of barriers to treatment and premature termination from child therapy. *Journal of Consulting and Clinical Psychology*, *65*, 453–463.

Keijsers, L., Frijns, T., Branje, S., & Meeus, W. (2009). Developmental links of adolescent disclosure, parental solicitation, and control with delinquency: Moderation by parental support. *Developmental Psychology*, *45*(5), 1314–1327.

Kelley, M., French, A., Bountress, K., Keefe, H., Schroeder, V., Streer, K., ... Gumienny, L. (2007). Parentification and family responsibility in the family of origin of adult children of alcoholics. *Addictive Behaviors*, *32*(4), 675–685.

Kelley, S. J. (1990). Parental distress response to sexual abuse and ritualistic abuse of children in day-care centers. *Nursing Research*, *39*, 25–29.

Kelly, A. E., & McKillop, K. L. (1996). Consequences of revealing personal secrets. *Psychological Bulletin*, *120*, 450–465.

Kelly, P. J., Owen, S. V., Peralez-Dieckmann, E., & Martinez, E. (2007). Health interventions with girls in the juvenile justice system. *Women's Health Issues*, *17*(4), 227–236. doi:10.1016/j.whi.2007.03.005

Kendall-Tackett, K., Williams, L., & Finkelhor, D. (1993). Impact of sexual abuse on children: A review and synthesis of recent empirical studies. *Psychological Bulletin*, *113*, 164–180.

Kennedy, G., Judd, T., Dalgarno, B., & Waycott, J. (2010). Beyond natives and immigrants: Exploring types of net generation students. *Journal of Computer Assisted Learning*, *26*(5), 332–343.

Kerkorian, D., McKay, M., & Bannon, W. M., Jr. (2006). Seeking help a second time: Parents'/caregivers' characterizations of previous experiences with mental health services for their children and perceptions of barriers to future use. *American Journal of Orthopsychiatry*, *76*(2), 161–166.

Kerns, K. A., & Aspelmeier, J. E. (2001). Parent-child attachment and monitoring in middle childhood. *Journal of Family Psychology*, *15*(1), 69–81.

Kerr, M., & Stattin, H. (2000). What parents know, how they know it, and several forms of adolescent adjustment: Further support for a reinterpretation of monitoring. *Developmental Psychology*, *36*, 366–380.

Kerr, M., Stattin, H., & Trost, K. (1999). To know you is to trust you: Parents' trust is rooted in child disclosure of information. *Journal of Adolescence*, *22*(6), 737–752.

Kessler, R. C., Avenevoli, S., Costello, E. J., Georgiades, K., Green, J. G., Gruber, M. J., … Merikangas, K. R. (2012). Prevalence, persistence, and sociodemographic correlates of DSM-IV disorders in the National Comorbidity Survey Replication Adolescent Supplement. *Archives of General Psychiatry*, *69*(4), 372–380. doi:10.1001/archgenpsychiatry.2011.160

Kilpatrick, D. G., Acierno, R., Saunders, B., Resnick, H. S., Best, C. L., & Schnurr, P. P. (2000). Risk factors for adolescent substance abuse and dependence: Data from a national sample. *Journal of Consulting and Clinical Psychology*, *68*(1), 19–30. doi:10.1037/0022-006X.68.1.19

Kilpatrick, D. G., Ruggiero, K. J., Acierno, R., Saunders, B. E., Resnick, H. S., & Best, C. L. (2003). Violence and risk of PTSD, major depression, substance abuse/dependence, and comorbidity: Results from the National Survey of Adolescents. *Journal of Consulting & Clinical psychology*, *71*(4), 692–700.

Kilroy, S. J., Egan, J., Maliszewska, A., & Sarma, K. M. (2014). "Systemic trauma": The impact on parents whose children have experienced sexual abuse. *Journal of Child Sexual Abuse: Research, Treatment, & Program Innovations for Victims, Survivors, & Offenders*, *23*(5), 481–503. doi:10.1080/10538712.2014.920458

Kim, K., Trickett, P. K., & Putnam, F. W. (2010). Childhood experiences of sexual abuse and later parenting practices among non-offending mothers of sexually abused and comparison girls. *Child Abuse & Neglect*, *34*(8), 610–622. doi:10.1016/j.chiabu.2010.01.007

King, C. A., Hovey, J. D., Brand, E., & Wilson, R. (1997). Suicidal adolescents after hospitalization: Parent and family impacts on treatment follow-through. *Journal of the American Academy of Child & Adolescent Psychiatry*, *36*(1), 85–93. doi:10.1097/00004583-199701000-00021

Kirsch, V., Wilhelm, F. H., & Goldbeck, L. (2011). Psychophysiological characteristics of PTSD in children and adolescents: A review of the literature. *Journal of Traumatic Stress*, *24*(2), 146–154.

Kitts, R. (2005). Gay adolescents and suicide: Understanding the association. *Adolescence*, *40*(159), 621–628.

Klein, M. (2012). Teens, parents face off over Facebook. Retrieved from http://usatoday30.usatoday.com/tech/news/story/2012-01-22/facebook-parents-teens/52743092/1

Klettke, B., & Simonis, S. (2011). Attitudes regarding the perceived culpability of adolescent and adult victims of sexual assault. *ACSSA Aware*, *26*, 7–12.

Kliethermes, M., & Wamser, R. (2012). Adolescents with complex trauma. In J. A. Cohen, A. Mannarino, & E. Deblinger (Eds.), *Trauma-focused CBT for children and adolescents: Treatment applications* (pp. 175–196). New York, NY: Guilford Press.

Knutsson-Medin, L., Edlund, B., & Ramklint, M. (2007). Experiences in a group of grown-up children of mentally ill parents. *Journal of Psychiatric & Mental Health Nursing*, *14*(8), 744–752. doi:10.1111/j.1365-2850.2007.01181.x

Kolmes, K., & Taube, D. O. (2014). Seeking and finding out clients on the Internet: Boundary considerations in cyberspace. *Professional Psychology: Research and Practice*, *45*(1), 3–10.

Kolmes, K., & Taube, D. O. (under review). Client discovery of therapist personal information online.

Korchmaros, J. D., Ybarra, M. L., Langhinrichsen-Rohling, J., Boyd, D., & Lenhart, A. (2013). Perpetration of teen dating violence in a networked society. *Cyberpsychology, Behavior, and Social Networking*, *16*(8), 561–567. doi:10.1089/cyber.2012.0627

Koren, P., & DeChillo, N. (1995). Empowering families whose children have emotional disorders. *Focal Point: A National Bulletin on Family Support and Children's Mental Health*, *9*(1), 1–4.

Kourany, R. F., Garber, J., & Tornusciolo, G. (1990). Improving first appointment attendance rates in child psychiatry outpatient clinics. *Journal of the American Academy of Child & Adolescent Psychiatry*, *29*(4), 657–660.

Kouyoumdjian, H., Perry, A. R., & Hansen, D. J. (2009). Nonoffending parent expectations of sexually abused children: Predictive factors and influence on children's recovery. *Journal of Child Sexual Abuse*, *18*(1), 40–60. doi:10.1080/10538710802584627

Kovarsky, R. S. (1989). Loneliness and disturbed grief: A comparison of parents who lost a child to suicide or accidental death. *Archives of Psychiatric Nursing*, *3*(2), 86–96.

Kowal, A. K., & Kramer, L. (1997). Children's perceptions of parental differential treatment. *Child Development*, *68*, 113–126.

Kowal, A. K., Kramer, L., Krull, J. L., & Crick, N. (2002). Children's perceptions of the fairness of parental preferential treatment and their socioemotional well-being. *Journal of Family Psychology*, *16*(3), 297–306.

Kowal, A. K., Krull, J. L., & Kramer, L. (2004). How the differential treatment of siblings is linked with parent-child relationship quality. *Journal of Family Psychology*, *18*(4), 658–665. doi:10.1037/0893-3200.18.4.658

Krell, H. L., & Okin, R. L. (1984). Countertransference issues in child abuse and neglect cases. *American Journal of Forensic Psychiatry*, *5*(1), 7–16.

Krishnakumar, A., & Buehler, M. M. (2000). Interparental conflict and parenting behaviors: A meta-analytic review. *Family Relations: Journal of Applied Family and Child Studies*, *49*, 25–44.

Kübler-Ross, E., & Kessler, D. (2005). *On grief and grieving: Finding the meaning of grief through the five stages of loss*. New York, NY: Simon & Schuster.

L'Abate, L. (2009). The drama triangle: An attempt to resurrect a neglected pathogenic model in family therapy theory and practice. *American Journal of Family Therapy*, *37*(1), 1–11. doi:10.1080/01926180701870163

Lackie, B. (1999). Trauma, invisibility and loss: Multiple metaphors of parentification. In N. Chase (Ed.), *Burdened children: Theory, research, and treatment of parentification* (pp. 141–153). Thousand Oaks, CA: Sage.

Laghi, F., D'Alessio, M., Pallini, S., & Baiocco, R. (2009). Attachment representations and time perspective in adolescence. *Social Indicators Research*, *90*, 181–194.

Laible, D. J., Carlo, G., & Raffaelli, M. (2000). The differential relations of parent and peer attachment to adolescent adjustment. *Journal of Youth and Adolescence*, *29*, 45–59.

Lambert, M. J., & Ogles, B. M. (2004). The efficacy and effectiveness of psychotherapy. In M. Lambert (Ed.), *Bergin and Garfield's handbook of psychotherapy and behavior change* (5th ed., pp. 139–193). New York, NY: John Wiley & Sons.

Lampis, J. A., Agus, M., & Cacciarru, B. (2014). Quality of family relationships as protective factors of eating disorders: An investigation amongst Italian teenagers. *Applied Research and Quality of Life*, *9*(2), 309–324.

Landolt, M. A., Vollrath, M., Ribi, K., Gnehm, H. E., & Sennhauser, F. H. (2003). Incidence and associations of parental and child posttraumatic stress symptoms in pediatric patients. *Journal of Child Psychology & Psychiatry & Allied Disciplines*, *44*(8), 1199–1207. doi:10.1111/1469-7610.00201

Landreth, G. (2012). *Play therapy: The art of the relationship*. New York, NY: Brunner & Routledge.

Langstrom, N., Rahman, Q., Carlstrom, E., & Lichtenstein, P. (2010). Genetic and environmental effects on same-sex sexual behavior: A population study of twins in Sweden. *Archives of Sexual Behavior*, *39*, 75–80.

LaSala, M. C. (2000). Lesbian, gay men, and their parents: Family therapy for the coming-out crisis. *Family Process*, *39*, 67–81.

LaSala, M. C. (2010). *Coming out, coming home: Helping families adjust to a gay or lesbian child*. New York, NY: Columbia University.

Lau, A., & Takeuchi, D. (2001). Cultural factors in help-seeking for child behavior problems: Value orientation, affective responding, and severity appraisals among Chinese-American parents. *Journal of Community Psychology*, *29*(6), 675–692.

Lee, C.-H., Moak, S., & Walker, J. T. (2016). Effects of self-control, social control, and social learning on sexting behavior among South Korean youths. *Youth & Society*, *48*(2), 242–264.

Leedom, L. J., Bass, A., & Almas, L. H. (2013). The problem of parental psychopathy. *Journal of Child Custody: Research, Issues, and Practices*, *10*(2), 154–184. doi:10.1080/15379418.2013.796268

Lehavot, K., Barnett, J. E., & Powers, D. (2010). Psychotherapy, professional relationships, and ethical considerations in the MySpace generation. *Professional Psychology: Research and Practice*, *41*, 160–166.

Lehman, S. J., & Koerner, S. S. (2002). Family financial hardship and adolescent girls' adjustment: The role of maternal disclosure of financial concerns. *Merrill-Palmer Quarterly*, *48*(1), 1.

Lerner, M. (1980). *The belief in a just world: A fundamental delusion*. New York, NY: Plenum.

Levi, B. H., Brown, G., & Erb, C. (2006). Reasonable suspicion: A pilot study of pediatric residents. *Child Abuse & Neglect*, *30*(4), 345–356.

Levy, M. (1998). A helpful way to conceptualize and understand reenactments. *The Journal of Psychotherapy Practice*, *7*, 227–235.

Lewinsohn, P. M., Pohde, P., Klein, D. N., & Seeley, J. R. (1999). Natural course of adolescent major depressive disorder. *Journal of the American Academy of Child & Adolescent Psychiatry*, *38*, 56–63.

Li, T., & Chan, D. K.-S. (2012). How anxious and avoidant attachment affect romantic relationship quality differently: A meta-analytic review. *European Journal of Social Psychology*, *42*, 406–419.

Li, X., Feigelman, S., & Stanton, B. (2000). Perceived parental monitoring and health risk behaviors among urban low-income African-American children and adolescents. *Journal of Adolescent Health*, *27*, 43–48.

Libo, L. M., & Griffith, C. R. (1996). Developing mental health programs in areas lacking professional facilities: The community consultant approach in New Mexico. *Community Mental Health Journal*, *2*, 163–169.

Lickel, B., Schmader, T., & Hamilton, D. L. (2003). A case of collective responsibility: Who else was to blame for the Columbine high school shootings? *Personality and Social Psychology Bulletin*, *29*, 194–204.

Lilenfeld, L. R., Kaye, W. H., Greeno, C. G., Merikangas, K. R., Plotnicov, K., Pollice, C., ... Nagy, L. (1998). A controlled family study of anorexia nervosa and bulimia nervosa: Psychiatric disorders in first-degree relatives and effects of proband comorbidity. *Archives of General Psychiatry*, *55*(7), 603–610.

Lilliengren, P., Falkenström, F., Sandell, R., Mothander, P. R., & Werbart, A. (2015). Secure attachment to therapist, alliance, and outcome in psychoanalytic psychotherapy with young adults. *Journal of Counseling Psychology*, *62*(1), 1–13. doi:10.1037/cou0000044

Lindhout, I., Markus, M., Hoogendijk, T., Borst, S., Maingay, R., Spinhoven, P., ... Boer, F. (2006). Childrearing style of anxiety-disordered parents. *Child Psychiatry & Human Development*, *37*(1), 89–102. doi:10.1007/s10578-006-0022-9

Ling, R. (2004). *The mobile connection: The cell phone's impact on society*. San Francisco, CA: Morgan Kauffman.

Ling, R., & Yttri, B. (2002). Hyper-coordination via mobile phones in Norway. In J. E. Katz & M. Aakhus (Eds.), *Perpetual contact: Mobile communication, private talk, public performance* (pp. 139–169). Cambridge, UK: Cambridge University Press.

Ling, R., & Yttri, B. (2006). Control, emancipation, and status: The mobile telephone in teens' parental and peer relationships. In R. Kraut, M. Brynin, & S. Kiesler (Eds.), *Computers, phones, and the Internet: Domesticating information technology* (pp. 219–234). New York, NY: Oxford University Press.

Lingiardi, V., Tanzilli, A., & Colli, A. (2015). Does the severity of psychopathological symptoms mediate the relationship between patient personality and therapist response? *Psychotherapy*, *52*(2), 228–237. doi:10.1037/a0037919

Lipton, M. (1997). The effect of the primary caretaker's distress on the sexually abused child: A comparison of biological and foster parents. *Child & Adolescent Social Work Journal*, *14*(2), 115–127. doi:10.1023/A:1024505216535

Liu, Y. (2007). Paternal/maternal attachment, peer support, social expectations of peer interaction, and depressive symptoms. *Adolescence*, *41*, 705–721.

Liz Claiborne Inc. (2007). Tech abuse in teen relationships study. Retrieved from http://www.loveisrespect.org/wp-content/uploads/2009/03/liz-claiborne-2007-tech-relationship-abuse.pdf

Lloyd-Richardson, E. E., Perrine, N., Dierker, L., & Kelley, M. L. (2007). Characteristics and functions of non-suicidal self-injury in a community sample of adolescents. *Psychological Medicine*, *37*, 1183–1192.

Lobbestael, J., Arntz, A., & Wiers, R. W. (2008). How to push someone's buttons: A comparison of four anger-induction methods. *Cognition and Emotion*, *22*(2), 353–373. doi:10.1080/02699930701438285

Logan, D. E., & King, C. A. (2001). Parental facilitation of adolescent mental health services utilization: A conceptual and empirical review. *Clinical Psychology: Science and Practice*, *8*(3), 319–333.

Lopez-Fernandez, O., Honrubia-Serrano, L., Freixa-Blanxart, M., & Gibson, W. (2014). Prevalence of problematic mobile phone use in British adolescents. *Cyberpsychology, Behavior, and Social Networking*, *17*(2), 91–98. doi:10.1089/cyber.2012.0260

Lothen-Kline, C., Howard, D. E., Hamburger, E. K., Worrell, K. D., & Boekeloo, B. O. (2003). Truth and consequences: Ethics, confidentiality, and disclosure in adolescent longitudinal prevention research. *Journal of Adolescent Health*, *33*(5), 385–394.

Lowes, L., Gregory, J. W., & Lyne, P. (2005). Newly diagnosed childhood diabetes: A psychosocial transition for parents? *Journal of Advanced Nursing*, *50*(3), 253–261. doi:10.1111/j.1365-2648.2005.03388.x

Luthar, S. S., & Becker, B. E. (2002). Privileged but pressured? A study of affluent youth. *Child Development*, *73*(5), 1593–1610. doi:10.1111/1467-8624.00492

Lyman, E. L., & Luthar, S. S. (2014). Further evidence on the "costs of privilege": Perfectionism in high-achieving youth at socioeconomic extremes. *Psychology in the Schools*, *51*(9), 913–930. doi:10.1002/pits.21791

Lyon, M. E., Benoit, M., O'Donnell, R., Getson, P. R., Silber, T., & Walsh, T. (2000). Assessing African American adolescents' risk for suicide attempts: Attachment theory. *Adolescence*, *35*, 121–134.

Maccoby, E. E., & Martin, J. A. (1983). Socialization in the context of the family: Parent child interaction. In P. H. Mussen (Ed.), *Handbook of child psychology, 4th Edition* (Vol. 4, pp. 1–101). New York, NY: Wiley.

Macfie, J., & Swan, S. A. (2009). Representations of caregiver-child relationship and of the self, and emotion regulation in the narratives of young children whose mothers have borderline personality disorder. *Development and Psychopathology*, *21*, 993–1011.

MacGregor, H. A., & Elliot, A. J. (2005). The shame of failure: Examining the link between fear of failure and shame. *Personality and Social Psychology Bulletin*, *31*, 218–231.

Madden, M., Cortesi, S., Gasser, U., Lenhart, A., & Duggan, M. (2012). Parents, teens, and online privacy. Pew Internet and American Life Project. Retrieved from http://pewinternet.org/Reports/2012/Teens-and-Privacy.aspx

Madge, C., Meek, J., Weelens, J., & Hooley, T. (2009). Facebook, social interaction and informal learning at university: "It is more for socialising and talking to friends about work than for actually doing work." *Learning, Media, and Technology*, *34*, 141–155.

Maercker, A., & Mehr, A. (2006). What if victims read a newspaper report about their victimization? A study on the relationship to PTSD symptoms in crime victims. *European Psychologist, 11*(2), 137–142.

Mahlstedt, D., & Kenny, L. (1993). Female survivors of dating violence and their social networks. *Feminism and Psychology, 3*(3), 319–333.

Maimon, D., Browning, C. R., & Brooks-Gunn, J. (2010). Collective efficacy, family attachment, and urban adolescent suicide attempts. *Journal of Health and Social Behavior, 51*, 307–324.

Main, M., & Solomon, J. (1990). Procedures for identifying infants as disorganized/disoriented during the Ainsworth Strange Situation. In M. T. Greenberg, E. M. Cicchetti, & E. M. Cummings (Eds.), *Attachment in the preschool years* (pp. 121–160). Chicago, IL: University of Chicago Press.

Maine, S., Shute, R., & Martin, G. (2001). Educating parents about youth suicide: Knowledge, response to suicidal statements, attitudes, and intentions to help. *Suicide and Life-Threatening Behavior, 31*, 320–333.

Malawista, K. L. (2004). Rescue fantasies in child therapy: Countertransference/transference enactments. *Child and Adolescent Social Work Journal, 21*(4), 373–386.

Mallinckrodt, B., & Jeong, J. (2015). Meta-analysis of client attachment to therapist: Associations with working alliance and client pretherapy attachment. *Psychotherapy, 52*(1), 134–139. doi:10.1037/a0036890

Mammen, O., Kolko, D., & Pilkonis, P. (2003). Parental cognitions and satisfaction: Relationship to aggressive parental behavior in child physical abuse. *Child Maltreatment, 8*(4), 288–301. doi:10.1177/1077559503257112

Manion, I. G., McIntyre, J., Firestone, P., Ligezinska, M., Ensom, R., & Wells, G. (1996). Secondary traumatization in parents following the disclosure of extrafamilial child sexual abuse: Initial effects. *Child Abuse & Neglect, 20*(11), 1095–1109.

Mannarino, A., Cohen, J. A., & Berman, S. R. (1994). The Children's Attributions and Perceptions Scale: A new measure of sexual abuse-related factors. *Journal of Clinical Child Psychology, 23*, 204–211.

Mannarino, A., Cohen, J. A., Deblinger, E., & Steer, R. (2007). Self-reported depression in mothers of children who have experienced sexual abuse. *Journal of Psychopathology and Behavioral Assessment, 29*(3), 203–210.

Manning, W. D., Giordano, P. C., & Longmore, M. A. (2006). Hooking up: The relationship contexts of "nonrelationship" sex. *Journal of Adolescent Research, 21*, 459–483.

Maples, J. L., & Walker, R. L. (2014). Consolidation rather than termination: Rethinking how psychologists label and conceptualize the final phase of psychological treatment. *Professional Psychology: Research and Practice, 45*(2), 104–110. doi:10.1037/a0036250

Marano, H. E. (2010, October). How college freshman have changed. *The New York Times*.

Margolis, H. (1991). Listening: The key to problem solving with angry parents. *School Psychology International, 12*(4), 329–347. doi:10.1177/0143034391124005

Mark, B. S. (1998). Countertransference issues in treating parents of child and adolescent patients. *Family Therapy, 25*(2), 97–109.

Marshall, J. (2014). When should you come between a teenager and her phone? Social media and adolescent development. Retrieved from http://www.childmind.org/en/posts/articles/2014-8-19-when-come-between-teens-and-phones

Martin, D. J., Garske, J. P., & Davis, M. K. (2000). Relation of the therapeutic alliance with outcome and other variables: A meta-analytic review. *Journal of Consulting and Clinical Psychology*, *68*, 438–450.

Martin, J., Romas, M., Medford, M., Leffert, N., & Hatcher, S. L. (2006). Adult helping qualities preferred by adolescents. *Adolescence*, *41*(161), 127–140.

Martin, K. A., Hutson, D. J., Kazyak, E., & Scherrer, K. S. (2010). Advice when children come out: The cultural "tool kits" of parents. *Journal of Family Issues*, *31*(7), 960–991. doi:10.1177/0192513X09354454

Marx, J. A., & Gelso, C. J. (1987). Termination of individual counseling in a university counseling center. *Journal of Counseling Psychology*, *34*, 3–9.

Massachusetts Department of Education. (2009). Massachusetts youth risk behavior survey. Retrieved from http://www.mass.gov/clgy/publications.htm

Mayseless, O., & Scharf, M. (2009). Too close for comfort: Inadequate boundaries with parents and individuation in late adolescent girls. *American Journal of Orthopsychiatry*, *79*, 191–202.

McCann, I. L., & Pearlman, L. A. (1990). Vicarious traumatization: A framework for understanding the psychological effects of working with victims. *Journal of Traumatic Stress*, *3*(1), 131–149.

McCourt, J., & Peel, J. C. F. (1998). The effects of child sexual abuse on the protecting parent(s): Identifying a counselling response. *Counselling Psychology Quarterly*, *11*(3), 283.

McElroy, L. P., & McElroy, R. A. (1991). Countertransference issues in the treatment of incest families. *Psychotherapy: Theory, Research, Practice, Training*, *28*(1), 48–54. doi:10.1037/0033-3204.28.1.48

McHale, S. M., Updegraff, K. A., Jackson-Newsom, J., Tucker, C. J., & Crouter, A. C. (2000). When does parents' differential treatment have negative implications? *Social Development*, *9*, 149–172.

McIntosh, J., & Drapeau, C. (2012). *U.S.A. suicide 2010: Official final data*. Washington, DC: American Association of Suicidality.

McIntosh, J., MacDonald, F., & McKeganey, N. (2005). The reasons why children in their pre and early teenage years do or do not use illegal drugs. *International Journal of Drug Policy*, *16*(4), 254–261. doi:10.1016/j.drugpo.2005.05.005

McKee, M. D., O'Sullivan, L. F., & Weber, C. M. (2006). Perspectives on confidential care for adolescent girls. *Annals of Family Medicine*, *4*, 519–526.

McLeod, B. D., & Weisz, J. R. (2005). The Therapy Process Observational Coding System Alliance Scale: Measure characteristics and prediction of outcome in usual clinical practice. *Journal of Consulting and Clinical Psychology*, *73*, 323–333.

McWilliams, N. (1994). *Psychoanalytic diagnosis*. New York, NY: Guilford Press.

Mears, C. L. (2005). Experiences of Columbine parents: Finding a way to tomorrow (unpublished doctoral dissertation). University of Denver, Colorado.

Mechanic, K., & Barry, C. (2015). Adolescent grandiose and vulnerable narcissism: Associations with perceived parenting practices. *Journal of Child & Family Studies*, *24*(5), 1510–1518. doi:10.1007/s10826-014-9956-x

Meichenbaum, D. (2007). Self-care for Trauma Psychotherapists and Caregivers: Individual, Social and Organizational Interventions. Paper presented at the Melissa Institute 11th Annual Conference, Coral Gables, FL. http://www.melissainstitute.org/handouts.html-Family07

Meiser-Stedman, R., Smith, P., Bryant, R., Salmon, K., Yule, W., Dalgleish, T., & Nixon, R. D. (2009). Development and validation of the Child Post-Traumatic Cognitions Inventory (CPTCI). *Journal of Child Psychology and Psychiatry*, *50*(4), 432–440.

Mekos, D., Hetherington, E. M., & Reiss, D. (1996). Sibling differences in problem behaviors: The role of differential treatment in nondivorced and remarried families. *Child Development*, *67*, 148–165.

Melton, G. (2005). Mandated reporting: A policy without reason. *Child Abuse & Neglect*, *29*(1), 9–18.

Merikangas, K. R., He, J. P., Burnstein, M., Swanson, S., Avenevoli, S., Cui, L., … Swendsen, J. (2010). Lifetime prevalence of mental disorders in U.S. adolescents: Results from the National Comorbidity Survey Replication–Adolescent Supplement (NCS-A). *Journal of the American Academy of Child & Adolescent Psychiatry*, *49*(10), 980–989.

Merriam Webster Online. (n.d.). Google (Def. 1). Retrieved from http://www.merriam-webster.com/dictionary/google

Meyer, D. C., & Phillips, W. M. (1990). No safe place: Parental alcoholism and adolescent suicide. *American Journal of Psychotherapy*, *44*(4), 552–562.

Mikulincer, M., & Shaver, P. R. (2007). *Attachment in adulthood: Structure, dynamics, and change*. New York, NY: Guilford Press.

Miles, A. (2005). Ending violence in teen dating relationships: A resource guide for parents and pastors. Minneapolis, MN: Augsberg Books.

Milevsky, A., Schlechter, M., Netter, S., & Keehn, D. (2007). Maternal and parental parenting styles in adolescents: Associations with self-esteem, depression, and life-satisfaction. *Journal of Child and Family Studies, 16*, 39–47.

Miller, D. J., & Thelen, M. H. (1987). Confidentiality in psychotherapy: History, issues, and research. *Psychotherapy: Theory, Research, Practice, Training*, *24*(4), 704–711.

Miller, L. (2003). Family therapy of terroristic trauma: Psychological syndromes and treatment strategies. *American Journal of Family Therapy, 31*, 257–280.

Milliken, J. P. (2001). Disenfranchised mothers: Caring for an adult child with schizophrenia. *Health Care for Women International*, *22*(1–2), 149–166.

Milner, J. S. (2000). Social information processing and child physical abuse: Theory and research. In D. J. Hansen (Ed.), *Nebraska symposium on motivation: Vol. 46. Motivation and child physical maltreatment* (pp. 39–84). Lincoln, NE: University of Nebraska Press.

Minuchin, S., & Fishman, H. C. (1981). *Family therapy techniques*. Cambridge, MA: Harvard University Press.

Mishna, F., Saini, M., & Solomon, S. (2009). Ongoing and online: Children and youth's perceptions of cyber bullying. *Child and Youth Services Review*, *31*(12), 1222–1228.

Mmari, K., Roche, K., Sudhinaraset, M., & Blum, R. (2009). When a parent goes off to war: Exploring the issues faced by adolescents and their families. *Youth and Society*, *40*(4), 455–475.

Mohr, J. J., & Fassinger, R. E. (2003). Self-acceptance and self-disclosure of sexual orientation in lesbian, gay, and bisexual adults: An attachment perspective. *Journal of Counseling Psychology*, *50*(4), 482–495. doi:10.1037/0022-0167.50.4.482

Mojtabai, R., & Olfson, M. (2008). Parental detection of youth self-harm behavior. *Suicide and Life-Threatening Behavior*, *38*(1), 60–73.

Molinari, L., Everri, M., & Fruggeri, L. (2010). Family microtransitions: Observing the process of change in families with adolescent children. *Family Process*, *49*(2), 236–250. doi:10.1111/j.1545-5300.2010.01320.x

Montgomery, C., Frisk, J. E., & Craig, L. (2008). The effects of perceived parenting style on the propensity for illicit drug use: The importance of parental warmth and control. *Drug and Alcohol Review*, *27*, 640–649.

Moore, G. F., Rothwell, H., & Segrott, J. (2010). An exploratory study of the relationship between parental attitudes and behaviour and young people's consumption of alcohol. *Substance Abuse Treatment, Prevention, and Policy*, *5*. doi:10.1186/1747-597X-5-6

Moran, G., & Diamond, G. M. (2008). Generating nonnegative attitudes among parents of depressed adolescents: The power of empathy, concern, and positive regard. *Psychotherapy Research*, *18*(1), 97–107. doi:10.1080/10503300701408325

Moran, G., Diamond, G. M., & Diamond, G. S. (2005). The relational reframe and parents' problem constructions in attachment-based family therapy. *Psychotherapy Research*, *15*(3), 226–235. doi:10.1080/10503300512331387780

Moran, P., Bifulco, A., Ball, C., Jacobs, C., & Benaim, K. (2002). Exploring psychological abuse in childhood. I. Developing a new interview scale. *Bulletin of the Menninger Clinic*, *66*, 213–240.

Moretti, M. M., Holland, R., & Peterson, S. (1994). Long term outcome of an attachment-based program for conduct disorder. *Canadian Journal of Psychiatry*, *39*, 380–390.

Morrissey-Kane, E., & Prinz, R. J. (1999). Engagement in child and adolescent treatment: The role of parental cognitions and attributions. *Clinical Child and Family Psychology Review*, *2*(3), 183–198.

Moses, T. (2010). Exploring parents' self-blame in relation to adolescents' mental disorders. *Family Relations: An Interdisciplinary Journal of Applied Family Studies*, *59*(2), 103–120.

Moss, H. B., Lynch, K. G., Hardie, T. L., & Baron, D. A. (2002). Family functioning and peer affiliation in children of fathers with antisocial personality disorder and substance dependence: Associations with problem behaviors. *The American Journal of Psychiatry*, *159*(4), 607–614.

Moyer, D., & Sandoz, E. (2015). The role of psychological flexibility in the relationship between parent and adolescent distress. *Journal of Child & Family Studies*, *24*(5), 1406–1418. doi:10.1007/s10826-014-9947-y

Muehlenkamp, J. J., Claes, L., Havertape, L., & Plener, P. L. (2012). International prevalence of adolescent non-suicidal self-injury and deliberate self-harm. *Child Adolescent Psychiatry and Mental Health, 6*, 10. doi:10.1186/1753-2000-6-10

Muehlenkamp, J., Hoff, E. R., Licht, J.-G., Azure, J. A., & Hasenzahl, S. J. (2008). Rates of non-suicidal self-injury: A cross-sectional analysis of exposure. *Current Psychology: A Journal for Diverse Perspectives on Diverse Psychological Issues, 27*(4), 234–241. doi:10.1007/s12144-008-9036-8

Mulligan, J., MacCulloch, R., Good, B., & Nicholas, D. B. (2012). Transparency, hope, and empowerment: A model for partnering with parents of a child with autism spectrum disorder at diagnosis and beyond. *Social Work in Mental Health, 10*(4), 311–330. doi:10.1080/15332985.2012.664487

Munoz Sastre, M. T., Olivari, C., Sorum, P. C., & Mullet, E. (2014). Minors' and adults' views about confidentiality. *Vulnerable Children and Youth Studies, 9*(2), 97–103.

Murrell, A. R., Wilson, K. G., LaBorde, C. T., Drake, C. E., & Rogers, L. J. (2008). Relational responding to parents. *The Behavior Analyst Today, 9*(3–4), 196–214.

Murtonen, K., Suomalainen, L., Haravuori, H., & Marttunen, M. (2012). Adolescents' experiences of psychosocial support after traumatization in a school shooting. *Child and Adolescent Mental Health, 17*, 23–30.

Myrick, A. C., & Green, E. J. (2013). A play-based treatment paradigm for nonoffending caretakers: Evidence-informed secondary trauma treatment. *International Journal of Play Therapy, 22*(4), 193–206. doi:10.1037/a0034560

Myrick, A. C., Green, E. J., & Crenshaw, D. (2013). The influence of divergent parental attachment styles on adolescent maturation: Implications for family counseling practitioners. *The Family Journal, 22*(1), 35–42. doi:10.1177/1066480713491217

Nadler, A., & Fisher, J. D. (1986). The role of threat to self-esteem and perceived control in recipient reaction to help: Theory development and empirical validation. *Advances in Experimental Social Psychology, 19*, 81–122.

Naidu, T., & Behari, S. (2010). The parent-child-therapist alliance: A case study using a strategic approach. *Journal of Child and Adolescent Mental Health, 22*(1), 41–50.

Nanda, M. B. R. (2012). Parental psychological control and childhood anxiety: The mediating role of perceived lack of control. *Journal of Child & Family Studies, 21*(4), 637–645. doi:10.1007/s10826-011-9516-6

National Child Traumatic Stress Network. (2007). Complex trauma. Retrieved from http://www.nctsn.org/trauma-types/complex-trauma

National Institute on Drug Abuse (NIDA). (2014). High school and youth trends. Retrieved from http://www.drugabuse.gov/publications/drugfacts/high-school-youth-trends

Navarre, E. (1987). Psychological maltreatment: The core component of child abuse. In M. R. Brassard, R. Germain, & S. N. Hart (Eds.), *Psychological maltreatment of children and youth* (pp. 45–58). New York, NY: Pergamon.

Neal, J., & Frick-Horbury, D. (2001). The effects of parenting styles and childhood attachment patterns on intimate relationships. *Journal of Instructional Psychology, 28*, 178–183.

Neger, E. N., & Prinz, R. J. (2015). Interventions to address parenting and parental substance abuse: Conceptual and methodological considerations. *Clinical Psychology Review, 39*, 71–82. doi:10.1016/j.cpr.2015.04.004

Nelson, J., O'Brien, M., Blankson, A., Calkins, S., & Keane, S. (2009). Family stress and parental responses to children's negative emotions: Tests of the spillover, crossover, and compensatory hypothesis. *Journal of Family Psychology, 23*, 671–679.

Neria, Y., DiGrande, L., & Adams, B. G. (2011). Posttraumatic stress disorder following the September 11, 2001, terror attacks: A review of the literature among highly exposed populations. *American Psychologist, 66*, 429–446.

Newman, B. S., & Muzzonigro, P. G. (1993). The effects of traditional family values on the coming out process of gay male adolescents. *Adolescence, 28*, 213–226.

Newman, L. K., Stevenson, C. S., Bergman, L. R., & Boyce, P. (2007). Borderline personality disorder, mother-infant interaction and parenting perceptions: Preliminary findings. *Royal Australian and New Zealand College of Psychiatrists, 41*, 598–605.

Nixon, M. K., & Heath, N. L. (2009). Self-injury in youth: The essential guide to assessment and intervention. New York, NY: Routledge/Taylor & Francis Group.

Nixon, M. K., Cloutier, P., & Jansson, S. M. (2008). Nonsuicidal self-harm in youth: A population-based survey. *Canadian Medical Association Journal, 178*(3), 306–312. doi:10.1503/cmaj.061693

NoBullying.com. (2015). Cyberbullying examples. Retrieved from http://nobullying.com/cyberbullying-examples/

Nock, M. K., & Favazza, A. (2009). Nonsuicidal self-injury: Definition and classification. In M. K. Nock (Ed.), *Understanding non-suicidal self-injury: Origins, assessment, and treatment* (pp. 9–18). Washington, DC: American Psychological Association.

Noronha, L. M. (2000). Parental response to the suicide attempts of adolescents: A narrative analysis. (61), ProQuest Information & Learning, US. Retrieved from http://search.ebscohost.com/login.aspx?direct=true&db=psyh&AN=2000-95021-036&site=ehost-live&scope=site

Norton, J. L. (1998). *Parent perspectives on factors influencing child mental health treatment*. University of Colorado.

Norwood, A., & Murphy, C. (2012). What forms of abuse correlate with PTSD symptoms in partners of men being treated for intimate partner violence? *Psychological Trauma: Theory, Research, Practice, and Policy, 4*(6), 596–604. doi:10.1037/a0025232

Nowell, D., & Spruill, J. (1993). If it's not absolutely confidential, will information be disclosed? *Professional Psychology: Research and Practice, 24*(3), 367–369.

Nursten, J. (1997). The end as a means to growth—within a social work relationship. *Journal of Social Work Practice, 11*(2), 73–80.

Oates, R. K., Tebbutt, J., Swanston, H., Lynch, D. L., & O'Toole, B. I. (1998). Prior sexual abuse in mothers of sexually abused children. *Child Abuse & Neglect, 22*(11), 1113–1118. doi:10.1016/S0145-2134(98)00091-X

Ocampo, B. W., Shelley, G. A., & Jaycox, L. H. (2007). Latino teens talk about help seeking and help giving in relation to dating violence. *Violence Against Women, 13*(2), 172–189. doi:10.1177/1077801206296982

O'Connell, K. L. (2012). Child and adolescent suicide. *Journal of Child and Adolescent Psychiatric Nursing, 25*(3), 111–112. doi:10.1111/j.1744-6171.2012.00333.x

Olfson, M., Gameroff, M. J., Marcus, S. C., & Waslick, B. D. (2003). Outpatient treatment of child and adolescent depression in the United States. *Archives of General Psychiatry, 60*, 1236–1242.

O'Reilly, M. (2006). Should children be seen and not heard? An examination of how children's interruptions are treated in family therapy. *Discourse Studies, 8*(4), 549–566.

O'Reilly, M. (2008). "What value is there in children's talk?" Investigating family therapist's interruptions of parents and children during the therapeutic process. *Journal of Pragmatics, 40*, 507–524.

O'Reilly, M. (2014). Blame and accountability in family therapy: Making sense of therapeutic spaces discursively. *Qualitative Psychology, 1*(2), 163–177. doi:10.1037/qup0000011

O'Reilly, M. (2015). "We're here to get you sorted": Parental perceptions of the purpose, progression, and outcomes of family therapy. *Journal of Family Therapy, 37*, 322–342.

O'Reilly, M., & Parker, N. (2013). "You can take a horse to water but you can't make it drink": Exploring children's engagement and resistance in family therapy. *Contemporary Family Therapy: An International Journal, 35*(3), 491–507.

O'Reilly, M., & Parker, N. (2014). "She needs a smack in the gob": Negotiating what is appropriate talk in front of children in family therapy. *Journal of Family Therapy, 36*(3), 287–307. doi:10.1111/j.1467-6427.2012.00595.x

Oreo, A., & Ozgul, S. (2007). Grief experiences of parents coping with an adult child with problem substance use. *Addiction Research & Theory, 15*(1), 71–83. doi:10.1080/16066350601036169

Oudekerk, B. A., Guarnera, L. A., & Reppucci, N. D. (2014). Older opposite-sex romantic partners, sexual risk, and victimization in adolescence. *Child Abuse & Neglect, 38*(7), 1238–1248. doi:10.1016/j.chiabu.2014.03.009

Ougrin, D. (2012). Commentary: Self-harm in adolescents: The best predictor of death by suicide? Reflections on Hawton et al. (2012). *Journal of Child Psychology and Psychiatry, 53*(12), 1220–1221. doi:10.1111/j.1469-7610.2012.02622.x

Owens, C., Lambert, H., Donovan, J., & Lloyd, K. R. (2005). A qualitative study of help seeking and primary care consultation prior to suicide. *Journal of General Practice, 55*, 503–509.

Owens, P. L., Hoagwood, K., Horwitz, S. M., Leaf, P. J., Poduska, J. M., Kellam, S. G., & Ialongo, N. S. (2002). Barriers to children's mental health services. *Journal of the American Academy of Child & Adolescent Psychiatry, 30*, 624–630.

Pace, G. T., & Shafer, K. (2015). Parenting and depression: Differences across parental roles. *Journal of Family Issues, 36*(8), 1001–1021.

Padilla-Walker, L. M., & Nelson, L. J. (2012). Black hawk down? Establishing helicopter parenting as a distinct construct from other forms of parental control during emerging adulthood. *Journal of Adolescence, 35*, 1177–1190. doi:10.1016/j.adolescence.2012.03.007

Padilla-Walker, L. M., Coyne, S. M., & Fraser, A. M. (2012). Getting a high-speed family connection: Associations between family media use and family connection. *Family Relations: An Interdisciplinary Journal of Applied Family Studies, 61*(3), 426–440. doi:10.1111/j.1741-3729.2012.00710.x

Paul, E., McManus, B., & Hayes, A. (2000). "Hook-ups": Characteristics and correlates of college students' spontaneous and anonymous sexual experiences. *Journal of Sex Research*, *37*, 76–88.

Pearlman, L. A., & Saakvitne, K. W. (1995). *Trauma and the therapist: Countertransference and vicarious traumatization in psychotherapy with incest survivors*. New York, NY: W. W. Norton and Company.

Pearlman, M. Y., Schwalbe, K. D. A., & Cloitre, M. (2010). *Grief in childhood: Fundamentals of treatment in clinical practice*. Washington, DC: American Psychological Association.

Penfold, P. S. (1995). Mendacious moms or devious dads? Some perplexing issues in child custody/sexual abuse allegation disputes. *The Canadian Journal of Psychiatry / La Revue canadienne de psychiatrie*, *40*(6), 337–341.

Peris, T. A., Goecke-Morey, M. C., Cummings, E. M., & Emery, R. E. (2008). Marital conflict and support seeking by parents in adolescence: Empirical support for the parentification construct. *Journal of Family Psychology*, *22*(3), 633–642.

Peterson, J. (2010). A qualitative comparison of parent and adolescent views regarding substance use. *Journal of School Nursing*, *26*(1), 53–64. doi:10.1177/1059840509355586

Pettifor, J., & Sawchuck, T. (2006). Psychologists' perceptions of ethically troubling incidents across international borders. *International Journal of Psychology*, *41*, 216–225.

Pettigrew, J. (2009). Text messaging and connectedness within close interpersonal relationships. *Marriage and Family Review*, *45*, 697–716.

Phares, V., Ehrbar, L. A., & Lum, J. J. (1996). Parental perceptions of the development and treatment of children's and adolescents' emotional/behavioral problems. *Family Behavior Therapy*, *18*, 19–36.

Phillips, M. J., & Ancis, J. R. (2008). The process of identity development as the parent of a lesbian or gay male. *Journal of LGBT Issues in Counseling*, *2*(2), 126–158.

Piko, B. F., & Kovács, E. (2010). Do parents and school matter? Protective factors for adolescent substance use. *Addictive Behaviors*, *35*(1), 53–56. doi:10.1016/j.addbeh.2009.08.004

Pinsof, W. M. (1995). *Integrative problem-centered therapy*. New York, NY: Basic Books.

Plante, L. G. (2006). Helping adolescents with self-injurious behavior: Cutting in developmental context. In T. G. Plante (Ed.), *Mental disorders of the new millennium: Behavioral issues* (Vol. 1, pp. 189–207). Westport, CT: Praeger/Greenwood.

Pölkki, P., Ervast, S.-A., & Huupponen, M. (2004). Coping and resilience of children of a mentally ill parent. *Social Work in Health Care*, *39*(1/2), 151.

Pollak, J., & Levy, S. (1989). Countertransference and faulure to report child abuse and neglect. *Child Abuse & Neglect*, *13*, 515–522.

Ponnet, K., Mortelmans, D., Wouters, E., Van Leeuwen, K., Bastaits, K., & Pasteels, I. (2013). Parenting stress and marital relationship as determinants of mothers' and fathers' parenting. *Personal Relationships*, *20*(2), 259–276. doi:10.1111/j.1475-6811.2012.01404.x

Pope, K. S., & Tabachnick, B. G. (1993). Therapists' anger, hate, fear, and sexual feelings: National survey of therapist responses, client characteristics, critical events, formal complaints, and training. *Professional Psychology: Research and Practice, 24*(2), 142–152.

Powers, J. L., & Eckenroade, J. (1988). The maltreatment of adolescents. *Child Abuse & Neglect, 12*, 189–199.

Prensky, M. (2001). Digital natives, digital immigrants. *On the Horizon, 9*(5), 1–6.

Quintana, S. M., & Holahan, W. (1992). Termination in short-term counseling: Comparison of successful and unsuccessful cases. *Journal of Counseling Psychology, 39*, 299–305.

Racusin, R., & Felsman, J. K. (1986). Reporting child abuse: The ethical obligation to inform parents. *Journal of the American Academy of Child Psychiatry, 25*(4), 485–489.

Rae, W. A. (2001). Common teen-parent problems. In C. E. Walker & M. C. Roberts (Eds.), *Handbook of clinical child psychology, 3rd edition* (pp. 621–637). New York, NY: Wiley.

Raissian, K. M., Dierkhising, C. B., Geiger, J. M., & Schelbe, L. (2014). Child maltreatment reporting patterns and predictors of substantiation: Comparing adolescents and younger children. *Child Maltreatment, 19*(1), 3–16.

Ransdell, S., Kent, B., Gaillard-Kenney, S., & Long, J. (2011). Digital immigrants fare better than difital natives due to social reliance. *British Journal of Educational Technology, 42*(6), 931–938.

Raphael, H., Clarke, G., & Kumar, S. (2006). Exploring parents' responses to their child's deliberate self-harm. *Health Education, 106*(1), 9–20.

Rappoport, A. (2005). Co-narcissism: How we accommodate narcissistic parents. *The Therapist, 16*(2), 36–48.

Raviv, A., Raviv, A., Propper, A., & Fink, A. S. (2003). Mothers' attitudes toward seeking help for their children from school and private psychologists. *Professional Psychology: Research and Practice, 34*(1), 95–101.

Raviv, A., Sharvit, K., Raviv, A., & Rosenblat-Stein, S. (2008). Mothers' and fathers' reluctance to seek psychological help for their children. *Journal of Child and Family Studies, 18*(2), 151–162. doi:10.1007/s10826-008-9215-0

Raviv, A., Sills, R., Raviv, A., & Wilansky, P. (2000). Adolescents' help-seeking behaviour: The difference between self- and other-referral. *Journal of Adolescence, 23*(6), 721–740.

Rayburn, N. R., Jaycox, L. H., McCaffrey, D. F., Ulloa, E. C., Zander-Cotugno, M., Marshall, G. N., & Shelley, G. A. (2007). Reactions to dating violence among Latino teenagers: An experiment utilizing the articulated thoughts in simulated situations paradigm. *Journal of Adolescence, 30*(6), 893–915. doi:10.1016/j.adolescence.2006.11.005

Regehr, C. (1990). Parental responses to extrafamilial child sexual assault. *Child Abuse and Neglect, 14*, 113–120.

Reid, W. H., & Gacono, C. (2000). Treatment of antisocial personality, psychopathy, and other characterologic antisocial syndromes. *Behavioral Sciences & the Law, 18*(5), 647–662. doi:10.1002/1099-0798(200010)18:5<647::AID-BSL407>3.0.CO;2-O

Reinelt, E., Stopsack, M., Aldinger, M., Ulrich, I., Grabe, H. J., & Barnow, S. (2013). Longitudinal transmission pathways of borderline personality disorder symptoms: From mother to child. *Psychopathology*, *47*(1), 10–16.

Reis, B., & Saewyc, E. (1999). *Eighty-three thousand youth: Selected findings of eight population-based studies as they pertain to anti-gay harassment and the safety and well-being of sexual minority students*. Seattle, WA: Safe Schools Coalition of Washington.

Rejiester, N. (2015). Perception of alienation from parents and peers during the coming out process for lesbian, gay, and bisexual individuals and self-reported attachment classifications: A preliminary investigation of the relationship between the attachment system and rejection due to sexual orientation. (76), ProQuest Information & Learning, US. Retrieved from http://search.ebscohost.com/login.aspx?direct=true&db=psyh&AN=2015-99140-098&site=ehost-live&scope=site

Repetti, R. L., & Wood, J. (1997). Effects of daily stress at work on mothers' interactions with preschoolers. *Journal of Family Psychology*, *11*, 900–1008.

Renner, L., & Whitney, S. (2010). Examining symmetry in intimate partner violence among young adults using socio-demographic characteristics. *Journal of Family Violence*, *25*, 91–106.

Ribak, R. (2009). Remote control, umbilical cord and beyond: The mobile phone as a transitional object. *British Journal of Developmental Psychology*, *27*(1), 183–196. doi:10.1348/026151008X388413

Richman, J. (1986). *Family therapy for suicidal people*. New York, NY: Springer.

Richmond, M. B. (1992). Countertransference problems in dealing with severely disturbed parents: Their potential value for understanding the patient. *Residential Treatment for Children & Youth*, *9*(4), 61–80.

Ridge, S. R., & Feeney, J. A. (1998). Relationship history and relationship attitudes in gay males and lesbians: Attachment style and gender differences. *Australian and New Zealand Journal of Psychiatry*, *32*, 848–859.

Ringler, L. L., & Hayden, D. C. (2000). Adolescent bereavement and social support: Peer loss compared to other losses. *Journal of Adolescent Research, 15*, 209–230.

Robins, E., Gassner, S., Kayes, J., WIlkinson, R. H., & Murphy, G. E. (1959). The communication of suicidal intent. *American Journal of Psychiatry*, *115*, 724–733.

Robinson, A. L., Strahan, E., Girz, L., Wilson, A., & Boachie, A. (2013). "I know I can help you": Parental self-efficacy predicts adolescent outcomes in family-based therapy for eating disorders. *European Eating Disorders Review*, *21*(2), 108–114.

Robinson, L. H. (1990). In defense of parents. In S. C. Feinstein, A. H. Esman, J. G. Looney, G. H. Orvin, J. L. Schimel, A. Z. Schwartzberg, A. D. Sorosky, & M. Sugar (Eds.), *Adolescent psychiatry: Developmental and clinical studies, Vol. 17* (pp. 36–50). Chicago, IL: University of Chicago Press.

Rodriguez, C. M. (2010). Parent-child aggression: Association with child abuse potential and parenting styles. *Violence & Victims*, *25*, 728–741.

Rodriguez, C. M. (2013). Analog of parental empathy: Association with physical child abuse risk and punishment intentions. *Child Abuse and Neglect, 37*, 493–99.

Rodriguez, C. M., & Eden, A. M. (2008). Disciplinary style and child abuse potential: Association with indicators of positive functioning in children with behavior problems. *Child Psychiatry and Human Development, 39*(2), 123–136.

Rodriguez, C. M., & Tucker, M. C. (2011). Behind the cycle of violence, beyond abuse history: A brief report on the association of parental attachment to physical child abuse potential. *Violence & Victims, 26*(1), 246–254.

Rogers, P., Davies, M., & Cottam, L. J. (2010). Perpetrator coercion, victim resistance and respondent gender: Their impact on blame attributions in a hypothetical child sexual abuse case. *Journal of Aggression, Conflict & Peace Research, 2*(3), 25.

Rogers, P., Josey, N., & Davies, M. G. (2007). Victim age, attractiveness and abuse history as factors in the perception of a hypothetical child sexual abuse case. *Journal of Sexual Aggression, 13*(2), 121–137.

Rogers, R. W. (1975). A protection motivation theory of fear appeals and attitude change. *Journal of Psychology, 91*, 93–114.

Ronningstam, E. (2012). Alliance building and narcissistic personality disorder. *Journal of Clinical Psychology: In Session, 68*(8), 943–953.

Rose, H. D., & Cohen, K. (2010). The experiences of young carers: A meta-synthesis of qualitative findings. *Journal of Youth Studies, 13*(4), 473–487. doi:10.1080/13676261003801739

Rosen, L. D. (2007). *Me, MySpace, and I*. New York, NY: Palgrave Macmillan.

Rosenbaum, M., & Richman, J. (1970). Suicide: The role of hostility and death wishes from the family and significant others. *The American Journal of Psychiatry, 126*(11), 1652–1655.

Rosenberg, L. (2009). Family therapy and resistant parents: The child cannot wait. Retrieved from http://www.psychotherapy.net/article/family-therapy-resistant-parents

Rossberg, J. I., Karterud, S., Pedersen, G., & Friis, S. (2010). Psychiatric symptoms and countertransference feelings: An empirical investigation. *Psychiatry Research, 178*, 191–195.

Roth, G., Assor, A., Niemiec, C. P., Ryan, R. M., & Deci, E. L. (2009). The emotional and academic consequences of parental conditional regard: Comparing conditional positive regard, conditional negative regard, and autonomy support as parenting practices. *Developmental Psychology, 45*, 1119–1142.

Rothman, E. F., MIller, E., Terpeluk, A., Glauber, A., & Randel, J. (2011). The proportion of U.S. parents who talk with their adolescent children about dating abuse. *Journal of Adolescent Health, 49*(2), 216–218.

Rothman, E. F., Sullivan, M., Keyes, S., & Boehmer, U. (2012). Parents' supportive reactions to sexual orientation disclosure associated with better health: Results from a population-based survey of LGB adults in Massachusetts. *Journal of Homosexuality, 59*(2), 186–200. doi:10.1080/00918369.2012.648878

Rothschild, B. (2006). *Help for the helper: The psychophysiology of compassion fatigue and vicarious trauma*. New York, NY: W. W. Norton and Company.

Rubin, K. H., Burgess, K. B., & Hastings, P. D. (2002). Stability and social-behavioral consequences of toddlers' inhibited temperament and parenting behaviors. *Child Development, 73*, 483–495.

Rudd, M. D., Joiner, T., & Rajab, M. H. (2001). *Treating suicidal behavior: An effective, time-limited approach*. New York, NY: Guilford Press.

Rudy, D., Awong, T., & Lambert, M. (2008). Parental psychological control and authoritarianism in Chinese-Canadian and European-Canadian cultural groups: Their meanings and implications for university students' adjustment. *Journal of Comparative Family Studies*, *39*(4), 471–490.

Ruscio, A. M. (2001). Predicting the childrearing practices of mothers sexually abused in childhood. *Child Abuse and Neglect*, *25*, 369–387.

Russo, D. M. (2015). The effects of a history of childhood sexual abuse on countertransference, vicarious traumatization, and positive self-transformation, in therapists who treat sexually abused children. (75), ProQuest Information & Learning, US. Retrieved from http://search.ebscohost.com/login.aspx?direct=true&db=psyh&AN=2015-99080-512&site=ehost-live&scope=site

Ryan, C., Huebner, D., Diaz, R. M., & Sanchez, J. (2009). Family rejection as a predictor of negative health outcomes in White and Latino lesbian, gay, and bisexual young adults. *Pediatrics*, *123*, 346–352.

Ryan, R. M., & Deci, E. L. (2000). Self-determination theory and the facilitation of intrinsic motivation, social development, and well-being. *American Psychologist*, *55*, 68–78.

Saakvitne, K. W., & Pearlman, L. A. (1996). *Transforming the pain: A workbook on vicarious traumatization*. London, UK: W. W. Norton and Company.

Saakvitne, K. W., Gamble, S., Pearlman, L. A., & Lev, B. (2000). *Risking connection: A training curriculum for working with survivors of childhood abuse*. Lutherville, MD: Sidran Press.

Saathoff-Wells, T., Culp, R. E., & Yancey, C. T. (2005). Expectancies for sexually abused children: Evidence of perceiver bias. *Journal of Child and Family Studies*, *14*, 487–503.

Sabbath, J. C. (1969). The suicidal adolescent: The expendable child. *Journal of the American Academy of Child Psychiatry*, *8*(2), 272–285. doi:10.1016/S0002-7138(09)61906-3

Sabina, C., Cuevas, C. A., & Rodriguez, R. M. (2014). Who to turn to? Help-seeking in response to teen dating violence among Latinos. *Psychological Violence*, *4*(3), 348–362. doi:10.1037/a0035037

Safran, J. D., & Muran, J. C. (2000). *Negotiating the therapeutic alliance: A relational treatment guide*. New York, NY: Guilford Press.

Saint-Jacques, M.-C., Drapeau, S., Lessard, G., & Beaudoin, A. (2006). Parent involvement practices in child protection: A matter of know-how and attitude. *Child & Adolescent Social Work Journal*, *23*(2), 196–215. doi:10.1007/s10560-005-0042-5

Salloum, A., Stover, C., Swaidan, V., & Storch, E. (2015). Parent and child PTSD and parent depression in relation to parenting stress among trauma-exposed children. *Journal of Child & Family Studies*, *24*(5), 1203–1212. doi:10.1007/s10826-014-9928-1

Saltzman, L. E., Fanslow, J. L., McMahon, P. M., & Shelley, G. A. (2002). *Intimate partner violence surveillance: Uniform definitions and recommended data elements*. Atlanta, GA: National Center for Injury Prevention and Control, Centers for Disease Control and Prevention.

Salzinger, S., Rosario, M., Feldman, R. S., & Ng-Mak, D. S. (2007). Adolescent suicidal behavior: Associations with preadolescent physical abuse and selected risk and protective factors. *Journal of the American Academy of Child & Adolescent Psychiatry, 46*, 859–866.

Sandberg, D. A., Suess, E. A., & Heaton, J. L. (2010). Attachment anxiety as a mediator of the relationship between interpersonal trauma and posttraumatic symptomatology among college women. *Journal of Interpersonal Violence, 25*, 33–49.

Santa-Sosa, E. J., Steer, R. A., Deblinger, E., & Runyon, M. K. (2013). Depression and parenting by nonoffending mothers of children who experienced sexual abuse. *Journal of Child Sexual Abuse, 22*(8), 915–930. doi:10.1080/10538712.2013.841309

Savin-Williams, R. C. (2001). *Mom, dad. I'm gay. How families negotiate coming out*. Washington, DC: American Psychological Association.

Savin-Williams, R. C. (2005). *The new gay teenager*. Cambridge, MA: Harvard University Press.

Schaeffer, C. M., Alexander, P. C., Bethke, K., & Kretz, L. S. (2005). Predictors of child abuse potential among military parents: Comparing mothers and fathers. *Journal of Family Violence, 20*(2), 123–129. doi:10.1007/s10896-005-3175-6

Schaffer, M., Clark, S. J., & Jeglic, E. (2009). The role of empathy and parenting style in the development of antisocial behaviors. *Crime and Delinquency, 55*, 586–599.

Scheeringa, M. S., & Zeanah, C. H. (2001). A relational perspective on PTSD in early childhood. *Journal of Traumatic Stress, 14*(4), 799–815.

Schimel, J. L. (1974). Two alliances in the treatment of adolescents: Toward a working alliance with parents and a therapeutic alliance with the adolescent. *Journal of the American Academy of Psychoanalysis, 2*(3), 243–253.

Schindler, A., & Bröning, S. (2015). A review on attachment and adolescent substance abuse: Empirical evidence and implications for prevention and treatment. *Substance Abuse, 36*(3), 304–313. doi:10.1080/08897077.2014.983586

Schinke, S. P., Fang, L., & Cole, K. C. A. (2008). Substance abuse among early adolescent girls: Risk and protective factors. *Journal of Adolescent Health, 43*, 191–194.

Schleider, J. L., Ginsburg, G. S., Keeton, C. P., Weisz, J. R., Birmaher, B., Kendall, P. C., … Walkup, J. T. (2015). Parental psychopathology and treatment outcome for anxious youth: Roles of family functioning and caregiver strain. *Journal of Consulting and Clinical Psychology, 83*(1), 213–224. doi:10.1037/a0037935

Schnitzer, G., Loots, G., Escudero, V., & Schechter, I. (2011). Negotiating the pathways into care in a globalizing world: Help-seeking behaviour of ultra-Orthodox Jewish parents. *International Journal of Social Psychiatry, 57*(2), 153–165.

Schonbucher, V., Maier, T., Mohler-Kuo, M., Schnyder, U., & Landolt, M. A. (2012). Disclosure of child sexual abuse by adolescents: A qualitative in-depth study. *Journal of Interpersonal Violence, 27*(17), 3486–3513.

Schope, R. D. (2002). The decision to tell: Factors influencing the disclosure of sexual orientation by gay men. *Journal of Gay and Lesbian Social Services: Issues in Practice, Policy, and Research, 14*, 1–22.

Schwartz, R. (2000). Relationships of shame, anger, and Gestalt resistances. (60), ProQuest Information & Learning, US. Retrieved from http://search.ebscohost.com/login.aspx?direct=true&db=psyh&AN=2000-95002-313&site=ehost-live&scope=site

Schwartz, R. C. (2000). Psychotherapeutic assessment and treatment of antisocial personality disorder. *Annals of the American Psychotherapy Association*, *4*(3), 6.

Schwartz, K. A., Pyle, S. A., Dowd, M. D., & Sheehan, K. (2010). Attitudes and beliefs of adolescents and parents regarding adolescent suicide. *Pediatrics*, *125*(2), 221–227.

Schwarz, E. D., & Kowalski, J. M. (1991). Malignant memories: PTSD in children and adults after a school shooting. *Journal of the American Academy of Child and Adolescent Psychiatry, 30*, 936–944.

Sears, H. A., Byers, E. S., & Price, E. L. (2007). The co-occurrence of adolescent boys' and girls' use of psychologically, physically, and sexually abusive behaviours in their dating relationships. *Journal of Adolescence*, *30*(3), 487–504. doi:10.1016/j.adolescence.2006.05.002

Segrin, C., Givertz, M., Swaitkowski, P., & Montgomery, N. (2015). Overparenting is associated with child problems and a critical family environment. *Journal of Child and Family Studies*, *24*(2), 470–479.

Shafii, M., & Shafii, S. L. (Eds.). (2001). *School violence: Assessment, management, prevention*. Washington, DC: American Psychiatric Publishing.

Shamoo, T. K., & Patras, P. G. (1990). *I want to kill myself: Helping your child cope with depression and suicidal thoughts*. Lexington, MA: Lexington Books.

Shanley, D. C., Reid, G. J., & Evans, B. (2008). How parents seek help for children with mental health problems. *Administration and Policy in Mental Health*, *35*(3), 135–146. doi:10.1007/s10488-006-0107-6

Shaver, K. G. (1985). *The attribution of blame: Causality, responsibility, and blameworthiness*. New York, NY: Springer-Verlag.

Shaw, D. (2010). Enter ghosts: The loss of intersubjectivity in clinical work with adult children of pathological narcissists. *Psychoanalytic Dialogues*, *20*, 46–59.

Shedler, J. (2010). The efficacy of psychodynamic psychotherapy. *American Psychologist, 65*(2), 98–109.

Sheehan, G., & Noller, P. (2002). Adolescent's perceptions of differential parenting: Links with attachment style and adolescent adjustment. *Personal Relationships*, *9*(2), 173–190. doi:10.1111/1475-6811.00011

Shelton, K. H., & van den Bree, M. B. M. (2010). The moderating effects of pubertal timing on the longitudinal associations between parent-child relationship quality and adolescent substance abuse. *Journal of Research on Adolescence*, *20*, 1044–1064.

Shepard, S. M. (1995). Parental support, family life events and teen suicide attempt. (56), ProQuest Information & Learning, US. Retrieved from http://search.ebscohost.com/login.aspx?direct=true&db=psyh&AN=1995-95024-061&site=ehost-live&scope=site

Shirk, S. R., Karver, M. S., & Brown, R. (2011). The alliance in child and adolescent psychotherapy. *Psychotherapy*, *48*, 17–24.

Shirk, S. R., Karver, M. S., Handelsman, J. B., Fields, S., & Bickman, L. (2006). Meta-analysis of therapeutic relationship variables in youth and family therapy: The evidence for different relationship variables in the child and adolescent treatment outcome literature. *Clinical Psychology Review*, *26*, 50–65.

Shneidman, E. (1987). A psychological approach to suicide. In G. R. Vanden Box & B. K. Bryant (Eds.), *Cataclysms, crises, and catastrophies: Psychology in action* (pp. 147–183). Washington, DC: American Psychological Association.

Shopper, M. (2013). Parental alienation: The creation of a false reality. In L. Gunsberg & P. Hymowitz (Eds.), *A handbook of divorce and custody: Forensic, developmental, and clinical perspectives* (pp. 109–125). Hoboken, NJ: Taylor and Francis.

Shulman, S. R. (1999). Termination of short-term and long-term psychotherapy: Patients' and therapists' affective reactions and therapists' technical management (attachment style, therapy model). (60), ProQuest Information & Learning, US. Retrieved from http://search.ebscohost.com/login.aspx?direct=true&db=psyh&AN=1999-95024-247&site=ehost-live&scope=site

Shuman, T. H. (2000). The relationship of countertransference reactions and/or ethnicity on compliance with mandatory child abuse reporting statutes. (61), ProQuest Information & Learning, US. Retrieved from http://search.ebscohost.com/login.aspx?direct=true&db=psyh&AN=2000-95016-058&site=ehost-live&scope=site

Silverman, J. G., Raj, A., Mucci, L. A., & Hathaway, J. E. (2001). Dating violence against adolescent girls and associated substance use, unhealthy weight control, sexual risk behavior, pregnancy, and suicidality. *JAMA: Journal of the American Medical Association, 286*(5), 572–579. doi:10.1001/jama.286.5.572

Sim, L., Adrian, M., Zeman, J., Cassano, M., & Friedrich, W. N. (2009). Adolescent deliberate self-harm: Linkages to emotion regulation and family emotional climate. *Journal of Research on Adolescence, 19*(1), 75–91.

Simons, R. L., Lin, K.-H., & Gordon, L. C. (1998). Socialization in the family of origin and male dating violence: A prospective study. *Journal of Marriage and the Family, 60*(2), 467–478.

Siskind, D. (2013). Psychotherapy with children and parents during divorce. In L. Gunsberg & P. Hymowitz (Eds.), *A handbook and divorce and custody: Forensic, developmental, and clinical perspectives* (pp. 331–342). Hoboken, NJ: Taylor and Francis.

Skiba, D., Monroe, J., & Wodarski, J. S. (2004). Adolescent substance use: Reviewing the effectiveness of prevention strategies. *Social Work, 49*, 343–353.

Smetana, J., & Metzger, A. (2008). Don't ask, don't tell (your mom and dad): Disclosure and nondisclosure in adolescent-parent relationships. In M. Kerr, H. Stattin, & R. C. M. Engels (Eds.), *What can parents do? New insights into the role of parents in adolescents' problem behavior* (pp. 65–87). Chichester: John Wiley & Sons.

Smetana, J., Campione-Barr, N., & Daddis, C. (2004). Developmental and longitudinal antecedents of family decision-making: Defining health behavioral autonomy for African American adolescents. *Child Development, 75*, 1–17.

Smith, D. M., & Donnelly, J. (2001). Adolescent dating violence: A multi-systemic approach of enhancing awareness in educators, parents, and society. *Journal of Prevention & Intervention in the Community, 21*(1), 53.

Smith, N. B., Kouros, C. D., & Meuret, A. E. (2014). The role of trauma symptoms in nonsuicidal self-injury. *Trauma Violence Abuse, 15*(1), 41.

Smith, S. G., & Cook, S. L. (2008). Disclosing sexual assault to parents: The influence of parental messages about sex. *Violence Against Women, 14*, 1326–1348.

Soenens, B., Vansteenkiste, M., Duriez, B., & Goossens, L. (2006). In search of the sources of psychologically controlling parenting: The role of parental separation anxiety and parental maladaptive perfectionism. *Journal of Research on Adolescence, 16*(4), 539–559.

Solomon, A. (2012). *Far from the tree: Parents, children, and the search for identity*. New York, NY: Scribner.

Sourander, A., Aromaa, M., Pihlakoski, L., Haavisto, A., Rautava, P., Helenius, H., & Sillanpää, M. (2006). Early predictors of deliberate self-harm among adolescents. A prospective follow-up study from age 3 to age 15. *Journal of Affective Disorders, 93*(1–3), 87–96. doi:10.1016/j.jad.2006.02.015

Southam-Gerow, M. A., Kendall, P. C., & Weersing, V. R. (2001). Examining outcome variability: Correlates of treatment response in a child and adolescent anxiety clinic. *Journal of Clinical Child Psychology, 30*, 422–436.

Speltz, M., DeKlyen, M., Greenberg, M., & Dryden, M. (1995). Clinic referral for oppositional defiant disorder: Relative significance of attachment and behavioral variables. *Journal of Abnormal Child Psychology, 23*, 487–507.

Spriggs, A. L., Halpern, C. T., & Martin, S. L. (2009). Continuity of adolescent and early adult partner violence victimisation: Association with witnessing violent crime in adolescence (English). *Journal of Epidemiology and Community Health, 63*(9), 741–748.

Stacey, J., & Biblarz, T. (2001). (How) does the sexual orientation of parents matter? *American Sociological Review, 66*, 159–183.

Starr, S., Campbell, L. R., & Herrick, C. (2002). Factors affecting use of the mental health system by rural children. *Issues in Mental Health Nursing, 23*, 291–304.

Stattin, H., & Kerr, M. (2000). Parental monitoring: A reinterpretation. *Child Development, 71*, 1072–1085.

Stauffer, L. B., & Deblinger, E. (1996). Cognitive behavioral groups for nonoffending mothers and their young sexually abused children: A preliminary treatment outcome study. *Child Maltreatment, 1*, 65–76.

Steinberg, L. (2001). We know some things: Parent-adolescent relationships in retrospect and prospect. *Journal of Research on Adolescence, 11*, 1–19.

Steinberg, L., Blatt-Eisengart, I., & Cauffman, E. (2006). Patterns of competence and adjustment among adolescents from authoritative, authoritarian, indulgent, and neglectful homes: A replication in a sample of serious juvenile offenders. *Journal of Research on Adolescence, 16*(1), 47–58. doi:10.1111/j.1532-7795.2006.00119.x

Steinberg, L., Lamborn, S. D., Darling, N., & Mounts, N. S. (1994). Over-time changes in adjustment and competence among adolescents from authoritative, authoritarian, indulgent, and neglectful families. *Child Development, 65*(3), 754–770.

Stelter, R. L., & Halberstadt, A. G. (2011). The interplay between parental beliefs about children's emotions and parental stress impacts children's attachment security. *Infant and Child Development, 20*(3), 272–287. doi:10.1002/icd.693

Sternberg, K. J., Lamb, M. E., Guterman, E., Abbott, C. B., & Dawud-Noursi, S. (2005). Adolescents' perceptions of attachments to their mothers and fathers in families with histories of domestic violence: A longitudinal perspective. *Child Abuse & Neglect, 29*(8), 853–869. doi:10.1016/j.chiabu.2004.07.009

Stith, S. M., Liu, T., Davies, C., Boykin, E. L., Adler, M. C., Harris, J. M., … Dees, J. E. M. E. G. (2009). Risk factors in child maltreatment: A meta-analytic review of the literature. *Aggression and Violent Behavior, 14*, 13–29.

Stoltenborgh, M., Bakermans-Kranenburg, M. J., Alink, L. R. A., & Van Ijzendoorn, M. H. (2012). The universality of childhood emotional abuse: A meta-analysis of worldwide prevalence. *Journal of Aggression, Maltreatment & Trauma*, *21*(8), 870–890. doi:10.1080/10926771.2012.708014

Stone, M. H. (1973). The parental factor in adolescent suicide. *International Journal of Child Psychotherapy*, *2*(2), 163–201.

Stouthamer-Loeber, M., Loeber, R., van Kammen, W., & Zhang, Q. (1995). Uninterrupted delinquent careers: The timing of parental help-seeking and juvenile court contact. *Studies on Crime & Crime Prevention*, *4*(2), 236–251.

Strickland-Clark, L., Campbell, D., & Dallos, R. (2000). Children's and adolescents' views on family therapy. *Journal of Family Therapy*, *22*, 324–341.

Strohmaier, H., Murphy, M., & DeMatteo, D. (2014). Youth sexting: Prevalence rates, driving motivations, and the deterrent effects of legal consequences. *Sexuality Research and Public Policy*, *11*, 245–255.

Sullivan, J. R., Ramirez, E., Rae, W. A., Razo, N. R., & George, C. A. (2002). Factors contributing to breaking confidentiality with adolescent clients: A survey of pediatric psychologists. *Professional Psychology: Research and Practice*, *33*(4), 396–401.

Sunseri, P. (2003). Predicting treatment termination due to running away among adolescents in residential care. *Residential Treatment for Children & Youth*, *21*, 43–60.

Swahn, M. H., & Potter, L. B. (2001). Factors associated with the medical severity of suicide attempts in youths and young adults. *Suicide and Life-Threatening Behavior*, *32*(Suppl), 21–29. doi:10.1521/suli.32.1.5.21.24214

Swanson, A. J., & Schaefer, C. E. (1993). *Children in residential treatment*. New York, NY: Von Norstrand Reinhold.

Swift, J. K., & Greenberg, R. P. (2015). Assist in planning for appropriate termination. In J. K. Swift & R. P. Greenberg (Eds.), *Premature termination in psychotherapy: Strategies for engaging clients and improving outcomes* (pp. 93–104). Washington, DC: American Psychological Association.

Swift, J. K., Greenberg, R. P., Whipple, J. L., & Kominiak, N. (2012). Practice recommendations for reducing premature termination in therapy. *Professional Psychology: Research and Practice*, *43*(4), 379–387. doi:10.1037/a0028291

Tabak, S. J., & Klettke, B. (2014). Mock jury attitudes towards credibility, age, and guilt in a fictional child sexual assault scenario. *Australian Journal of Psychology*, *66*, 47–55.

Taffel, R. (2005). *Breaking through to teens: Psychotherapy for the new adolescence*. New York, NY: Guilford Press.

Tamrouti-Makkink, I. D., Dubas, J. S., Gerris, J. R. M., & van Aken, M. A. G. (2004). The relation between the absolute level of parenting and differential parental treatment with adolescent siblings' adjustment. *Journal of Child Psychology and Psychiatry*, *45*(8), 1397–1406. doi:10.1111/j.1469-7610.2004.00331.x

Tavkar, P., & Hansen, D. J. (2011). Interventions for families victimized by child sexual abuse: Clinical issues and approaches for child advocacy center-based services. *Aggression and Violent Behavior*, *16*, 188–199. doi:10.1016/j.avb.2011.02.005

Taylor, L., Adelman, H., & Kaser-Boyd, N. (1986). The origin climate questionnaire as a toll for studying psychotherapeutic process. *Journal of Child and Adolescent Psychotherapy*, *3*, 10–16.

Tebb, K. P. (2011). Forging partnerships with parents while delivering adolescent confidential health services: A clinical paradox. *Journal of Adolescent Health*, *49*(4), 335–336. doi:10.1016/j.jadohealth.2011.08.005

Tebb, K. P., Hernandez, L. K., Shafer, M.-A., Chang, F., Eyre, S. L., & Otero-Sabogal, R. (2012). Understanding the attitudes of Latino parents toward confidential health services for teens. *Journal of Adolescent Health*, *50*(6), 572–577. doi:10.1016/j.jadohealth.2011.10.008

Tebb, K. P., Pollack, L. M., Millstein, S., Otero-Sabogal, R., & Wibbelsman, C. J. (2014). Mothers' attitudes toward adolescent confidential services: Development and validation of scales for use in English- and Spanish-speaking populations. *Journal of Adolescent Health*, *55*, 341–346.

Temple, J. R., Paul, J. A., van den Berg, P., Le, V. D., McElhany, A., & Temple, B. W. (2012). Teen sexting and its association with sexual behaviors. *Archives of Pediatrics & Adolescent Medicine*, *166*, 828–833.

Thompson, K. L., & Gullone, E. (2008). Prosocial and antisocial behaviors in adolescents: An investigation into associations with attachment and empathy. *Anthrozoos: A Multidisciplinary Journal of the Interactions of People & Animals*, *21*, 123–137.

Thomson, S., Marriott, M., Telford, K., Law, H., McLaughlin, J., & Sayal, K. (2014). Adolescents with a diagnosis of anorexia nervosa: Parents' experience of recognition and deciding to seek help. *Clinical Child Psychology and Psychiatry*, *19*(1), 43–57. doi:10.1177/1359104512465741

Thoresen, S., Jensen, T. K., & Dyb, G. (2014). Media participation and mental health in terrorist attack survivors. *Journal of Traumatic Stress, 27*, 639–646.

Timmons, K. A., Selby, E. A., Lewinsohn, P. M., & Joiner, T. E. (2011). Parental displacement and adolescent suicidality: Exploring the role of failed belonging. *Journal of Clinical Child and Adolescent Psychology*, *40*(6), 807–817. doi:10.1080/15374416.2011.614584

Tishby, O., Turel, M., Gumble, O., Pinus, U., Lavy, S. B., Winokour, M., & Sznajderman, S. (2000). Help-seeking attitudes among Israeli adolescents. *Adolescence*, *36*(142), 249–264.

Tobin, J. J. (2000). Adolescent suicide attempters in the year following hospitalization: Does the parent-child relationship predict symptom relapse and recurrent suicidality? (61), ProQuest Information & Learning, US. Retrieved from http://search.ebscohost.com/login.aspx?direct=true&db=psyh&AN=2000-95020-085&site=ehost-live&scope=site

Tokić, A., & Pećnik, N. (2011). Parental behaviors related to adolescents' self-disclosure: Adolescents' views. *Journal of Social and Personal Relationships*, *28*(2), 201–222.

Tolin, D. F., & Foa, E. B. (2006). Sex differences in trauma and posttraumatic stress disorder: A quantitative review of 25 years of research. *Psychological Bulletin*, *132*, 959–992.

Tolou-Shams, M., Hadley, W., Conrad, S. M., & Brown, L. K. (2012). The role of family affect in juvenile drug court offenders' substance use and HIV risk. *Journal of Child and Family Studies*, *21*(3), 449–456. doi:10.1007/s10826-011-9498-4

Torry, Z. D., & Billick, S. B. (2011). Implications of antisocial parents. *Psychiatric Quarterly*, *82*(4), 275–285. doi:10.1007/s11126-011-9169-z

Tritt, A. M., & Pryor, J. E. (2005). The relationship between perceived marital conflict, attitudes towards parents, and parenting styles experienced by adolescents. *Journal of Family Studies, 11*(2), 284–296. doi:10.5172/jfs.327.11.2.284

Troister, T., & Holden, R. R. (2010). Comparing psychache, depression, and hopelessness in their associations with suicidality: A test of Shneidman's theory of suicide. *Personality and Individual Differences, 49*(7), 689–693. doi:10.1016/j.paid.2010.06.006

Trost, K., Biesecker, G., Stattin, H., & Kerr, M. (2007). Not wanting parents' involvement: Sign of autonomy or sign of problems? *European Journal of Developmental Psychology, 4*(3), 314–331. doi:10.1080/17405620601008980

Turner, H. A., Finkelhor, D., Ormrod, R., Hamby, S., Leeb, R. T., Mercy, J. A., & Holt, M. (2012). Family context, victimization, and child trauma symptoms: Variations in safe, stable, and nurturing relationships during early and middle childhood. *American Journal of Orthopsychiatry, 82*, 209–219.

Turney, D., & Tanner, K. (2001). Working with neglected children and their families. *Journal of Social Work Practice, 15*, 193–204.

Ulloa, E. C., Martinez-Arango, N., & Hokoda, A. (2014). Attachment anxiety, depressive symptoms, and adolescent dating violence perpetration: A longitudinal mediation analysis. *Journal of Aggression, Maltreatment & Trauma, 23*(6), 652–669. doi:10.1080/10926771.2014.920452

Ungar, M., Theron, L., & Didkowsky, N. (2011). Adolescents' precocious and developmentally appropriate contributions to their families' well-being and resilience in five countries. *Family Relations, 60*(2), 231–246.

Updegraff, J. A., Silver, R. C., & Holman, E. (2008). Searching for and finding meaning in collective trauma: Results from a national longitudinal study of the 9/11 terrorist attacks. *Journal of Personality and Social Psychology, 95*, 709–722.

US Department of Health and Human Services, A. o. C., Youth, and Families. (2006). *Child maltreatment 2004*. Washington, DC.

US Department of Health and Human Services. (2003). *Children's bureau, child maltreatment 2001: Reports from the states to the nation child abuse and neglect data system*. Washington, DC.

Vakili, S., Currie, S., & el-Guebaly, N. (2009). Evaluating the utility of drug testing in an outpatient addiction program. *Addictive Disorders & Their Treatment, 8*(1), 22–32. doi:10.1097/ADT.0b013e318166efc4

Valentino, K., Berkowitz, S., & Stover, C. S. (2010). Parenting behaviors and post-traumatic symptoms in relation to children's symptomatology following a traumatic event. *Journal of Traumatic Stress, 23*(3), 403–407. doi:10.1002/jts.20525

van der Vorst, H., Engels, R. C. M., Meeus, W., Devokic, M., & Vermulst, A. (2006). Parental attachment, parental control, and early development of alcohol use: A longitudinal study. *Psychology of Addictive Behaviors, 20*, 107–116.

Van Parys, H., & Rober, P. (2013). Trying to comfort the parent: A qualitative study of children dealing with parental depression. *Journal of Marital & Family Therapy, 39*(3), 330–345. doi:10.1111/j.1752-0606.2012.00304.x

Vanden Abeele, M., Campbell, S. W., Eggermont, S., & Roe, K. (2014). Sexting, mobile porn use, and peer group dynamics: Boys' and girls' self-perceived popularity, need for popularity, and perceived peer pressure. *Media Psychology, 17*, 6–33.

Vandenbosch, H., & Cleemput, V. K. (2009). Cyberbullying among youngsters: Profiles of bullies and victims. *New Media Society, 11*(8), 1349–1371.

Vander Stoep, A., McCauley, E., Flynn, C., & Stone, A. (2009). Thoughts of death and suicide in early adolescence. *Suicide and Life-Threatening Behavior, 39*, 599–613.

VanFleet, R. (2004). *Overcoming Resistance: Engaging Parents in Play Therapy* [DVD]. Boiling Springs, PA: Play Therapy Press.

Vasterman, P., Yzermans, J., & Dirkzwager, A. (2005). The role of the media and media hypes in the aftermath of disasters. *American Journal of Epidemiology, 27*, 107–114.

Vaughn, C. E. (1989). Annotation: Expressed emotion in family relationships. *Journal of Child Psychology & Psychiatry, 35*(2), 365–376.

Veenstra, G. J., & Scott, C. G. (1993). A model for using time out as an intervention technique with families. *Journal of Family Violence, 8*(1), 71–87. doi:10.1007/BF00986994

Venable, W. M., & Thompson, B. (1998). Caretaker psychological factors predicting premature termination of children's counseling. *Journal of Counseling and Development, 76*(3), 286–293.

Violato, C., & Arato, J. (2004). Childhood attachment and adolescent suicide: A stepwise discriminant analysis in a case-comparison study. *Individual Differences Research, 2*, 162–168.

Vivona, J. M. (2000). Parental attachment styles of late adolescents: Qualities of attachment relationships and consequences for adjustment. *Journal of Counseling Psychology, 47*, 316–329.

Wainright, J. L., Russell, S. T., & Patterson, C. J. (2004). Psychosocial adjustment, school outcomes, and romantic relationships of adolescents with same-sex parents. *Child Development, 75*, 886–898.

Waizenhofer, R. N., Buchanan, C. M., & Jackson-Newsom, J. (2004). Mothers' and fathers' knowledge of adolescents' daily activities: Its sources and its links with adolescent adjustment. *Journal of Family Psychology, 18*, 348–360.

Walker, M., Moreau, D., & Weissman, M. M. (1990). Parents' awareness of children's suicide attempts. *American Journal of Psychiatry, 147*, 1364–1366.

Wall, J. C., & Levy, A. J. (1994). Treatment of noncustodial fathers: Gender issues and clinical dilemmas. *Child & Adolescent Social Work Journal, 11*(4), 295–313.

Wallach, L. (1997). Informing clients of limits to confidentiality associated with child welfare: Will informed clients talk freely? (57), ProQuest Information & Learning, US. Retrieved from http://search.ebscohost.com/login.aspx?direct=true&db=psyh&AN=1997-95006-160&site=ehost-live&scope=site

Wallerstein, J. S. (1985). The overburdened child: Some long-term consequences of divorce. *Social Work, 30*(2), 116–123.

Wallin, P. (2012). Building your online presence as an expert. In C. E. Stout (Ed.), *Getting better at private practice* (pp. 196–213). Hoboken, NJ: John Wiley & Sons.

Walsh, C., MacMillan, H., & Jamieson, E. (2002). The relationship between parental psychiatric disorder and child physical and sexual abuse: Findings from the Ontario Health Supplement. *Child Abuse & Neglect, 26*(1), 11–22. doi:10.1016/S0145-2134(01)00308-8

Waters, E., Kondo-Ikemura, K., Posada, G., & Richters, J. E. (1991). Learning to love: Mechanisms and milestones. In M. Gunnar (Ed.), *Minnesota Symposium on Child Psychology* (pp. 217–255). Hillsdale, NJ: Erlbaum.

Webster, S. W., O'Toole, R., O'Toole, A. W., & Lucal, B. (2005). Overreporting and underreporting of child abuse: Teachers' use of professional discretion. *Child Abuse & Neglect, 29*(11), 1281–1296.

Wedig, M. M., & Nock, M. K. (2007). Parental expressed emotion and adolescent self-injury. *Journal of the American Academy of Child & Adolescent Psychiatry, 46*(9), 1171–1178. doi:10.1097/chi.0b013e3180ca9aaf

Weigle, P., & Reid, D. (2014). Helping parents promote healthy and safe computer habits. *Adolescent Psychiatry, 4*(2), 92–97. doi:10.2174/221067660402140709120835

Weiner, I. (1992). *Psychological disturbance in adolescence* (2nd ed.). Oxford, England: Wiley.

Weinstein, B., Levine, M., Kogan, N., Harkavy-Friedman, J., & Miller, J. M. (2002). Mental health professionals' experiences reporting suspected child abuse and maltreatment. *Child Abuse & Neglect, 24*(10), 1317–1328.

Weissman, M. M., Markowitz, J. C., & Klerman, G. L. (2000). *Comprehensive guide to interpersonal therapy*. New York, NY: Basic Books.

Weisz, A. N., Tolman, R. M., Callahan, M. R., Saunders, D. G., & Black, B. M. (2007). Informal helpers' responses when adolescents tell them about dating violence or romantic relationship problems. *Journal of Adolescence, 30*(5), 853–868. doi:10.1016/j.adolescence.2006.09.004

Wekerle, C., Leung, E., Wall, A.-M., MacMillan, H., Boyle, M., Trocme, N., & Waechter, R. (2009). The contribution of childhood emotional abuse to teen dating violence among child protective services-involved youth. *Child Abuse & Neglect, 33*(1), 45–58. doi:10.1016/j.chiabu.2008.12.006

Wekerle, C., Wolfe, D. A., Hawkins, D. L., Pittman, A. L., Glickman, A., & Lovald, B. E. (2001). Childhood maltreatment, posttraumatic stress symptomatology, and adolescent dating violence: Considering the value of adolescent perceptions of abuse and a trauma mediational model. *Development and Psychopathology, 13*(4), 847–871.

Wells, K. C., & Albano, A. M. (2005). Parent involvement in CBT treatment of adolescent depression: Experiences in the Treatment for Adolescents with Depression Study (TADS). *Cognitive and Behavioral Practice, 12*(2), 209–220.

White, M. K., Godley, S. H., & Passetti, L. L. (2004). Adolescent and parent perceptions of outpatient substance abuse treatment: A qualitative study. *Journal of Psychoactive Drugs, 36*(1), 65–74.

Whiteside, R. G. (1993). Making a referral for family therapy: The school counselor's role. *Elementary School Guidance & Counseling, 27*(4), 273–279. Retrieved from http://search.ebscohost.com/login.aspx?direct=true&db=psyh&AN=1993-39409-001&site=ehost-live&scope=site

Whitlock, J., Eckenrode, J., & Silverman, D. (2006). Self-injurious behaviors in a college population. *Pediatrics, 117*(6), 1939–1948.

Wiederhold, B. K. (2012). As parents invade Facebook, teens tweet more. *Cyberpsychology, Behavior, and Social Networking, 15*(8), 385–385. doi:10.1089/cyber.2012.1554

Williams, J. (2006). How social myths about childhood, motherhood, and medicine affect the detection of subtle developmental problems in young children. *Contemporary Nurse*, *23*(2), 274–287.

Willoughby, B. L. B., Doty, N. D., & Malik, N. M. (2008). Parental reactions to their child's sexual orientation disclosure: A family stress perspective. *Parenting: Science and Practice*, *8*(1), 70–91. doi:10.1080/15295190701830680

Willoughby, B. L. B., Malik, N. M., & Lindahl, K. M. (2006). Parental reactions to their sons' sexual orientation disclosures: The roles of family cohesion, adaptability, and parenting style. *Psychology of Men & Masculinity*, *7*(1), 14–26. doi:10.1037/1524-9220.7.1.14

Wills, T. A., Sandy, J. M., Yaeger, A., & Shinar, O. (2001). Family risk factors and adolescent substance use: Moderation effects for temperament dimensions. *Developmental Psychology*, *37*(3), 283–297. doi:10.1037/0012-1649.37.3.283

Wisdom, J. P., Cavaleri, M., Gogel, L., & Nacht, M. (2011). Barriers and facilitators to adolescent drug treatment: Youth, family, and staff reports. *Addiction Research & Theory*, *19*(2), 179–188.

Wiseman, M., & McBride, M. (1998). Increasing the attendance rate for first appointments at child and family psychiatry clinics: An opt-in system. *Child Psychology & Psychiatry Review*, *3*(2), 68–71.

Wolak, J., Finkelhor, D., & Mitchell, K. S. (2004). Internet-initiated sex crimes against minors: Implications for prevention based on findings from a national study. *Journal of Adolescent Health*, 35, 424.e411–424.e420.

Wolak, J., Finkelhor, D., Mitchell, K. J., & Ybarra, M. L. (2010). Online "predators" and their victims: Myths, realities, and implications for prevention and treatment. *Psychology of Violence, 1*, 13–35.

Wolf, M. E., Ly, U., Hobart, M. A., & Kemic, M. A. (2003). Barriers to seeking police help for intimate partner violence (English). *Journal of Family Violence*, *18*(2), 121–129.

Wolfradt, U., Hempel, S., & Miles, J. N. V. (2003). Perceived parenting styles, depersonalisation, anxiety and coping behaviour in adolescents. *Personality and Individual Differences*, *34*(3), 521–532. doi:10.1016/S0191-8869(02)00092-2

Wood, S. L., & Sommers, M. S. (2011). Consequences of intimate partner violence on child witnesses: A systematic review of the literature. *Journal of Child and Adolescent Psychiatric Nursing*, *24*(4), 223–236. doi:10.1111/j.1744-6171.2011.00302.x

Woodruff-Borden, J., Morrow, C., Bourland, S., & Cambron, S. (2002). The behavior of anxious parents: Examining mechanisms of transmission of anxiety from parent to child. *Journal of Clinical Child & Adolescent Psychology*, *31*(3), 364.

Woolgar, M., & Murray, L. (2010). The representation of fathers by children of depressed mothers: Refining the meaning of parentification in high-risk samples. *Journal of Child Psychology & Psychiatry*, *51*(5), 621–629.

World Health Organization (WHO). (1999). *Report of the consultation on child abuse prevention, 29–31 March 1999, WHO, Geneva*. Geneva, Switzerland: Author.

Wright, E. M., Fagan, A. A., & Pinchevsky, G. M. (2013). The effects of exposure to violence and victimization across life domains on adolescent substance use. *Child Abuse & Neglect*, *37*(11), 899–909. doi:10.1016/j.chiabu.2013.04.010

Wu, P., Hoven, C. W., Bird, H. R., Moore, R. E., Cohen, P., Alegria, M., … Roper, M. T. (1999). Depressive and disruptive disorders and mental health service utilization in children and adolescents. *Journal of the American Academy of Child & Adolescent Psychiatry, 38*, 1081–1090.

Yahav, R., & Sharlin, S. A. (2002). Blame and family conflict: Symptomatic children as scapegoats. *Child & Family Social Work, 7*(2), 91–98. doi:10.1046/j.1365-2206.2002.00231.x

Yan, Z. (2008). Useful resources, important messages: The explosion of parenting books on adolescents and social networking sites. *Journal of Applied Developmental Psychology, 29*(6), 472–474. doi:10.1016/j.appdev.2008.07.006

Yap, M. B. H., Wright, A., & Jorm, A. F. (2011). The influence of stigma on young people's help-seeking intentions and beliefs about the helpfulness of various sources of help. *Social Psychiatry and Psychiatric Epidemiology, 46*(12), 1257–1265.

Yarkovsky, N., & Timmons Fritz, P. A. (2014). Attachment style, early sexual intercourse, and dating aggression victimization. *Journal of Interpersonal Violence, 29*(2), 279–298. doi:10.1177/0886260513505143

Yates, T. M., Tracy, A. J., & Luthar, S. S. (2008). Nonsuicidal self-injury among "privileged" youths: Longitudinal and cross-sectional approaches to developmental process. *Journal of Consulting and Clinical Psychology, 76*(1), 52–62. doi:10.1037/0022-006X.76.1.52

Ybarra, M. L., Mitchell, K. S., Finkelhor, D., & Wolak, J. (2007). Internet prevention messages: Are we targeting the right online behaviors? *Archives of Pediatrics & Adolescent Medicine, 161*, 138–145.

Yip, K.-s. (2005). A multi-dimensional perspective of adolescents' self-cutting. *Child and Adolescent Mental Health, 10*(2), 80–86. doi:10.1111/j.1475-3588.2005.00122.x

Yip, K.-s., Ngan, M., & Lam, I. (2003). A qualitative study of parental influence on and response to adolescents' self-cutting in Hong Kong. *Families in Society: Journal of Contemporary Social Services, 84*(3), 405–416. doi:10.1606/1044-3894.129

Yoast, R. A., Fleming, M., & Balch, G. I. (2007). Reactions to a concept for physician intervention in adolescent alcohol use. *Journal of Adolescent Health, 41*(1), 35–41. doi:10.1016/j.jadohealth.2007.02.008

Young, A. M., Grey, M., & Boyd, C. J. (2009). Adolescents' experiences of sexual assault by peers: Prevalence and nature of victimization occurring within and outside of school. *Journal of Youth and Adolescence, 38*(8), 1072–1083. doi:10.1007/s10964-008-9363-y

Younstrom, E., Loeber, R., & Stouthamer-Loeber, M. (2000). Patterns and correlates of agreement between parent, teacher, and male adolescent ratings of externalizing and internalizing problems. *Journal of Consulting and Clinical Psychology, 68*, 1038–1050.

Zalewski, M., Stepp, S. D., Scott, L. N., Whalen, D. J., Beeney, J. F., & Hipwell, A. E. (2014). Maternal borderline personality disorder symptoms and parenting of adolescent daughters. *Journal of Personality Disorders, 28*(4), 541–554. doi:10.1521/pedi_2014_28_131

Zavis, A. (2010). Gay and homeless: In plain sight, a largely hidden population. *The Los Angeles Times*. Retrieved from http://articles.latimes.com/2010/dec/12/local/la-me-gay-homeless-20101212

Zeratsion, H., Dalsklev, M., Bjertness, E., Lien, L., Haavet, O. R., Halvorsen, J. A., … Claussen, B. (2013). Parental divorce in late adolescence does not seem to increase mental health problems: A population study from Norway. *BMC Public Health, 13*(1), 1–5. doi:10.1186/1471-2458-13-413

Zhang, J., & Li, Z. (2013). The association between depression and suicide when hopelessness is controlled for. *Comprehensive Psychiatry, 54*(7), 790–796.

Zimmer-Gembeck, M. J., Ducat, W., & Collins, W. A. (2011). Autonomy development during adolescence. In B. B. Brown & M. J. Prinstein (Eds.), *Encyclopedia of adolescence* (pp. 66–76). New York, NY: Academic Press.

Zoroglu, S. S., Tuzan, U., Sar, V., Tutkun, H., Savas, H. A., Ozturk, M., … Kora, M. E. (2003). Suicide attempt and self-mutilation among Turkish high school students in relation with abuse, neglect, and dissociation. *Psychiatry & Clinical Neurosciences, 57*, 119–126.

Zwaanswijk, M., van der Ende, J., Verhaak, P. F. M., Bensing, J. M., & Verhulst, F. C. (2007). The different stages and actors involved in the process leading to the use of adolescent mental health services. *Clinical Child Psychology and Psychiatry, 12*(4), 567–582.

Zwaanswijk, M., Verhaak, P. F. M., Bensing, J. M., van der Ende, J., & Verhulst, F. C. (2003). Help seeking for emotional and behavioural problems in children and adolescents: A review of recent literature. *European Child & Adolescent Psychiatry, 12*(4), 153–161.

Zyrek, E., Gencoz, F., Bergman, Y., & Lester, D. (2009). Suicidality, problem-solving skills, attachment style, and hopelessness in Turkish students. *Death Studies, 33*, 815–827.

Name Index

Subject Index

www.ingramcontent.com/pod-product-compliance
Ingram Content Group UK Ltd.
Pitfield, Milton Keynes, MK11 3LW, UK
UKHW012036150926
475560UK00001B/42

9 781442 250000